Ventricular Tachycardia in Structural Heart Disease

Editors

AMIN AL-AHMAD
FRANCIS E. MARCHLINSKI

CARDIAC ELECTROPHYSIOLOGY CLINICS

www.cardiacEP.theclinics.com

Consulting Editors
RANJAN K. THAKUR
ANDREA NATALE

March 2017 • Volume 9 • Number 1

ELSEVIER

1600 John F. Kennedy Boulevard • Suite 1800 • Philadelphia, Pennsylvania, 19103-2899

http://www.theclinics.com

CARDIAC ELECTROPHYSIOLOGY CLINICS Volume 9, Number 1
March 2017 ISSN 1877-9182, ISBN-13: 978-0-323-50974-9

Editor: Stacy Eastman
Developmental Editor: Susan Showalter

Cardiac Electrophysiology Clinics (ISSN 1877-9182) is published quarterly by Elsevier Inc., 360 Park Avenue South, New York, NY 10010-1710. Months of issue are March, June, September, and December. Subscription prices are $215.00 per year for US individuals, $331.00 per year for US institutions, $236.00 per year for Canadian individuals, $373.00 per year for Canadian institutions, $299.00 per year for international individuals, $399.00 per year for international institutions and $100.00 per year for US, Canadian and international students/residents. To receive student/resident rate, orders must be accompanied by name of affiliated institution, date of term, and the signature of program/residency coordinator on institution letterhead. Orders will be billed at individual rate until proof of status is received. Foreign air speed delivery is included in all Clinics subscription prices. All prices are subject to change without notice. **POSTMASTER:** Send address changes to Cardiac Electrophysiology Clinics, Elsevier Health Sciences Division, Subscription Customer Service, 3251 Riverport Lane, Maryland Heights, MO 63043. **Customer Service: 1-800-654-2452 (US and Canada). From outside of the US and Canada, call 314-477-8871. Fax: 314-447-8029. E-mail: JournalsCustomerService-usa@elsevier.com (for print support); JournalsOnlineSupport-usa@elsevier.com (for online support).**

Reprints. For copies of 100 or more of articles in this publication, please contact the Commercial Reprints Department, Elsevier Inc., 360 Park Avenue South, New York, NY 10010-1710. Tel.: 212-633-3874; Fax: 212-633-3820; E-mail: reprints@elsevier.com.

Cardiac Electrophysiology Clinics is covered in *MEDLINE/PubMed (Index Medicus).*

Contributors

CONSULTING EDITORS

RANJAN K. THAKUR, MD, MPH, MBA, FACC, FHRS
Professor of Medicine and Director, Arrhythmia Service, Thoracic and Cardiovascular Institute, Sparrow Health System, Michigan State University, Lansing, Michigan

ANDREA NATALE, MD, FACC, FHRS, FESC
Department of Cardiology, Texas Cardiac Arrhythmia Institute, St. David's Medical Center; Department of Biomedical Engineering, Cockrell School of Engineering; Department of Internal Medicine, Dell Medical School, University of Texas, Austin, Texas; Department of Cardiology, MetroHealth Medical Center, Case Western Reserve University School of Medicine, Cleveland, Ohio; Atrial Fibrillation and Arrhythmia Center, California Pacific Medical Center, San Francisco, California; Division of Cardiology, Stanford University, Stanford, California; Interventional Electrophysiology, Scripps Clinic, La Jolla, California

EDITORS

AMIN AL-AHMAD, MD
Texas Cardiac Arrhythmia Institute, St. David's Medical Center, Austin, Texas

FRANCIS E. MARCHLINSKI, MD
Richard T. and Angela Clark President's Distinguished Professor of Medicine, Director of Electrophysiology Laboratory, Hospital of the University of Pennsylvania, Director of Electrophysiology, University of Pennsylvania Health System, University of Pennsylvania, Philadelphia, Pennsylvania

AUTHORS

AMIN AL-AHMAD, MD
Texas Cardiac Arrhythmia Institute, St. David's Medical Center, Austin, Texas

ARASH ARYANA, MS, MD
Vice Chair, Department of Cardiology and Cardiovascular Surgery, Mercy General

Hospital, Dignity Health Heart and Vascular Institute, Sacramento, California

FRANK BOGUN, MD
Associate Professor, Division of Electrophysiology, Department of Internal Medicine, University of Michigan Health System, Ann Arbor, Michigan

JASON S. BRADFIELD, MD
Assistant Professor of Medicine, Director,
Specialized Program for Ventricular
Tachycardia, UCLA Cardiac Arrhythmia
Center, David Geffen School of Medicine at
University of California, Los Angeles, California

DAVID F. BRICEÑO, MD
Division of Cardiovascular Disease, Montefiore
Medical Center, Albert Einstein College of
Medicine, Bronx, New York

J. DAVID BURKHARDT, MD
Texas Cardiac Arrhythmia Institute, St. David's
Medical Center, Austin, Texas

ARNAUD CHAUMEIL, MD
Bordeaux University Hospital, LIRYC Institute,
INSERM 1045, Bordeaux University, France

GHASSEN CHENITI, MD
Bordeaux University Hospital, LIRYC Institute,
INSERM 1045, Bordeaux University, France

**KARIN K.M. CHIA, MBBS (Hons), PhD,
FRACP, FHRS**
Department of Cardiology, Consultant
Cardiologist and Cardiac Electrophysiologist,
Royal North Shore Hospital, The University of
Sydney, Sydney, North South Wales, Australia

HUBERT COCHET, MD, PhD
Bordeaux University Hospital, LIRYC Institute,
INSERM 1045, Bordeaux University, France

ANDRÉ D'AVILA, MD, PhD
Director, Cardiac Arrhythmia Service, Instituto
de Pesquisa em Arritmia Cardiaca, Hospital
Cardiologico – Florianopolis, Florianopolis,
Santa Catarina, Brazil

GOPI DANDAMUDI, MD
Assistant Professor of Clinical Medicine,
Department of Medicine, Krannert Institute of
Cardiology, Indiana University School of
Medicine, Indianapolis, Indiana

CHRISTIAN DE CHILLOU, MD, PhD
Professor of Cardiology, University Hospital
Nancy; INSERM-IADI, U947, Vandoeuvre
lès-Nancy, France

ARNAUD DENIS, MD
Bordeaux University Hospital, LIRYC Institute,
INSERM 1045, Bordeaux University, France

NICOLAS DERVAL, MD
Bordeaux University Hospital, LIRYC
Institute, INSERM 1045, Bordeaux University,
France

LUIGI DI BIASE, MD, PhD
Division of Cardiovascular Disease, Montefiore
Medical Center, Albert Einstein College of
Medicine, Bronx, New York; Department of
Cardiology, Texas Cardiac Arrhythmia
Institute, St. David's Medical Center;
Department of Biomedical Engineering,
Cockrell School of Engineering, University
of Texas, Austin, Texas; Arrhythmia
Services, Department of Clinical and
Experimental Medicine, University of Foggia,
Foggia, Italy

SRINIVAS R. DUKKIPATI, MD
Assistant Professor, Helmsley
Electrophysiology Center, Division of
Cardiology, Department of Medicine, Icahn
School of Medicine at Mount Sinai, New York,
New York

ANTONIO FRONTERA, MD
Bordeaux University Hospital, LIRYC
Institute, INSERM 1045, Bordeaux University,
France

FERMIN C. GARCIA, MD
Clinical Cardiac Electrophysiology,
Cardiovascular Medicine Division, Hospital of
the University of Pennsylvania, Philadelphia,
Pennsylvania

CAROLA GIANNI, MD, PhD
Department of Cardiology, Texas Cardiac
Arrhythmia Institute, St. David's Medical
Center, Austin, Texas; Department of Clinical
Sciences and Community Health, University of
Milan, Milan, Italy

MICHEL HAISSAGUERRE, MD
Bordeaux University Hospital, LIRYC Institute,
INSERM 1045, Bordeaux University, France

MELEZE HOCINI, MD
Bordeaux University Hospital, LIRYC Institute,
INSERM 1045, Bordeaux University, France

HENRY H. HSIA, MD, FACC, FHRS
Chief, Arrhythmia Service, Veterans
Administration Medical Center, San Francisco,
Health Sciences Clinical Professor of Medicine,
University of California, San Francisco, San
Francisco, California

RAHUL JAIN, MD, MPH
Assistant Professor of Clinical Medicine,
Department of Medicine, Krannert Institute of
Cardiology, Roudebush VA Medical Center,
Indiana University School of Medicine,
Indianapolis, Indiana

PIERRE JAIS, MD
Bordeaux University Hospital, LIRYC Institute,
INSERM 1045, Bordeaux University, France

THOMAS R. KAMBUR, MD
Fellow in Electrophysiology, Department of
Medicine, Krannert Institute of Cardiology,
Indiana University School of Medicine,
Indianapolis, Indiana

SAURABH KUMAR, BSc(Med), MBBS, PhD
Arrhythmia Service, Cardiovascular Division,
Department of Medicine, Brigham and
Women's Hospital, Harvard Medical School,
Boston, Massachusetts

RAKESH LATCHAMSETTY, MD
Assistant Professor, Division of
Electrophysiology, Department of Internal
Medicine, University of Michigan Health
System, Ann Arbor, Michigan

JACKSON J. LIANG, DO
Electrophysiology Section, Division of
Cardiology, Hospital of the University of
Pennsylvania, Philadelphia, Pennsylvania

RONALD LO, MD, FACC, FHRS
Electrophysiology and Arrhythmia Service,
Veterans Administration Medical Center-Loma
Linda, Associate Professor of Medicine, Loma
Linda University, Loma Linda, California

ISABELLE MAGNIN-POULL, MD
Department of Cardiology, University Hospital
Nancy; INSERM-IADI, U947, Vandoeuvre
lès-Nancy, France

GREGOIRE MASSOULLIE, MD
Bordeaux University Hospital, LIRYC Institute,
INSERM 1045, Bordeaux University, France

JOHN M. MILLER, MD
Professor, Department of Medicine, Krannert
Institute of Cardiology, Director, Clinical
Cardiac Electrophysiology, Indiana University
School of Medicine, Indiana University,
Indianapolis, Indiana

MARC A. MILLER, MD
Assistant Professor, Helmsley
Electrophysiology Center, Division of
Cardiology, Department of Medicine, Icahn
School of Medicine at Mount Sinai, New York,
New York

SANGHAMITRA MOHANTY, MD, MS
Department of Cardiology, Texas Cardiac
Arrhythmia Institute, St. David's Medical
Center; Department of Internal Medicine, Dell
Medical School, University of Texas, Austin,
Texas

DANIELE MUSER, MD
Electrophysiology Section, Division of
Cardiology, Hospital of the University of
Pennsylvania, Philadelphia, Pennsylvania

ANDREA NATALE, MD, FACC, FHRS, FESC
Department of Cardiology, Texas Cardiac
Arrhythmia Institute, St. David's Medical
Center; Department of Biomedical
Engineering, Cockrell School of Engineering;
Department of Internal Medicine, Dell Medical
School, University of Texas, Austin, Texas;
Department of Cardiology, MetroHealth
Medical Center, Case Western Reserve
University School of Medicine, Cleveland,
Ohio; Atrial Fibrillation and Arrhythmia Center,
California Pacific Medical Center, San
Francisco, California; Division of Cardiology,
Stanford University, Stanford, California;
Interventional Electrophysiology, Scripps
Clinic, La Jolla, California

CHANDRASEKAR PALANISWAMY, MD
Assistant Professor, Division of Cardiology,
Department of Medicine, University of
California San Francisco Fresno Medical
Education Program, Fresno, California

RAJEEV K. PATHAK, MBBS, PhD
Clinical Cardiac Electrophysiology,
Cardiovascular Medicine Division, Hospital of
the University of Pennsylvania, Philadelphia,
Pennsylvania

VIVEK Y. REDDY, MD
Professor, Helmsley Electrophysiology Center,
Division of Cardiology, Department of
Medicine, Icahn School of Medicine at Mount
Sinai, New York, New York

JORGE ROMERO, MD
Division of Cardiovascular Disease, Montefiore
Medical Center, Albert Einstein College of
Medicine, Bronx, New York

FREDERIC SACHER, MD, PhD
Bordeaux University Hospital, LIRYC Institute,
INSERM 1045, Bordeaux University, France

PASQUALE SANTANGELI, MD, PhD
Electrophysiology Section, Division of
Cardiology, Hospital of the University of
Pennsylvania, Philadelphia, Pennsylvania

JEAN-MARC SELLAL, MD
Department of Cardiology, University Hospital
Nancy; INSERM-IADI, U947, Vandoeuvre
lès-Nancy, France

KALYANAM SHIVKUMAR, MD, PhD
Professor of Medicine and Radiology, Director,
UCLA Cardiac Arrhythmia Center and EP
Programs, Director and Chief, Interventional
CV Programs, Director, Adult Cardiac
Catheterization Laboratories, UCLA Cardiac
Arrhythmia Center, David Geffen School of
Medicine at University of California, Los
Angeles, Los Angeles, California

WILLIAM G. STEVENSON, MD
Arrhythmia Service, Cardiovascular Division,
Department of Medicine, Brigham and
Women's Hospital, Harvard Medical School,
Boston, Massachusetts

MASATERU TAKIGAWA, MD
Bordeaux University Hospital, LIRYC Institute,
INSERM 1045, Bordeaux University, France

USHA B. TEDROW, MD, MSc
Arrhythmia Service, Cardiovascular Division,
Department of Medicine, Brigham and
Women's Hospital, Harvard Medical School,
Boston, Massachusetts

NATHANIEL THOMPSON, MD
Bordeaux University Hospital, LIRYC Institute,
INSERM 1045, Bordeaux University, France

CHINTAN TRIVEDI, MD, MPH
Texas Cardiac Arrhythmia Institute, St. David's
Medical Center, Austin, Texas

PEDRO A. VILLABLANCA, MSc, MD
Division of Cardiovascular Disease, Montefiore
Medical Center, Albert Einstein College of
Medicine, Bronx, New York

ADRIANUS P. WIJNMAALEN, MD, PhD
Department of Cardiology, Leiden University
Medical Center, Leiden, The Netherlands

KATJA ZEPPENFELD, MD, PhD
Department of Cardiology, Leiden University
Medical Center, Leiden, The Netherlands

Contents

The 12-lead electrocardiogram (ECG) during ventricular tachycardia (VT) in patients with structural heart disease contains information that helps to narrow the electrophysiologist's search for target sites for ablation. Although replacement of myocardium by scar might be expected to produce variability in the spread of activation during VT, nonetheless reasonably consistent ECG patterns exist that can regionalize exit sites from VT circuits in up to 75% of cases. Most experience with this comes from patients with prior myocardial infarction, but a growing body of data exists concerning patients with nonischemic cardiomyopathies.

Ablation of ventricular tachycardia (VT) in the setting of structural heart disease, previously reserved for highly experienced specialized centers, is being performed at more centers internationally as cardiac electrophysiologists gain advanced training. Interventional cardiac electrophysiologists need a high level of anatomic knowledge to guide a procedure that can carry significant risk. Understanding cardiac anatomy improves the chance of procedural success and also the likelihood of appropriate decision making if complications are encountered. This article focuses on selected anatomic regions where complex anatomy can be an impediment to successful VT ablation.

Ventricular arrhythmias are a significant cause of morbidity and mortality in patients with ischemic structural heart disease. Endocardial and epicardial mapping strategies include scar characterization, channel identification, and recording and ablation of late potentials and local abnormal ventricular activities. Catheter ablation along with new technology and techniques of bipolar ablation, needle catheter, and autonomic modulation may increase efficacy in difficult to ablate ventricular arrhythmias. Catheter ablation of ventricular arrhythmias seem to confer mortality and morbidity benefits in patients with ischemic heart disease.

Although catheter ablation has been successful in reducing the recurrence of ventricular tachycardia in patients with ischemic disease, outcomes in patients with nonischemic cardiomyopathy (NICM) have not met with the same results. Success is predicated on a methodical approach to diagnosis of disease type and identification of critical substrate, and the ablation strategies used. Cardiac MRI with delayed enhancement is able to identify areas of substrate involvement, particularly in situations when conventional catheter mapping is not able to do so. Radiofrequency needle, irrigated bipolar radiofrequency, and transcoronary alcohol ablation are effective and alternative techniques to endocardial and epicardial ablation.

Mapping during ventricular tachycardia (VT) aims to elucidate mechanism, describe myocardial propagation, and identify the origin and critical regions of VT that can be targeted for ablation, most commonly with radiofrequency ablation. Most VTs in structural heart disease are due to macro-reentry in and around scar. A combination of mapping techniques, including mapping to identify the arrhythmia substrate, activation sequence mapping, pace-mapping, and entrainment mapping, may be used to identify putative ablation targets. This review describes the principles of entrainment mapping as it pertains to catheter ablation of scar-related VT.

Most postinfarct ventricular tachycardias (VT) are sustained by a reentrant mechanism. The "protected isthmus" of the reentrant circuit is critical for the maintenance of VTs and the target for catheter ablation. In this article, the authors describe the technique of pace-mapping during sinus rhythm to unmask postinfarct VT isthmuses. A pace-mapping map should be considered as the surrogate of an activation map during VT, in both patients with a normal heart and patients with a structural heart disease. Pace mapping is useful to unmask VT isthmuses in patients with postinfarct reentrant VTs.

Ventricular arrhythmias are a frequent cause of mortality in patients with ischemic cardiomyopathy and nonischemic cardiomyopathy. Scar-related reentry represents the most common arrhythmia substrate in patients with recurrent episodes of sustained ventricular tachycardia (VT). Initial mapping of scar-related VT circuits is focused on identifying arrhythmogenic tissue. The substrate-based strategies include targeting late potentials, scar dechanneling, local abnormal ventricular activities, core isolation, and homogenization of the scar. Even though substrate-based strategies for VT ablation have shown promising outcomes for patients with structural heart disease related to ischemic cardiomyopathy, the data are scarce for patients with nonischemic substrates.

Carola Gianni, Sanghamitra Mohanty, Chintan Trivedi, Luigi Di Biase, Amin Al-Ahmad, Andrea Natale, and J. David Burkhardt

Ventricular tachycardia (VT) ablation is usually performed with an ablation catheter that delivers unipolar radiofrequency (RF) energy to eliminate the re-entry circuit responsible for VT. However, there are some instances when unipolar RF ablation fails, notably in VTs with a deep intramural origin, or cases in which epicardial access is not attainable due to prior cardiac surgery. To overcome these limitations, several alternative approaches have been used in clinical practice, including alcohol ablation or coil embolization, simultaneous unipolar or bipolar RF ablation, surgical ablation, or noninvasive ablation with stereotactic radiosurgery. This review article describes some of these alternative techniques.

Rajeev K. Pathak and Fermin C. Garcia

Endocardial and epicardial electroanatomical mapping and ablation is a safe and effective therapy in the treatment of right ventricle arrhythmias occurring in the setting of arrhythmogenic right ventricular cardiomyopathy (ARVD). Careful mapping and ablation plans must be tailored for each patient based on comorbidities and ventricular tachycardia morphologies. This review focuses on the catheter ablation for ventricular arrhythmias in patients with ARVD.

Adrianus P. Wijnmaalen and Katja Zeppenfeld

Radiofrequency catheter ablation (RFCA) is an important treatment modality to prevent ventricular tachycardia (VT) recurrence in patients with repaired congenital heart disease. Identification and ablation of anatomic isthmuses has improved acute ablation outcome with excellent VT-free survival in those with preserved biventricular function. Reports on RFCA for VT in patients with infiltrative disease are sparse and cardiac sarcoidosis seems to be the most prevalent cause for ventricular arrhythmia. Patients with active and ongoing inflammation are at high risk for VT recurrence. RFCA reduces the number of VT but often multiple procedures are required and long-term VT-free survival is unfavorable in those with left ventricular dysfunction.

Arash Aryana and André d'Avila

Over the last two decades, epicardial catheter ablation has evolved into a practical approach for treatment of ventricular tachycardia (VT). There are certain considerations when performing this procedure. First, presence of epicardial fat can diminish peak-to-peak electrogram amplitude and also impede radiofrequency energy delivery. Hence, epicardial VT ablation should be performed with cooled-tip radiofrequency using reduced irrigation flow within a relatively 'dry' pericardial milieu. Furthermore, catheter orientation is key when performing epicardial ablation. Lastly, hemo-pericardium remains the most common major adverse event of epicardial ablation and its presenting timeline may be used to identify the precise nature of this complication.

> Frequent premature ventricular complexes (PVCs) in patients with underlying structural heart disease, particular after myocardial infarction, can predict increased mortality. Use of antiarrhythmic medications to suppress PVCs in this setting can result in a further increase in mortality. High PVC burdens in patients with structural heart disease can cause or worsen cardiomyopathy and successful elimination of PVCs with catheter ablation can improve or, in some cases normalize, cardiac function. PVCs may also trigger more malignant ventricular arrhythmias, particularly in patients with previous myocardial infarction, and when identified can be mapped and ablated.

> This review discusses the role of hemodynamic support for catheter ablation of unstable ventricular tachycardia, using commercially available mechanical circulatory support devices (intra-aortic balloon pump, Impella, TandemHeart, extracorporeal membrane oxygenation) and analyzes the published clinical experience of the safety and efficacy of these devices during ventricular tachycardia ablation. Appropriate selection of patients, device-specific characteristics, and hemodynamic monitoring is also discussed.

> Catheter ablation is an increasingly used treatment option for patients with ventricular tachycardia (VT) in the setting of structural heart disease. Although there are extensive data from several retrospective studies as well as prospective non-randomized observational studies, there are limited data from relatively few randomized controlled trials, especially comparing VT ablation with antiarrhythmic drugs. In this review, the authors aim to summarize the major studies examining efficacy of VT ablation in patients with structural heart disease, discuss barriers to enrollment and completion of randomized clinical trials, and propose areas of future research in the field.

CARDIAC ELECTROPHYSIOLOGY CLINICS

THE CLINICS ARE AVAILABLE ONLINE!
Access your subscription at:
www.theclinics.com

CARDIAC ELECTROPHYSIOLOGY CLINICS

ISSUE OF RELATED INTEREST

Foreword
Ventricular Tachycardia Ablation

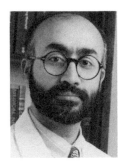
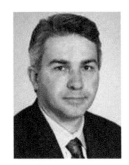

Ranjan K. Thakur, MD, MPH, MBA, FACC, FHRS   Andrea Natale, MD, FACC, FHRS, FESC
Consulting Editors

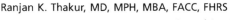

Ventricular arrhythmias and sudden cardiac death were the main focus of cardiac electrophysiology in its nascent years. As the cause of ventricular tachycardia (VT), its mechanisms and substrates became better understood, attempts at ablation were undertaken, first by using surgical techniques (endocardial resection ± cryoablation and ventricular exclusion) and then by using direct current shocks. Other energy sources, such as laser ablation, were also investigated, but later supplanted by radiofrequency (RF) ablation. Now, catheter-based RF ablation is the predominant method for VT ablation used worldwide.

VT ablation has evolved into a field by itself, with a body of literature that's vast, and there are experts who devote a major part of their clinical and research efforts to these arrhythmias.

This issue of *Cardiac Electrophysiology Clinics* focuses on VT ablation in patients with some form of structural heart disease. The editors have invited experts in the field to shed light on anatomic considerations during VT ablation and electrocardiographic and catheter localization of the VT ablation site using various techniques; each of these localizing techniques are discussed in detail, endocardial and epicardial

ablation as well as ablation in various types of heart disease.

We congratulate the editors and contributors for readable and practical reviews relevant to the clinical electrophysiologist. This issue of *Cardiac Electrophysiology Clinics* should be essential reading for clinicians in practice, because it provides a good review of relevant clinical matters, and for electrophysiology fellows in training, who are developing their foundational knowledge in electrophysiology.

Ranjan K. Thakur, MD, MPH, MBA, FACC, FHRS
Sparrow Thoracic and Cardiovascular Institute
Michigan State University
1200 East Michigan Avenue, Suite 580
Lansing, MI 48912, USA

Andrea Natale, MD, FACC, FHRS, FESC
Texas Cardiac Arrhythmia Institute
Center for Atrial Fibrillation at
St. David's Medical Center
1015 East 32nd Street, Suite 516
Austin, TX 78705, USA

E-mail addresses:
thakur@msu.edu (R.K. Thakur)
andrea.natale@stdavids.com (A. Natale)

Card Electrophysiol Clin 9 (2017) xiii
http://dx.doi.org/10.1016/j.ccep.2016.12.002
1877-9182/17/© 2016 Published by Elsevier Inc.

Preface

Ventricular Tachycardia in Structural Heart Disease

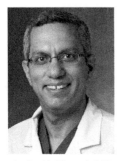
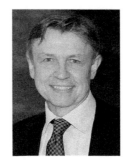

Amin Al-Ahmad, MD   Francis E. Marchlinski, MD

Editors

This issue of *Cardiac Electrophysiology Clinics* is focused on ventricular tachycardia in patients with structural heart disease. We are fortunate to have a group of experts and leaders in the field contribute the latest knowledge in this area. The issue begins with an article on electrocardiogram localization as well as an article on anatomic considerations, important when contemplating an ablative strategy for management of ventricular tachycardia patients.

Next, considerations specific to ablation in patients with ischemic heart disease as well as those with nonischemic heart disease are discussed. Techniques such as entrainment mapping, pace mapping, and substrate ablation are also covered in subsequent articles. In addition, an article is dedicated to techniques that may be useful when standard ablation is unsuccessful, such as surgical ablation and alcohol ablation.

Specific disease states that may have unique challenges are also discussed in an article on arrhythmogenic right ventricular dysplasia as well as an article on ablation of ventricular tachycardia in patients with congenital and infiltrative heart disease.

An article on the important aspects of epicardial ablation is also covered, as is premature ventricular contaction ablation in patients with structural heart disease, and the use of hemodynamic support during ablation procedures.

This issue is complete with an article detailing clinical trials in ventricular tachycardia ablation.

We are confident that this issue will be relevant to cardiac electrophysiologists and cardiac electrophysiology trainees as well as all clinicians interested in the management of ventricular tachycardia.

Amin Al-Ahmad, MD
Texas Cardiac Arrhythmia Institute
3000 North IH35, Suite 700
Austin, TX 78705, USA

Francis E. Marchlinski, MD
Hospital of the University of Pennsylvania
University of Pennsylvania Health System
University of Pennsylvania
3400 Spruce Street
9 Founders Pavilion
Philadelphia, PA 19104-4283, USA

E-mail addresses:
aalahmadmd@gmail.com (A. Al-Ahmad)
Francis.Marchlinski@uphs.upenn.edu
(F.E. Marchlinski)

http://dx.doi.org/10.1016/j.ccep.2016.12.001
1877-9182/17/© 2016 Published by Elsevier Inc.

cardiacEP.theclinics.com

Electrocardiographic Localization of Ventricular Tachycardia in Patients with Structural Heart Disease

John M. Miller, MD[a],*, Rahul Jain, MD, MPH[b],
Gopi Dandamudi, MD[c], Thomas R. Kambur, MD[c]

KEYWORDS

- Electrocardiogram • Ventricular tachycardia • Exit sites • Mapping

KEY POINTS

- In the presence of scar related to structural heart disease, common sense rules for localizing the source of ventricular complexes and ventricular tachycardia (VT) are not always valid.
- However, reasonably consistent 12-lead patterns of VT exist such that exit sites can be regionalized in up to 75% of VTs in patients with prior myocardial infarction.
- Exit sites of VTs with left bundle branch block (BBB) are more readily regionalized than are VTs with right BBB.
- The presence of a q wave (followed by an r wave) is a strong indicator of epicardial exit sites in non-ischemic cardiomyopathies.

INTRODUCTION

Before the advent of cardiac mapping techniques, the site of origin or source of ectopic complexes from the heart was a matter of interesting conjecture but lacked relevance. When therapeutic options became available, such as surgical ablation for treatment of Wolff–Parkinson–White syndrome and ventricular tachycardia (VT), mapping tools to locate areas responsible for arrhythmias quickly became important. Among these were the ability to correlate the surface electrocardiogram (ECG) during VT with an area in the heart at which ablation could eradicate it. With surgical ablation using a variety of methods, absolute precision of locating the arrhythmogenic tissue was not critical because these techniques (endocardial resection, extensive cryoablation) were able to remove or otherwise destroy large portions of abnormal tissue. With the subsequent development of catheter

Author Disclosures: Dr J.M. Miller reports having received honoraria from Medtronic, St. Jude Medical, Biotronik, Biosense Webster, Boston Scientific and has been a scientific advisor to Abbott/Topera (modest, <$10,000); Dr R. Jain has received honoraria from Biosense Webster; Dr G. Dandamudi has received honoraria from Medtronic and Biosense Webster; Dr T.R. Kambur has no disclosures to report.
[a] Department of Medicine, Krannert Institute of Cardiology, Indiana University School of Medicine, Indiana University, 1800 North Capitol Avenue, E-488, Indianapolis, IN 46202, USA; [b] Department of Medicine, Krannert Institute of Cardiology, Roudebush VA Medical Center, Indiana University School of Medicine, 1000 West 10th Street, Indianapolis, IN 46202, USA; [c] Department of Medicine, Krannert Institute of Cardiology, Indiana University School of Medicine, 1800 North Capitol Avenue, Indianapolis, IN 46202, USA
* Corresponding author.
E-mail address: jmiller6@iu.edu

cardiacEP.theclinics.com

ablation techniques, however, precision of localization was more important owing to the more limited amount of damage that could be effected by catheter as opposed to surgical ablation. In this article, we review the ECG features that indicate exit sites of wavefronts from VT reentrant circuits or foci, with an emphasis on patients with structural heart disease (SHD).

GENERAL PRINCIPLES

In patients without SHD, the QRS morphology during VT correlates well with the site of impulse formation (ie, a focus, causal in the vast majority of patients). In this setting, VT with right bundle branch block (RBBB) pattern (defined here as the latter portion of the QRS in lead V1 being a positive deflection) arise from the left ventricle (LV; thus the right ventricle [RV] is activated last), and left bundle branch block (LBBB) pattern VTs (with a negative deflection as the latter half of lead V1) arise from the RV. VTs with tall R waves in inferior leads arise from the anterior/superior aspects of the ventricles and those with R waves in leads 1 and aVL arise from the RV or septal aspect of the LV, and so forth. However, in the presence of SHD, these straightforward relationships between VT morphology and exit sites may be disrupted. This is because SHD in whatever form—myocardial infarction (MI), idiopathic cardiomyopathy (CM), Chagas disease, sarcoid, etc—is generally accompanied by replacement of some amount of myocardium with scar. This has 2 important effects on the QRS complex: first, myocardium that has been supplanted by scar no longer contributes to the contour of the QRS, and second, scar forms a barrier to propagation from 1 portion of the ventricle to another, slowing conduction and altering the QRS in sometimes unpredictable ways. Thus, the QRS complex during VT in a patient with SHD typically differs from VT exiting from a similar location in a patient without SHD by having (1) a lower QRS amplitude, (2) a wider QRS duration, and (3) notches in the QRS rather than smooth contours, indicating change in direction of the wavefront owing to diversion by scar (**Fig. 1**). It is perhaps surprising that, despite the presence of scar and its influence on conduction patterns in residual myocardium, there remains a reasonably consistent relationship between VT QRS morphology and region of exit to the remaining myocardium.

In contrast with the case with VT in the absence of SHD, most cases of VT in patients with SHD have a reentrant mechanism; thus, the cardiac site that is activated at the time of QRS onset in

these VTs corresponds with the exit from a circuit. As noted elsewhere, the exit site or region from a VT circuit is typically wider than the diastolic isthmus (which may be >1 cm away). The latter region, from which mid diastolic potentials are recorded during VT, is a more suitable target for ablation than the exit site in most cases, and although the diastolic corridor is near the exit site, they are not at the same location. Thus, in most cases of SHD, the QRS morphology in VT can direct attention to a region near which an appropriate ablation target site (the diastolic corridor) can be found, but usually not the actual ideal ablation target itself.

As noted, LBBB VTs in patients without SHD arise from the RV, RBBB VTs from the LV; however, in patients with the most common forms of SHD (prior MI and idiopathic CM), whereas RBBB VTs almost always exit from the LV, most LBBB VTs also exit from the LV (septum or <1 cm paraseptal). This seems to be related to more rapid spread of activation to and through the RV, which has less disease, than the LV, which has more scarring.

ISCHEMIC HEART DISEASE/PRIOR MYOCARDIAL INFARCTION

The most common setting in which VT occurs is after a prior extensive MI. Historically, myocardial regions damaged by anterior infarction (left anterior descending artery occlusion, usually proximal or mid vessel) include the apex, anterior, and often apical lateral walls and apical one-half of the interventricular septum. Regions damaged by inferior infarction (right or circumflex coronary occlusions) include the inferobasal free wall with variable extension laterally (to the obtuse margin in many cases) and basal septum. These areas are illustrated in **Fig. 2**. VT exit sites tend to occur within or at the periphery of these infarct regions, which are composed of very dense scar with endocardial sparing and "marbling" through the thinned walls with strands of surviving myocardium. Since the mid 1990s, reperfusion therapy has modified this pattern, resulting in varying degrees of myocardial salvage and thus less scar development. Infarction zones tend to be smaller than before the reperfusion era, but exit sites from VT circuits are generally similar.

The vast majority of VTs in post-MI patients are owing to reentry within endocardial circuits[1,2] (or, at least a portion is accessible on the endocardial surface) and exit sites; this suggests that endocardial catheter ablation should have a high likelihood of successful ablation in these cases. A very small proportion (<5%) of VTs have successful ablation

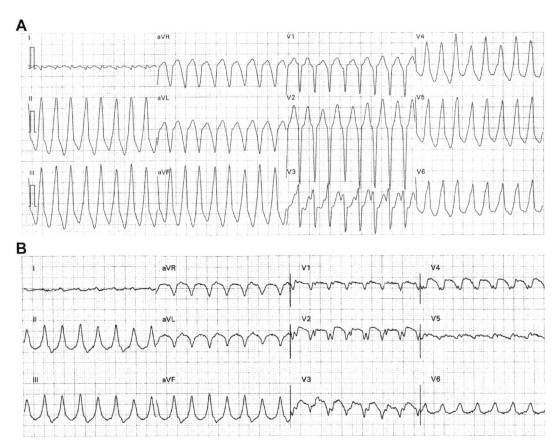

Fig. 1. Electrocardiographs showing ventricular tachycardia (VT) with similar morphologies from 2 different patients. (A) Right ventricular outflow tract VT in a patient without structural heart disease. (B) Left ventricular anterior septal VT in a patient with prior anterior myocardial infarction. Although the overall QRS contours are qualitatively similar in these 2 VTs, the complexes in B are of a lower amplitude, wider, and contain notches compared with the complexes in A, indicating the influence of scar on the complexes in B. LBBB, left bundle branch block.

sites that are uniquely epicardial (ie, not ablatable from an endocardial approach). Additionally, some patients with prior MI have a focal, rather than reentrant, source VT.[3]

Early efforts in endocardial catheter-based activation mapping of VT (sampling a large number of endocardial sites during VT, seeking those with electrograms preceding the QRS onset) showed that several similar VT morphologies from different patients had reasonably consistent exit sites in their respective ventricles[4]; the principle of pace mapping (matching a target QRS morphology with that resulting from pacing at various sites) developed from this process.[5] Based on data obtained during point-by-point activation mapping during surgical or catheter-based mapping and ablation procedures, and pace mapping during catheterization procedures, several algorithms have been developed to correlate VT QRS complexes with exit sites from VT circuits. These have also been tested

prospectively on additional sets of VTs by each respective set of authors. The overall sensitivity and specificity of these algorithms are reasonable, but rather than pinpointing an exact site at which ablation will eliminate VTs, they instead serve as a guide as to where initial mapping efforts should be directed (these areas must then be explored further with denser activation mapping to locate the diastolic corridor for optimal ablation). These algorithms have several similarities, but significant differences as well.

1. Miller and colleagues[6] (**Fig. 3**) divided the LV into 12 roughly similarly sized regions of 3 to 5 cm^2, and analyzed 182 VTs that had been mapped (catheter or surgically) according to infarct location (anterior or inferior); LBBB or RBBB morphology in lead V1; quadrant of frontal plane axis; and precordial R wave pattern (1 of 8 possibilities). An algorithm based on these features was then tested on

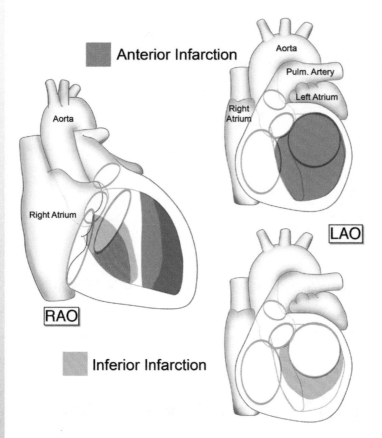

Fig. 2. Left ventricular regions affected by anterior (*red*) versus inferior (*blue*) infarctions. Ventricular tachycardia in such patients tends to exit from within or at the perimeter of the infarction zone. LAO, left anterior oblique; RAO, right anterior oblique.

110 additional VTs from 63 other patients and found to be 93% correct, when the algorithm could be applied (~75%). LBBB VTs and those related to prior inferior MI were more readily localized with this algorithm than VTs related to anterior MI or RBBB VTs.

2. Kuchar and colleagues[7] (**Fig. 4**) divided the LV into 3 different zones in each of 3 spatial axes for regionalization; ECGs obtained during pacing from different LV sites in 22 patients were then analyzed in a 3-step algorithm evaluating lead V4 (to regionalize in the basal-apical axis), then lead 2 (anterior–inferior axis), and finally lead V1 (septal–lateral axis). The algorithm developed from these data was tested in 44 VTs from 42 additional patients and was found to be correct or very nearly so in 75% of these VTs.

3. Segal and colleagues[8] (**Fig. 5**) divided the LV into 9 regions and used noncontact activation mapping in 121 VTs from 51 post-MI patients to develop an algorithm incorporating the bundle branch block pattern, then polarity of the inferior leads, followed by polarity in lead 1 and/or aVL, and finally (in some cases of RBBB VT), polarity in aVL and aVR. The algorithm thus derived was tested in an additional

17 VTs in 11 patients and, with this limited application, found to be correct in 93% of cases.

4. Yokokawa and colleagues[9] divided the LV into 10 regions and developed an algorithm based on digitized ECGs derived from pacing in scar areas of post-MI patients. This algorithm was applied to 58 VTs in which pace mapping was used to define the exit site. In the authors' hands, the new semiautomated algorithm indicated the correct anatomic region about 70% of the time and compared favorably to the algorithms of Miller and associates[6] and Segal and coworkers.[8]

There have been no studies that directly compared the accuracy of these different algorithms on the same VT dataset. Recent reviews of application of these algorithms as well as additional insights and explanations have been published by different groups.[10,11]

The ability to regionalize exit sites for VT has important implications for activation mapping, but can also aid in substrate mapping. If activation mapping cannot be performed during VT owing to hemodynamic instability, knowledge of the likely

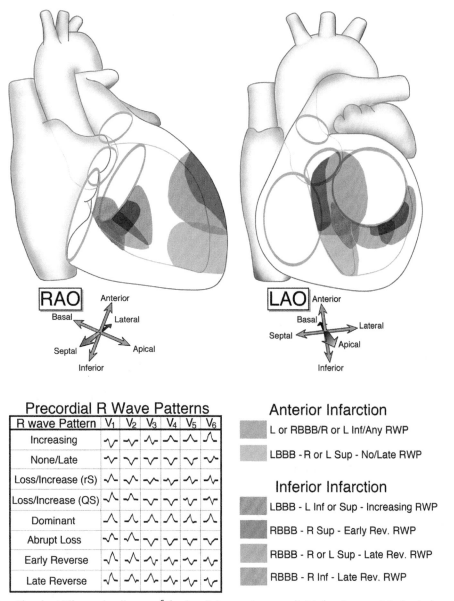

Fig. 3. Algorithm by Miller and colleagues[6] for localizing postmyocardial infarction ventricular tachycardia exit sites based on standard activation mapping. See text for details. Inf, inferior; L, left; LAO, left anterior oblique; LBBB, left bundle branch block; R, right; RAO, right anterior oblique; RBBB, right bundle branch block; RWP, R wave progression; Sup, superior.

VT exit site can direct the operator to ablate in that region and thus hope to eliminate critical portions of the VT circuit.

NONISCHEMIC CARDIOMYOPATHY

This heterogeneous group comprises a number of different disorders including hypertrophic CM, sarcoid CM, arrhythmogenic right (and/or left) ventricular dysplasia/CM, Chagas CM, and the largest group, namely, idiopathic dilated CM.

Because there are considerable differences among them, these disorders are considered separately.

Idiopathic Dilated Cardiomyopathy

The cause of myocardial scarring is obscure in this category (which may be the end result of several different pathologic processes). However, in many cases, scar distribution is predominantly basal (near valve orifices) and, although endocardial

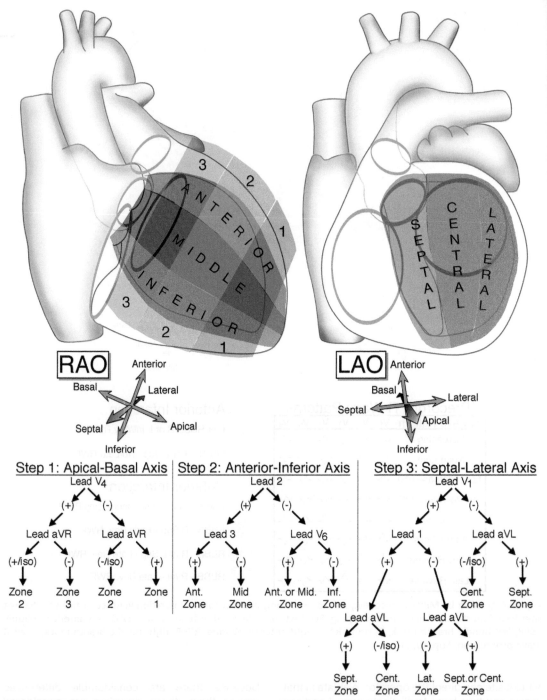

Fig. 4. Algorithm by Kuchar and colleagues[7] for localizing postmyocardial infarction ventricular tachycardia exit sites based on pacemapping. See text for details. LAO, left anterior oblique; RAO, right anterior oblique.

scar is usually present, mid myocardial and epicardial scarring are present to the degree that circuits and exits from these circuits are more common than in post-MI VTs. Because of the clustering of VT substrate near the cardiac base, large R waves are generally present in precordial leads. When this is not the case (ie, poor R wave progression during VT), the patient often has more extensive disease (extending to the apex) and should be evaluated carefully for significant worsening of heart failure that might require mechanical assistance or transplantation.[12]

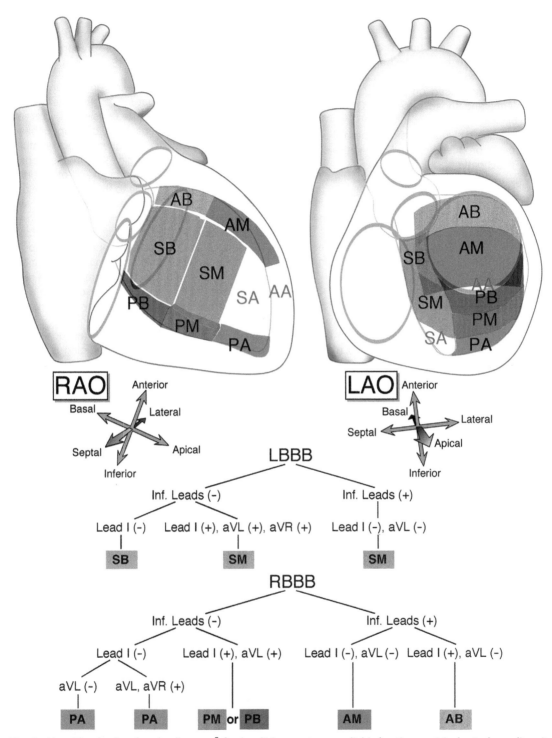

Fig. 5. Algorithm by Segal and colleagues[8] for localizing postmyocardial infarction ventricular tachycardia exit sites based on noncontact activation mapping. See text for details. Inf, inferior; LAO, left anterior oblique; RAO, right anterior oblique.

VTs in patients with idiopathic dilated CM tend to have substantial QRS notching or fragmentation and have among the widest QRS complexes. This is perhaps because of either the distribution of scar that delays myocardial propagation, or coexisting disease in the His-Purkinje system (HPS), which seems to mediate the spread of the wavefront once it is engaged. Delayed entry into the

HPS from an epicardial circuit/exit is also a likely cause.

Several criteria have been proposed to identify VTs that require epicardial mapping and ablation; these can be separated into 2 categories, namely, those based on interval/duration measurements and those based on QRS contours (**Fig. 6**).

Several interval indicators of epicardial sources have been proposed, based on analysis of LV VTs (RBBB pattern):

a. Pseudo delta wave of 34 ms or greater (measured from earliest QRS onset in any lead to the earliest rapid deflection in any precordial lead[13];
b. Intrinsicoid deflection in lead V2 of greater than 85 ms (measured from earliest QRS onset in any lead to peak in V2)[13];
c. Shortest RS complex interval of 121 ms or greater (measured from the earliest QRS onset in any lead to the nadir of the first S wave in any precordial lead)[13];
d. QRS duration of greater than 200 ms in any lead[13]; or

e. Maximum deflection index[14] of 0.55 or greater (the quotient of the interval from QRS onset to earliest R wave peak in precordial leads, divided by maximum QRS duration).

When 1 criterion suggests an epicardial process and others do not (as is often the case), it is unclear which should be considered "correct." As noted, these criteria were developed based on LV VTs and have not been found helpful in analyzing VTs of RV origin. With the exception of the maximum deflection index, all of the interval criteria are susceptible to the influence of antiarrhythmic drug effects that nonspecifically slow conduction and could prolong any of the "raw" or absolute interval measurements into the range that suggests the need for epicardial mapping and ablation. Only the maximum deflection index, using the patient's own QRS duration as a reference, does not seem to be altered by the effect of antiarrhythmic drugs. A corollary to this caution is that if the interval indices do not suggest epicardial pathology despite the presence of antiarrhythmic drugs, epicardial mapping is unlikely to be needed.

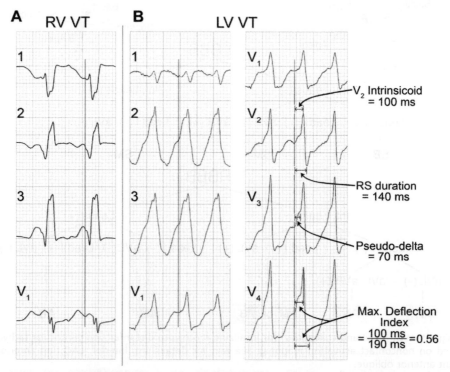

Fig. 6. Examples of electrocardiographic criteria suggesting an epicardial source of ventricular tachycardia (VT) in 2 patients with idiopathic dilated cardiomyopathy. In each panel, red lines denote onset of QRS complexes. In (*A*), a right ventricular (RV) VT shows a small q wave in lead 1 and q waves in the inferior leads. In (*B*), a left ventricular (LV) VT, a small q wave is seen in lead 1 in the center panel; duration indices are shown in the right panel. See text for details.

Several morphologic (QRS contour) indicators of epicardial sources in the presence of SHD have been proposed:

a. An initial q wave (followed by r wave) in lead 1 is a strong indicator of an epicardial source, especially in RBBB VTs with inferior axis (superior basal LV epicardium).[15] It likewise indicates an epicardial source in LBBB VTs arising from the anterior RV.[16]
b. QS in lead V2 in LBBB VTs correlates with an exit site in the anterior RV.[16]
c. An initial q wave (followed by an r wave) in inferior leads in LBBB VTs correlates with an exit site in the inferobasal RV.[17]

Of note, the criteria for epicardial sources of VT in cardiomyopathies have not been found to be useful in patients with prior MI.

Bundle branch reentry

Patients with idiopathic dilated CM often have significant disease in the HPS, leading to the appearance of LBBB on the sinus rhythm ECG. In a significant proportion of these patients (some authors suggest as high as 30%), reentry within the HPS is a cause of spontaneous VT. The majority of these have an LBBB appearance similar to that of the sinus rhythm ECG, but some manifest a typical RBBB appearance with either left anterior or posterior fascicular block; rarely, intrafascicular reentry is present with a variety of possible QRS duration and bundle branch block patterns. The key to diagnosis of bundle branch reentrant VT is recognition of the VT QRS complex as (1) nearly identical to the sinus rhythm complex (if LBBB) or (2) consistent with typical aberration patterns (if RBBB). Further diagnostic testing requires recordings from the HPS during VT (as discussed elsewhere).

Arrhythmogenic Right Ventricular Dysplasia/Cardiomyopathy

Because RV disease is a defining feature of this disorder, most VTs have LBBB patterns in V1. Very thick scar and epicardial circuits make endocardial ablation less effective than epicardial approaches. VTs typically exit from the inferior or inferolateral basal region near the tricuspid valve (with a leftward superior axis), or in the outflow tract region (with an inferior axis). QRS complexes in VT may be quite wide, reflecting several features that tend to prolong the QRS (far lateral [nonseptal] and often epicardial exits that are some distance from entry to the HPS, and extensive scar that slows conduction). Some patients have biventricular involvement, with RBBB patterns in V1 in VTs with LV exit sites. Multiple morphologies of VT

are common, an important feature distinguishing this disorder from benign RV outflow tract VT or other idiopathic RV VTs (in which patients rarely have >1 VT morphology).

Sarcoid Cardiomyopathy

Although no characteristic ECG morphologies have been described in patients with VT related to cardiac sarcoidosis, most have RV pathology with LBBB patterns in V1 that have a very delayed downstroke of the QS complex. Some patients have biventricular involvement in the granulomatous process, with RBBB patterns in V1 related to LV sources of VT. Multiple VT morphologies in each patient are the rule rather than the exception.[18] Some cases respond to immunosuppression. Distinction of cardiac sarcoidosis from arrhythmogenic right (and/or left) ventricular dysplasia/CM is important in that treatments may be very different [epicardial ablation required in most cases of arrhythmogenic right (and/or) left] ventricular dysplasia/CM, as well as the importance of restriction of exercise and genetic counseling, and immunosuppressive therapy in cardiac sarcoidosis). Wider QRS complexes during sinus rhythm, worse LV ejection fraction, and septal scar on cardiac MRI favor sarcoidosis,[19,20] but no distinguishing patterns during VT have been reported between these 2 disorders.

Chagasic Cardiomyopathy

Scarring and wall motion abnormalities in chronic Chagasic CM affect the inferolateral basal LV and apical LV most commonly; a typical VT morphology is RBBB with a rightward axis, exiting from the inferolateral LV. Some patients also have some degree of RV disease with resultant LBBB VTs.[21]

Hypertrophic Cardiomyopathy

VTs in this disorder may exit from the apical region (especially in the presence of an apical aneurysm). As such, VTs have small R waves or even QS complexes in the precordial leads, a superior axis, and either RBBB or LBBB pattern.[22] However, when there is no aneurysm, epicardial circuits and exit sites are common[23]; no characteristic ECG findings in these settings have been reported.

SUMMARY

In patients without SHD, the 12-lead ECG in VT often provides information that can localize the myocardial site of exit from a focus to within a small anatomic area (1-2 cm^2). In the presence of SHD, replacement of QRS-generating myocardium by scar tissue—from a variety of pathologic causes—alters routes of propagation in the remaining myocardium. Although this would be expected to introduce additional variables in the contour of the QRS complex during VT in these cases, it is still possible to at least regionalize exit sites based on information in the VT ECG in up to 75% of cases. This has important procedural implications, such as where to focus initial mapping efforts on the endocardium and whether to plan for pericardial access and epicardial mapping. Scar-based VT is most often owing to reentry, and thus the ECG during VT (that indicates the exit site from a circuit, not its mid diastolic corridor) does not point to a good ablation site but can help to narrow the search area for such sites.

REFERENCES

1. Josephson ME, Almendral JM, Buxton AE, et al. Mechanisms of ventricular tachycardia. Circulation 1987;75(4 Pt 2):III41–47.
2. Josephson ME, Horowitz LN, Farshidi A, et al. Recurrent sustained ventricular tachycardia. 1. Mechanisms. Circulation 1978;57(3):431–40.
3. Das MK, Scott LR, Miller JM. Focal mechanism of ventricular tachycardia in coronary artery disease. Heart Rhythm 2010;7(3):305–11.
4. Josephson ME, Horowitz LN, Waxman HL, et al. Sustained ventricular tachycardia: role of the 12-lead electrocardiogram in localizing site of origin. Circulation 1981;64(2):257–72.
5. Josephson ME, Waxman HL, Cain ME, et al. Ventricular activation during ventricular endocardial pacing. II. Role of pace-mapping to localize origin of ventricular tachycardia. Am J Cardiol 1982;50(1):11–22.
6. Miller JM, Marchlinski FE, Buxton AE, et al. Relationship between the 12-lead electrocardiogram during ventricular tachycardia and endocardial site of origin in patients with coronary artery disease. Circulation 1988;77(4):759–66.
7. Kuchar DL, Ruskin JN, Garan H. Electrocardiographic localization of the site of origin of ventricular tachycardia in patients with prior myocardial infarction. J Am Coll Cardiol 1989;13(4):893–903.
8. Segal OR, Chow AW, Wong T, et al. A novel algorithm for determining endocardial VT exit site from 12-lead surface ECG characteristics in human, infarct-related ventricular tachycardia. J Cardiovasc Electrophysiol 2007;18(2):161–8.
9. Yokokawa M, Liu TY, Yoshida K, et al. Automated analysis of the 12-lead electrocardiogram to identify the exit site of postinfarction ventricular tachycardia. Heart Rhythm 2012;9(3):330–4.
10. Josephson ME, Callans DJ. Using the twelve-lead electrocardiogram to localize the site of origin of ventricular tachycardia. Heart Rhythm 2005;2(4):443–6.
11. de Riva M, Watanabe M, Zeppenfeld K. Twelve-lead ECG of ventricular tachycardia in structural heart disease. Circ Arrhythm Electrophysiol 2015;8(4):951–62.
12. Frankel DS, Tschabrunn CM, Cooper JM, et al. Apical ventricular tachycardia morphology in left ventricular nonischemic cardiomyopathy predicts poor transplant-free survival. Heart Rhythm 2013;10(5):621–6.
13. Berruezo A, Mont L, Nava S, et al. Electrocardiographic recognition of the epicardial origin of ventricular tachycardias. Circulation 2004;109(15):1842–7.
14. Daniels DV, Lu YY, Morton JB, et al. Idiopathic epicardial left ventricular tachycardia originating remote from the sinus of Valsalva: electrophysiological characteristics, catheter ablation, and identification from the 12-lead electrocardiogram. Circulation 2006;113(13):1659–66.
15. Valles E, Bazan V, Marchlinski FE. ECG criteria to identify epicardial ventricular tachycardia in nonischemic cardiomyopathy. Circ Arrhythm Electrophysiol 2010;3(1):63–71.
16. Bazan V, Bala R, Garcia FC, et al. Twelve-lead ECG features to identify ventricular tachycardia arising from the epicardial right ventricle. Heart Rhythm 2006;3(10):1132–9.
17. Bazan V, Gerstenfeld EP, Garcia FC, et al. Site-specific twelve-lead ECG features to identify an epicardial origin for left ventricular tachycardia in the absence of myocardial infarction. Heart Rhythm 2007;4(11):1403–10.
18. Koplan BA, Soejima K, Baughman K, et al. Refractory ventricular tachycardia secondary to cardiac sarcoid: electrophysiologic characteristics, mapping, and ablation. Heart Rhythm 2006;3(8):924–9.
19. Dechering DG, Kochhauser S, Wasmer K, et al. Electrophysiological characteristics of ventricular tachyarrhythmias in cardiac sarcoidosis versus arrhythmogenic right ventricular cardiomyopathy. Heart Rhythm 2013;10(2):158–64.
20. Vasaiwala SC, Finn C, Delpriore J, et al. Prospective study of cardiac sarcoid mimicking arrhythmogenic right ventricular dysplasia. J Cardiovasc Electrophysiol 2009;20(5):473–6.
21. Sarabanda AV, Sosa E, Simoes MV, et al. Ventricular tachycardia in Chagas' disease: a comparison of clinical, angiographic, electrophysiologic and myocardial perfusion disturbances between patients presenting with either sustained or nonsustained forms. Int J Cardiol 2005;102(1):9–19.
22. Rodriguez LM, Smeets JL, Timmermans C, et al. Radiofrequency catheter ablation of sustained monomorphic ventricular tachycardia in hypertrophic cardiomyopathy. J Cardiovasc Electrophysiol 1997;8(7):803–6.
23. Santangeli P, Di Biase L, Lakkireddy D, et al. Radiofrequency catheter ablation of ventricular arrhythmias in patients with hypertrophic cardiomyopathy: safety and feasibility. Heart Rhythm 2010;7(8):1036–42.

Anatomy for Ventricular Tachycardia Ablation in Structural Heart Disease

Jason S. Bradfield, MD*, Kalyanam Shivkumar, MD, PhD

KEYWORDS

- Ventricular tachycardia • Ablation • Structural heart disease • Anatomy • Cardiomyopathy
- Septum • Papillary muscle • Epicardium

KEY POINTS

- Current ablation technology may have limits in the setting of diffuse or midmyocardial scar.
- The term septal is often inappropriately invoked in the outflow region.
- Aspects of the septal right ventricular outflow tract are not truly septal and perforation at that site enters the pericardial space.
- Successful epicardial mapping and ablation requires not just anatomic understanding of the epicardial surfaces of the heart, coronary venous and arterial system, and the pericardial reflections but also requires an understanding of gastrointestinal, diaphragmatic, and pleural anatomy in order to avoid complications.
- Intracavitary structural anatomy must be understood to avoid inadvertent damage (mitral valve apparatus) and to understand the best ablation techniques when these structures are involved in VT (papillary muscles, perivalvular fibrosis).

INTRODUCTION

Ventricular tachycardia (VT) radiofrequency ablation has become standard of care for VT either resistant to antiarrhythmic medication or if the patient prefers not to take antiarrhythmics.[1,2] Further, it seems that early referral may improve patient outcomes[3] and there may be a survival benefit,[4] which may lead physicians to more aggressively refer their patients for ablation and increase the volume of VT ablations performed. VT in the setting of structural heart disease, previously reserved for highly experienced specialized centers, is being performed at an increasing number of centers internationally as cardiac electrophysiologists gain advanced training.

Given the poor tolerance of induced VT in most patients, a substrate-based approach is often required.[5] This technique requires more extensive ablation than an activation mapping/entrainment approach that focuses on a single VT circuit. A substrate-based approach potentially targets current clinical VTs but also regions of slow conduction that may predispose to future VTs. Ablation of potential circuits often requires ablation in multiple segments/regions of the ventricles.

Given the likely increase in VT ablations performed and the use of substrate-based ablation, a comprehensive and detailed understanding of cardiac anatomy is essential for interventional cardiac electrophysiologists.[6–11] The importance of understanding anatomy is further escalated when dealing with patients with structural heart disease, in which understanding the normal anatomy along with anatomic variations that can occur in dilated, rotated, scarred, thinned,

Disclosures: None.
UCLA Cardiac Arrhythmia Center, David Geffen School of Medicine at UCLA, 100 Medical Plaza, Suite 660, Los Angeles, CA 90095, USA
* Corresponding author.
E-mail address: JBradfield@mednet.ucla.edu

hypertrophied, and/or aneurysmal hearts can be the difference between successful ablation and major complication. Whether patients have VT from ischemic cardiomyopathy (ICM) or non-ICM (NICM) (eg, idiopathic, arrhythmogenic right ventricular cardiomyopathy [ARVC], sarcoidosis, myocarditis, Chagas disease), the importance of understanding cardiac anatomy remains the same. The understanding of anatomy for any cardiac procedure, and specifically ablation, is best understood attitudinally[10,12] and relative to fluoroscopic views.[13]

PREPROCEDURE AND INTRAPROCEDURE IMAGING

Preprocedure imaging with contrast-enhanced computed tomography or cardiac MRI[14–18] has become a mainstay of VT ablation. Imaging can alert physicians to anatomic variation, but more commonly is used to better define potential arrhythmia substrates (scar/fibrosis). Nuclear imaging can add essential understanding of inflammatory substrates.[19] During mapping and ablation of VT, these imaging modalities can be fused with three-dimensional electroanatomic maps to aid anatomic understanding. The addition of intracardiac ultrasonography imaging can allow direct visualization of ablation substrates.[20,21] Techniques still in development, such as real-time MRI,[22] have the potential to further improve direct anatomic visualization during ablation. However, real-time imaging is still limited, and a clear understanding of anatomy and anatomic variation is essential to interpret imaging findings.

LIMITATIONS OF CURRENT ABLATION TECHNOLOGY

Although techniques have been described to affect distant substrates with local ablation,[23] in some anatomic regions, unipolar radiofrequency ablation lesions may not produce adequately deep lesions[24] to interrupt reentrant circuits or focal arrhythmias originating deep within the myocardium. Regions such as the interventricular septum and left ventricle (LV) summit can provide such a challenge. Ablation technology continues to develop, with externally irrigated ablation being the mainstay of current technology.

SEPTAL SUBSTRATES

Isolated septal scar[25] has been shown in patients with NICM, but septal scars can occur with ICM as well. In patients with NICM with VT, anteroseptal scars have been found to have higher recurrence rates then inferolateral scars,

possibly because of a higher prevalence of midmyocardial substrates.[26] Pace maps should be interpreted with caution in this region, because different outputs and exits sites, and whether or not the conduction system is captured, can vastly change QRS morphology and lead physicians astray. Septal substrates must often be approached with mapping and ablation of both the right and left sides of the septum in order to reach deep midmyocardial circuits or foci. Additional modalities such as alcohol septal ablation[27] and wire mapping/coil embolization[28] have been described to target these arrhythmias (**Fig. 1**).

Understanding the cardiac conduction system anatomy is essential to understanding septal substrates but also to avoid collateral damage whenever possible[29] (**Fig. 2**). In patients with previous anteroseptal infarcts, those with right bundle branch block (RBBB) tend to have larger scars then patients with left bundle branch block.[30] The first septal perforator provides blood flow to the right bundle and left anterior fascicle. Therefore, more challenging septal scars may be seen in patients with RBBB. This coronary anatomy is essential to understand in the setting of baseline conduction disease when considering alcohol sepal ablation or coil embolization. In certain situations, the conduction system might be a target for ablation, such as in bundle branch reentry tachycardia or fascicular tachycardia. In other situations, the conduction system may need to be sacrificed in order to successfully ablate intraseptal substrates.

Obtaining good catheter contact on the septum from a transseptal approach often requires a deflectable sheath such as the St. Jude Agilis (St. Jude, Austin, TX). Although nondeflectable sheaths can be used, transseptal access often directs the sheath preferentially to the lateral wall of the LV. Aggressive counterclockwise torque on the sheath can overcome this, but in a dilated ventricle adequate contact may not be possible without a deflectable sheath, particularly when the transseptal puncture is too posterior.

Once common misunderstanding about septal structures is that, when mapping substrates in the lower aspect of the right ventricular outflow tract (RVOT) and the catheter is pointed leftward or septally, the operator is without risk of perforation. However, this region is not truly septal. Over-aggressive manipulation can result in the catheter perforating into the pericardial space (**Fig. 3**). Septal in this instance is used as a way of describing catheter position with the tip pointing toward the LV, but no true septum exists at this level.

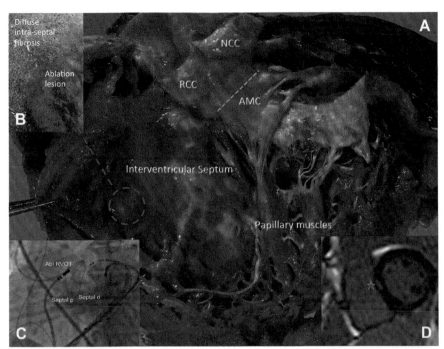

Fig. 1. (*A*) Pathologic specimen showing diffuse septal scar with superimposed ablation lesions (*red circle*) from a 65-year-old man who underwent orthotopic heart transplant. The patient had previously undergone endocardial and surgical epicardial VT ablation for recurrent VT storm. (*B*) Pathologic specimen from a site of ablation on the LV septum showing a confluent endocardial lesion but midmyocardial fibrosis that could not be reached. (*C*) Fluoroscopy of wire mapping technique to map midmyocardial substrates via the septal perforators. (*D*) MRI showing midmyocardial delayed enhancement (*asterisk*). ABL, ablation catheter; AMC, aortomitral continuity; NCC, noncoronary cusp; RCC, right coronary cusp; RVOT, right ventricular outflow tract; Septal d, septal perforator distal; Septal p, septal perforator proximal.

Septal substrate key points:

- Septal substrates are common in NICM
- Septal thickness may necessitate ablation on both sides of the septum
- A clear understanding of the conduction system anatomy decreases the risk of complete heart block
- Intraseptal substrates may be successfully ablated with current technology, or may require consideration of novel techniques such as alcohol septal ablation or coil embolization
- Not all areas described as septal fluoroscopically are truly septal and perforation in this septal region of the RVOT can lead to pericardial effusion and tamponade
- Deflectable sheaths allow improved contact when using a transseptal approach

LEFT VENTRICLE SUMMIT

The LV summit, defined as the region between the proximal aspects of the left anterior descending artery (LAD) and circumflex arteries, is the most superior and often the thickest portion of the LV.

Arrhythmias originating in this region can be extremely difficult to successfully ablate[31] (**Fig. 4**). The coronary venous system (end of the great cardiac vein and beginning of the anterior interventricular vein) can be accessed to attempt epicardial ablation, but small vessel caliber in this region in relation to ablation catheter diameter often limits power delivery. The thickness of this region cannot typically be overcome with the addition of percutaneous epicardial ablation because this region epicardially is by definition very close to the proximal coronary arteries and is additionally covered in fat, making successful lesion formation difficult. The exception is cases in which the origin is on the apical/distal side of the great cardiac vein/anterior interventricular vein junction, where, if epicardial fat is not prohibitive, there may be sites sufficiently far from coronary arteries.

The endocardial aspect of the LV summit can be approached either from a retrograde transaortic or transseptal approach. Midmyocardial circuits or foci in this region often require longer duration lesions at high power to have sufficient effect. In some cases, ablation of a deeper circuit or focus can be accomplished or aided

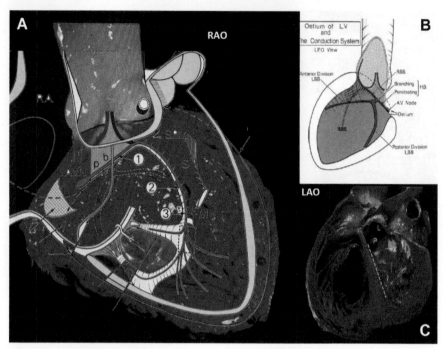

Fig. 2. (*A*) Right anterior oblique (RAO) view of the right ventricular septum with superimposed conduction system and other key anatomic landmarks. (*B*) The left-sided conduction system in a left posterior oblique view. (*C*) Pathologic specimen in left anterior oblique (LAO) view showing the slanted orientation of the septum. Numbers 1, 2, and 3 indicate the first, second and third segments of the right bundle. AVN, atrioventricular node; b, branching segment of His bundle; HB, his bundle; L, left coronary cusp; LBB, left bundle branch; M, moderator band; p, penetrating segment of His bundle; P, posterior coronary cusp; RBB, right bundle branch; SPM, superior papillary muscle. (*Courtesy of* Wallace A, MD, McAlpine Collection-UCLA Cardiac Arrhythmia Center, Los Angeles, CA; with permission.)

by ablation within the left coronary cusp.[32] Much like with septal substrates, pace maps should be interpreted with caution because of variable exit sites in this complex anatomic region. Newer techniques, such as wire mapping with coil embolization or alcohol ablation, can also be used in the LV summit, much like with intramural septal substrates.

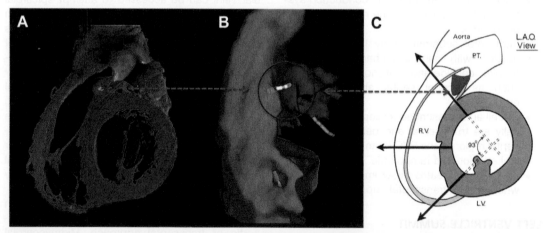

Fig. 3. Pathologic specimen (*A*) and schematic (*C*) of the interventricular septum in LAO view. The red arrows demarcate the region of the septal outflow that has no true septum and where perforation into the pericardium is a risk. A three-dimensional (3D) electroanatomic map (NavX, St. Jude, Austin, TX) (*B*) shows catheter perforation at this vulnerable site. Green, RV; PT, pulmonary artery; red, pericardial space; RV, right ventricle. (*Courtesy of* Wallace A, MD, McAlpine Collection-UCLA Cardiac Arrhythmia Center, Los Angeles, CA; with permission.)

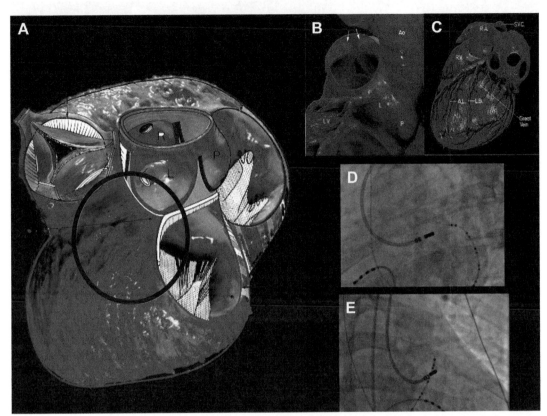

Fig. 4. (*A*) Pathologic specimen and schematic with demarcation of the LV summit region (*black circle*) with epicardial coronary arteries removed. (*B*) Pathologic specimen of the bifurcation of the left main coronary artery to form the LAD and circumflex arteries, which form the borders epicardially of the LV summit. (*C*) Pathologic specimen of the LV summit with coronary venous system present (dark vessels), showing the proximity of the great cardiac vein and anterior interventricular vein to the associated coronary arteries. (*D, E*) Ablation catheter position at the endocardial aspect of the LV summit via a retrograde aortic approach. Ablation at the endocardial LV summit often requires long lesions at high power with an irrigated tip catheter to achieved successful ablation. AL, anterolateral branch; LB, lateral branch; RA, right atrium; SVC, superior vena cava. (*Courtesy of* Wallace A, MD, McAlpine Collection-UCLA Cardiac Arrhythmia Center, Los Angeles, CA; with permission.)

LV summit key points:

- The LV summit is the thickest portion of myocardium in a normal heart. Circuits and foci in this region may be midmyocardial and require longer duration ablation and/or ablation from multiple sites to be effective.
- Percutaneous epicardial access in these cases is rarely warranted because proximity to proximal coronary arteries and epicardial fat limit ablation options in this region
- Although often approached from retrograde transaortic access, a transseptal approach in some cases allows more stable contact.

MITRAL-AORTIC VALVE APPARATUS/ PAPILLARY MUSCLES

A clear understanding of the complex anatomy of the aortic and mitral valve, the aortomitral continuity, valve chordae, and papillary muscles is essential to VT ablation (**Fig. 5**). The mitral apparatus/chordae can impede catheter movement when access to the LV is via a transseptal approach. Care must be taken to avoid entanglement[33] in these structures, and, when catheter movement feels impeded, force should not be used to release the catheter because this can cause chordal/papillary muscle rupture.[34]

VT originating from the periaortic valve tissue is common in idiopathic VT or PVCs. However, recent evidence suggests that a significant percentage of these cases are not idiopathic, but scar-related reentry.[35] Subaortic valve scar can be approached from a retrograde or transseptal approach. However, care must be taken to avoid the left-sided bundle of His below the right coronary cusp. VT originating from the aortomitral continuity (AMC) has been described in structural heart disease.[36] Although given the anatomic location and the fact that the AMC is a fibrous

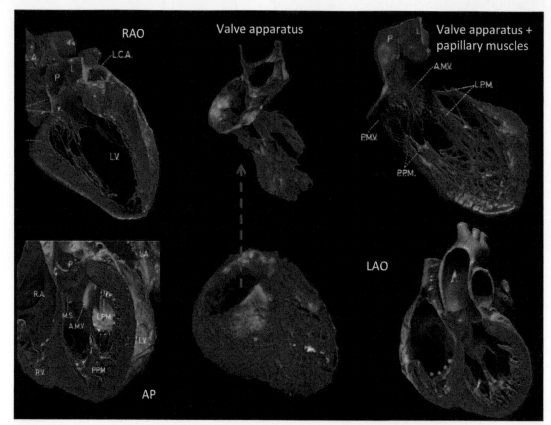

Fig. 5. Pathologic specimens of the mitral and aortic valve apparatus and the LV papillary muscles. RAO, anteroposterior, and LAO views are shown in addition to the complex anatomy of the valve apparatus and chordal structures. The arrow indicates removal of the valve apparatus from the left ventricle. AMV, anterior mitral valve leaflet; L, left coronary cusp; LA, left atrium; LCA, left coronary artery; LPM, anterolateral papillary muscle; P, noncoronary cusp; PMV, posterior mitral valve leaflet; PPM, posteromedial papillary muscle. (*Courtesy of* Wallace A, MD, McAlpine Collection-UCLA Cardiac Arrhythmia Center, Los Angeles, CA; with permission.)

structure, these arrhythmias may be an extension of LV summit VTs, as discussed earlier. Regardless of origin, targeting this region can be anatomically complex (see **Figs. 1** and **5**).

Structures within the cavity of both the LV and right ventricle (RV) can be the origin of focal and reentrant ventricular arrhythmias.[37] Although more frequently associated with idiopathic VT,[38,39] papillary muscles can also be involved in VT associated with structural heart disease.[40] Given the complex three-dimensional and intracavitary nature, electroanatomic maps of these structures can be confusing, because current electroanatomic mapping systems are built primarily to assess a single plane of activation. Catheter stability on papillary muscles can be a challenge and is more easily accomplished when ablating at the base of the muscle. Intracardiac echo catheter imaging can help ensure appropriate contact (**Fig. 6**).

Mitral apparatus/papillary muscle key points:

- Fluoroscopically and on three-dimensional mapping systems, ablation catheter position on papillary muscles appears intracavitary. Intracardiac echo imaging is essential to ensure good catheter contact in these cases and can often visualize lesion formation.
- Restricted catheter movement can be secondary to entanglement in mitral valve chordae. When not appropriately identified, chordal rupture is a risk.

EPICARDIAL MAPPING AND ABLATION

Epicardial circuits can be present in all VT substrates. However, they may be more common in certain NICM substrates such as Chagas disease and postmyocarditis.[41–43] Epicardial mapping may additionally be useful in hypertrophic cardiomyopathy (HCM) and myocardial noncompaction cases as well. In HCM, ablation on both the endocardial and epicardial surfaces may be needed because of the thickness of the ventricle (**Fig. 7**). In noncompaction, there is increased risk of perforation with endocardial catheter manipulation and obtaining epicardial access in

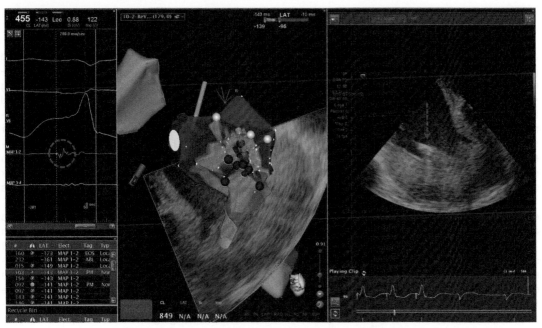

Fig. 6. Electroanatomic map and Cartosound (Carto, Biosense Webster, Irvine, CA) images from a 62-year-old woman with papillary muscle VT. (*Left*) Earliest ventricular signal (*circle*). (*Right*) Intracardiac echo of papillary muscle (*arrow*), with superimposed 3D electroanatomic activation map (earliest sites *red* and latest sites *purple*) and ablation sites (*red dots*) (*middle*).

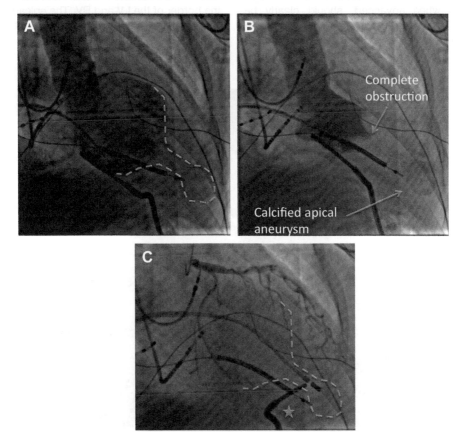

Fig. 7. Fluoroscopic images from a 58-year-old patient with apical hypertrophic cardiomyopathy who underwent VT ablation for recurrent implantable cardioverter-defibrillator (ICD) shocks. LV angiogram during diastole (*A*) shows severe apical obstruction with a small neck of access to the apex. The obstruction becomes complete during systole (*B*) on LV angiogram. The calcified apex of the LV can be seen in *B*. The endocardial ablation catheter is seen being advanced through the neck of the obstruction in *C*. Epicardial access was undertaken and the ablation catheter can be seen advancing through a long sheath to the inferior aspect of the region of obstruction (*star*).

advance may be wise, with epicardial ablation providing less theoretic risk (**Fig. 8**). Epicardial mapping and ablation are frequently required for ARVC; however, ARVC is covered in depth in another article in this series. In experienced hands, epicardial mapping and ablation are safe.[44,45] Regardless of the substrate, detailed epicardial mapping in combination with endocardial mapping can clarify complex three-dimensional anatomic substrates (**Fig. 9**).

Comprehensive anatomic understanding of the epicardium begins with a clear understanding of anatomy related to epicardial access (**Fig. 10**). This anatomy includes abdominal anatomy (liver, spleen, colon, vasculature, diaphragm), and the structures that must be avoided to ensure safe access. Initial subxiphoid approach should be superficial to avoid vital structures, then the depth of access can be adjusted based on whether an anterior or posterior approach is undertaken. In relation to the RV in right anterior oblique orientation, a basal approach should be avoided to minimize the risk of coronary artery or venous damage. The wire, when advanced, should clearly be extracardiac, which is easiest seen in the left anterior oblique (LAO) view tracking outside the left

heart border. A pericardiogram may be helpful to ensure free flow within the pericardial space. However, some centers have concern regarding contrast-induced adhesions if repeat epicardial access is needed in the future. When present, pericardial adhesions (see **Fig. 10**) may limit catheter movement and three-dimensional electroanatomic map formation. These adhesions can often be broken up with a deflectable catheter, but risk of bleeding increases, because the adhesions can be vascular.

When mapping epicardially on the anterior and lateral wall of the LV, consideration must be given to the phrenic nerve course.[46,47] Although the left phrenic nerve can often be visualized on preprocedure imaging, there can be variability from case to case, and high output pacing in possible at-risk regions is essential regardless of what preprocedure imaging shows.[48] When needed, balloon protection can be used to allow safe epicardial ablation (see **Fig. 8**). When mapping the anteroseptal epicardial region, clinicians must remember that the LAD does not demarcate the border of the LV and RV. The epicardial septal aspect of the LV extends rightward of the LAD in the LAO view (see **Fig. 9**).

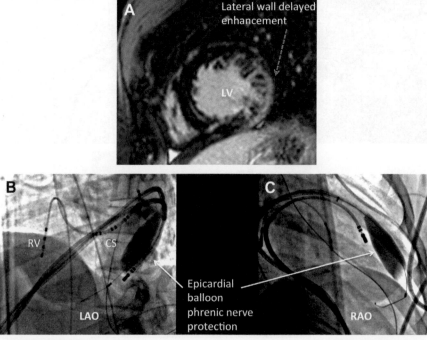

Fig. 8. (*A*) Left lateral MRI view of a 48-year-old patient with LV noncompaction with associated lateral wall delayed enhancement presenting with recurrent ICD shocks caused by VT. Endocardial ablation in the setting of noncompaction may carry increased perforation risk. Ablation of the lateral wall epicardially can be limited by risk of phrenic nerve damage. Epicardial balloon protection can be used to obviate this risk (*B, C*). CS, coronary sinus catheter; RV, RV catheter.

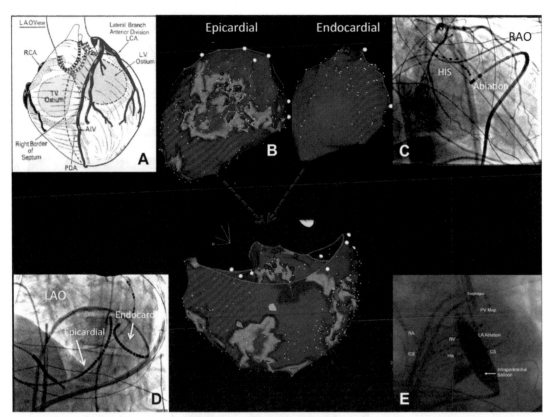

Fig. 9. Epicardial mapping can be essential to understanding complex substrates. An endocardial voltage map and the associated epicardial map are shown in (*B*) and superimposed. When mapping epicardially, clinicians should remember that the LV epicardium extends rightward of the LAD (*A*). Adjacent endocardial and epicardial high-density mapping (*D*) with multipolar catheters (2-2-2-2-2 duodecapolar, St. Jude, Austin, TX) can define critical substrates. In this case, 2 closely spaced duodecapolar catheters are placed directly across from one another in the LV apex in a patient with VT related to cardiac sarcoidosis. Esophageal protection is most often considered for atrial fibrillation ablation (*E*), but may be necessary for ablation of basal inferior LV substrates. When appropriate ablation sites are found on the epicardium, coronary angiography is critical to ensure a safe distance. A basal-lateral epicardial VT circuit is targeted (*C*) in a patient with NICM. AIV, anterior interventricular vein; HIS, HIS bundle catheter; ICE, intracardiac echo catheter; LAD, left anterior descending artery; PDA, posterior descending artery; PV, pulmonary vein; RA, right atrial catheter; RCA, right coronary artery; RV, RV catheter; TV, tricuspid valve.

The basal inferoposterior wall or crux of the heart is a complex region both endocardially and epicardially (**Fig. 11**). The 4 chambers of the heart are offset from each other, and therefore from the endocardium a portion of the LV can be reached for ablation from the right atrium (posterior-superior process).[49] However, the atrioventricular (AV) nodal artery, which can have variable origin, from the right or left coronary system, may be at risk during ablation in this region. When approaching this region epicardially, posterior branches of both the circumflex and right coronary arterial systems may be at risk, depending on location and coronary dominance. The esophagus can be at risk in this region and this should be considered when extensive epicardial ablation is considered (see **Fig. 9**). Although this region can be reached via the coronary venous system (middle cardiac vein), delivery of radiofrequency energy can be difficult because of impedance limitations.

Coronary Venous System

The coronary venous system anatomy is important to understand for VT ablation.[50–52] Although more often involved in idiopathic VT, the venous system can be involved in patients with structural heart disease or may be an access point for epicardial substrates if percutaneous epicardial access is not possible because of previous cardiac surgery or other limitations.

Epicardial Fat

Epicardial fat can be present throughout the pericardium, but predominates along the AV

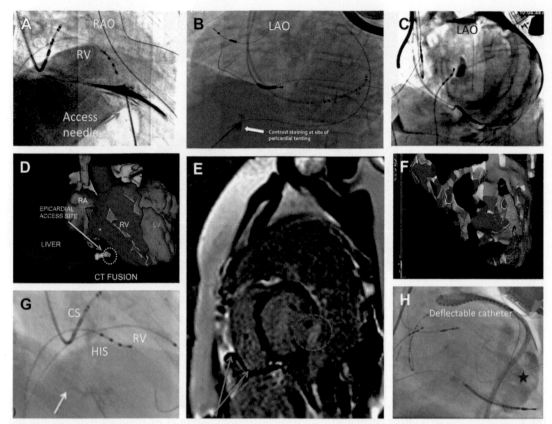

Fig. 10. Safe epicardial access to map epicardial or transmural substrates (*E, red circle*) requires understanding of cardiac as well as subdiaphragmatic anatomy. Epicardial access angle depends on whether an anterior or posterior approach is desired (*E, blue arrows*). Pericardial tenting of the access needle (*A*), followed by wire advancement along the left heart border (*B*) and a pericardiogram through a 5-French dilator before 8-French sheath advancement (*C*). A 3D electroanatomic map (*D*) (NavX, St. Jude, Austin, TX) with fusion with cardiac MRI including the liver shows the access site relative to those structures. Given the close proximity of the liver in (*D*), care must be taken to avoid hepatic access (*G*), where an unintentional hepatic angiogram is shown (*arrow*). Pericardial adhesions can limit epicardial access and mapping. Although adhesions (*blue star*) can be broken up with a deflectable catheter (*H*), full map construction may be limited (*F*). CT, computed tomography.

and interventricular grooves. There can be significant variability between patients in distribution and thickness, which makes generalized statements difficult. With regard to electrophysiology, epicardial fat is predominantly considered in the context of a potential impediment to successful epicardial ablation. However, epicardial fat characteristics have been associated with atrial fibrillation[53] and overall cardiac events.[54] Epicardial fat presence makes differentiation of local electrogram characteristics difficult[55] and can significantly attenuate ablation lesion formation. Ablation parameter adjustments can be made to attempt to overcome this limitation.[56] However, when unsuccessful, an open surgical approach with epicardial fat resection may be required.

Epicardial mapping and ablation key points:

- Successful epicardial access with minimal complications requires an understanding of subdiaphragmatic anatomy (liver, colon, vasculature, and so forth) in addition to cardiac anatomy.
- Understanding phrenic nerve and esophageal course is essential to minimize risk when ablating lateral and basal inferior substrates.
- The epicardial LV anterior wall extends rightward of the LAD. The LAD does not demarcate the RV and LV border.
- Epicardial crux VTs involve complex and variable coronary artery and venous anatomy and assessment of both the left and right coronary artery systems is essential before ablation is undertaken.

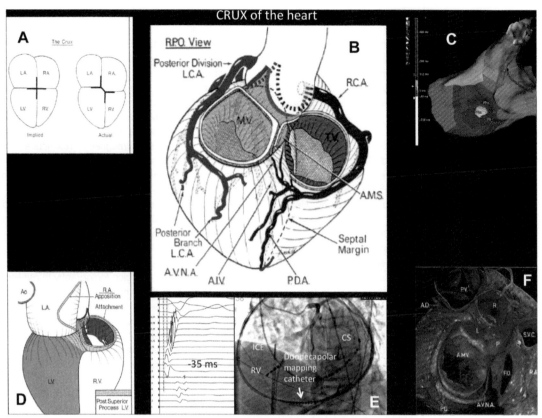

Fig. 11. The crux of the heart (*B*) is a complex anatomic region. Endocardially the atrioventricular (AV) relationship is offset (*A, D*) with a portion of the LV adjacent to the right atrium. This region, called the posterior-superior process (*D*), can be targeted for ablation from the RA; however, the AV nodal coronary branch can be at risk (*B, F*). When mapping VT originating epicardially from this region (*B, C*) the posterior branches of both the right and left coronary systems may be at risk. (*E*) Fluoroscopy and electrogram timing of an epicardial ablation site of a crux VT. An associated electroanatomic map (St. Jude, NavX, Austin, TX) showing the earliest site of activation (*white region*) of this focal VT is shown. AVNA, AVN artery; RCA, right coronary artery. (*Courtesy of* Wallace A, MD, McAlpine Collection-UCLA Cardiac Arrhythmia Center, Los Angeles, CA; with permission.)

- Ablation on epicardial fat, commonly seen at the base and along coronary distributions, may require longer lesions because of the insulating effects of the fat tissue.

troubleshoot, interpret, and adjust to complex electrical signals and three-dimensional electroanatomic map findings but also to complex anatomy.

DISCUSSION

Just as critical to the interventional cardiac electrophysiologist as understanding intracardiac signals and mapping and ablation strategies is having a detailed understanding of cardiac anatomy of the normal heart and how that anatomy can be altered in the setting of structural heart disease. However, although anatomy is learned during training, it is often learned secondarily and without sufficient focus. This lack of focus can lead to diminished success and increased complication risk when VT ablation is undertaken. Successful electrophysiologists must be able to

REFERENCES

1. Aliot EM, Stevenson WG, Almendral-Garrote JM, et al, European Heart Rhythm Association, European Society of Cardiology, Heart Rhythm Society. EHRA/HRS expert consensus on catheter ablation of ventricular arrhythmias: developed in a partnership with the European Heart Rhythm Association (EHRA), a registered branch of the European Society of Cardiology (ESC), and the Heart Rhythm Society (HRS); in collaboration with the American College of Cardiology (ACC) and the American Heart Association (AHA). Europace 2009;11: 771–817.

2. Pedersen CT, Kay GN, Kalman J, et al, Ep-Europace UK. EHRA/HRS/APHRS expert consensus on ventricular arrhythmias. Heart Rhythm 2014;11:e166–96.

3. Dinov B, Arya A, Bertagnolli L, et al. Early referral for ablation of scar-related ventricular tachycardia is associated with improved acute and long-term outcomes: results from the Heart Center of Leipzig ventricular tachycardia registry. Circ Arrhythm Electrophysiol 2014;7:1144–51.

4. Tung R, Vaseghi M, Frankel DS, et al. Freedom from recurrent ventricular tachycardia after catheter ablation is associated with improved survival in patients with structural heart disease: an International VT Ablation Center Collaborative Group study. Heart Rhythm 2015;12:1997–2007.

5. Jais P, Maury P, Khairy P, et al. Elimination of local abnormal ventricular activities: a new end point for substrate modification in patients with scar-related ventricular tachycardia. Circulation 2012;125: 2184–96.

6. Lachman N, Syed FF, Habib A, et al. Correlative anatomy for the electrophysiologist, part I: the pericardial space, oblique sinus, transverse sinus. J Cardiovasc Electrophysiol 2010;21:1421–6.

7. Lachman N, Syed FF, Habib A, et al. Correlative anatomy for the electrophysiologist, part II: cardiac ganglia, phrenic nerve, coronary venous system. J Cardiovasc Electrophysiol 2011;22:104–10.

8. Noheria A, DeSimone CV, Lachman N, et al. Anatomy of the coronary sinus and epicardial coronary venous system in 620 hearts: an electrophysiology perspective. J Cardiovasc Electrophysiol 2013;24:1–6.

9. Mori S, Spicer DE, Anderson RH. Revisiting the anatomy of the living heart. Circ J 2016;80:24–33.

10. Anderson RH, Loukas M. The importance of attitudinally appropriate description of cardiac anatomy. Clin Anat 2009;22:47–51.

11. Anderson RH. The time has come to describe cardiac structures as seen during life, and not as perceived in the autopsy room. Heart Rhythm 2015;12:515–6.

12. Anderson RH, Spicer DE, Hlavacek AJ, et al. Describing the cardiac components–attitudinally appropriate nomenclature. J Cardiovasc Transl Res 2013;6:118–23.

13. Farre J, Anderson RH, Cabrera JA, et al. Cardiac anatomy for the interventional arrhythmologist: I. terminology and fluoroscopic projections. Pacing Clin Electrophysiol 2010;33:497–507.

14. Andreu D, Ortiz-Perez JT, Boussy T, et al. Usefulness of contrast-enhanced cardiac magnetic resonance in identifying the ventricular arrhythmia substrate and the approach needed for ablation. Eur Heart J 2014;35:1316–26.

15. Aquaro GD, Pingitore A, Strata E, et al. Cardiac magnetic resonance predicts outcome in patients with premature ventricular complexes of left bundle branch block morphology. J Am Coll Cardiol 2010; 56:1235–43.

16. Fernandez-Armenta J, Berruezo A, Andreu D, et al. Three-dimensional architecture of scar and conducting channels based on high resolution ce-CMR: insights for ventricular tachycardia ablation. Circ Arrhythm Electrophysiol 2013;6:528–37.

17. Perazzolo Marra M, De Lazzari M, Zorzi A, et al. Impact of the presence and amount of myocardial fibrosis by cardiac magnetic resonance on arrhythmic outcome and sudden cardiac death in nonischemic dilated cardiomyopathy. Heart Rhythm 2014;11:856–63.

18. Piers SR, Tao Q, de Riva Silva M, et al. CMR-based identification of critical isthmus sites of ischemic and nonischemic ventricular tachycardia. JACC Cardiovasc Imaging 2014;7:774–84.

19. Tung R, Bauer B, Schelbert H, et al. Incidence of abnormal positron emission tomography in patients with unexplained cardiomyopathy and ventricular arrhythmias: the potential role of occult inflammation in arrhythmogenesis. Heart Rhythm 2015;12:2488–98.

20. Hussein A, Jimenez A, Ahmad G, et al. Assessment of ventricular tachycardia scar substrate by intracardiac echocardiography. Pacing Clin Electrophysiol 2014;37:412–21.

21. Rivera S, Ricapito Mde L, Tomas L, et al. Results of cryoenergy and radiofrequency-based catheter ablation for treating ventricular arrhythmias arising from the papillary muscles of the left ventricle, guided by intracardiac echocardiography and image integration. Circ Arrhythm Electrophysiol 2016; 9:e003874.

22. Rogers T, Lederman RJ. Interventional CMR: clinical applications and future directions. Curr Cardiol Rep 2015;17:31.

23. Komatsu Y, Daly M, Sacher F, et al. Endocardial ablation to eliminate epicardial arrhythmia substrate in scar-related ventricular tachycardia. J Am Coll Cardiol 2014;63:1416–26.

24. Berte B, Cochet H, Magat J, et al. Irrigated needle ablation creates larger and more transmural ventricular lesions compared with standard unipolar ablation in an ovine model. Circ Arrhythm Electrophysiol 2015; 8:1498–506.

25. Haqqani HM, Tschabrunn CM, Tzou WS, et al. Isolated septal substrate for ventricular tachycardia in nonischemic dilated cardiomyopathy: incidence, characterization, and implications. Heart Rhythm 2011;8:1169–76.

26. Oloriz T, Silberbauer J, Maccabelli G, et al. Catheter ablation of ventricular arrhythmia in nonischemic cardiomyopathy: anteroseptal versus inferolateral scar sub-types. Circ Arrhythm Electrophysiol 2014; 7:414–23.

27. Kumar S, Barbhaiya CR, Sobieszczyk P, et al. Role of alternative interventional procedures when

endo- and epicardial catheter ablation attempts for ventricular arrhythmias fail. Circ Arrhythm Electrophysiol 2015;8:606–15.

28. Tholakanahalli VN, Bertog S, Roukoz H, et al. Catheter ablation of ventricular tachycardia using intracoronary wire mapping and coil embolization: description of a new technique. Heart Rhythm 2013;10:292–6.

29. Anderson RH, Yanni J, Boyett MR, et al. The anatomy of the cardiac conduction system. Clin Anat 2009;22:99–113.

30. Strauss DG, Loring Z, Selvester RH, et al. Right, but not left, bundle branch block is associated with large anteroseptal scar. J Am Coll Cardiol 2013;62:959–67.

31. Yamada T, McElderry HT, Doppalapudi H, et al. Idiopathic ventricular arrhythmias originating from the left ventricular summit: anatomic concepts relevant to ablation. Circ Arrhythm Electrophysiol 2010;3:616–23.

32. Jauregui Abularach ME, Campos B, Park KM, et al. Ablation of ventricular arrhythmias arising near the anterior epicardial veins from the left sinus of Valsalva region: ECG features, anatomic distance, and outcome. Heart Rhythm 2012;9:865–73.

33. Kim KH, Choi KJ, Kim SH, et al. Ablation catheter entrapment by chordae tendineae in the mitral valve during ventricular tachycardia ablation. J Cardiovasc Electrophysiol 2012;23:218–20.

34. Rodriguez-Caulo E, Quintana E, Castella M. Iatrogenic anterior papillary muscle rupture. Rev Esp Cardiol (Engl Ed) 2013;66:63.

35. Nagashima K, Tedrow UB, Koplan BA, et al. Reentrant ventricular tachycardia originating from the periaortic region in the absence of overt structural heart disease. Circ Arrhythm Electrophysiol 2014;7:99–106.

36. Steven D, Roberts-Thomson KC, Seiler J, et al. Ventricular tachycardia arising from the aortomitral continuity in structural heart disease: characteristics and therapeutic considerations for an anatomically challenging area of origin. Circ Arrhythm Electrophysiol 2009;2:660–6.

37. Abouezzeddine O, Suleiman M, Buescher T, et al. Relevance of endocavitary structures in ablation procedures for ventricular tachycardia. J Cardiovasc Electrophysiol 2010;21:245–54.

38. Yamada T, Doppalapudi H, McElderry HT, et al. Electrocardiographic and electrophysiological characteristics in idiopathic ventricular arrhythmias originating from the papillary muscles in the left ventricle: relevance for catheter ablation. Circ Arrhythm Electrophysiol 2010;3:324–31.

39. Yokokawa M, Good E, Desjardins B, et al. Predictors of successful catheter ablation of ventricular arrhythmias arising from the papillary muscles. Heart Rhythm 2010;7:1654–9.

40. Bogun F, Desjardins B, Crawford T, et al. Post-infarction ventricular arrhythmias originating in papillary muscles. J Am Coll Cardiol 2008;51:1794–802.

41. Berte B, Sacher F, Cochet H, et al. Postmyocarditis ventricular tachycardia in patients with epicardial-only scar: a specific entity requiring a specific approach. J Cardiovasc Electrophysiol 2015;26:42–50.

42. Cano O, Hutchinson M, Lin D, et al. Electroanatomic substrate and ablation outcome for suspected epicardial ventricular tachycardia in left ventricular nonischemic cardiomyopathy. J Am Coll Cardiol 2009;54:799–808.

43. Daniels DV, Lu YY, Morton JB, et al. Idiopathic epicardial left ventricular tachycardia originating remote from the sinus of Valsalva: electrophysiological characteristics, catheter ablation, and identification from the 12-lead electrocardiogram. Circulation 2006;113:1659–66.

44. Sacher F, Roberts-Thomson K, Maury P, et al. Epicardial ventricular tachycardia ablation a multicenter safety study. J Am Coll Cardiol 2010;55:2366–72.

45. Tung R, Michowitz Y, Yu R, et al. Epicardial ablation of ventricular tachycardia: an institutional experience of safety and efficacy. Heart Rhythm 2013;10:490–8.

46. Sanchez-Quintana D, Cabrera JA, Climent V, et al. How close are the phrenic nerves to cardiac structures? Implications for cardiac interventionalists. J Cardiovasc Electrophysiol 2005;16:309–13.

47. Sanchez-Quintana D, Ho SY, Climent V, et al. Anatomic evaluation of the left phrenic nerve relevant to epicardial and endocardial catheter ablation: implications for phrenic nerve injury. Heart Rhythm 2009;6:764–8.

48. Fan R, Cano O, Ho SY, et al. Characterization of the phrenic nerve course within the epicardial substrate of patients with nonischemic cardiomyopathy and ventricular tachycardia. Heart Rhythm 2009;6:59–64.

49. Santangeli P, Hutchinson MD, Supple GE, et al. Right atrial approach for ablation of ventricular arrhythmias arising from the left posterior-superior process of the left ventricle. Circ Arrhythm Electrophysiol 2016;9(7).

50. Baman TS, Ilg KJ, Gupta SK, et al. Mapping and ablation of epicardial idiopathic ventricular arrhythmias from within the coronary venous system. Circ Arrhythm Electrophysiol 2010;3:274–9.

51. Mountantonakis SE, Frankel DS, Tschabrunn CM, et al. Ventricular arrhythmias from the coronary venous system: prevalence, mapping, and ablation. Heart Rhythm 2015;12:1145–53.

52. Kawamura M, Gerstenfeld EP, Vedantham V, et al. Idiopathic ventricular arrhythmia originating from the cardiac crux or inferior septum: epicardial idiopathic ventricular arrhythmia. Circ Arrhythm Electrophysiol 2014;7:1152–8.

53. Thanassoulis G, Massaro JM, O'Donnell CJ, et al. Pericardial fat is associated with prevalent atrial fibrillation: the Framingham Heart Study. Circ Arrhythm Electrophysiol 2010;3:345–50.

54. Cheng VY, Dey D, Tamarappoo B, et al. Pericardial fat burden on ECG-gated noncontrast CT in asymptomatic patients who subsequently experience adverse cardiovascular events. JACC Cardiovasc Imaging 2010;3:352–60.

55. Tung R, Nakahara S, Ramirez R, et al. Distinguishing epicardial fat from scar: analysis of electrograms using high-density electroanatomic mapping in a novel porcine infarct model. Heart Rhythm 2010;7: 389–95.

56. Aryana A, O'Neill PG, Pujara DK, et al. Impact of irrigation flow rate and intrapericardial fluid on cooled-tip epicardial radiofrequency ablation. Heart Rhythm 2016;13:1602–11.

Ventricular Tachycardia in Ischemic Heart Disease

Ronald Lo, MD, FHRS[a], Karin K.M. Chia, PhD, FRACP, FHRS[b], Henry H. Hsia, MD, FHRS[c,*]

KEYWORDS

- Ischemic heart disease • Ventricular tachycardia • Catheter ablation

KEY POINTS

- Ventricular arrhythmias are a significant cause of morbidity and mortality in patients with ischemic heart disease.
- Detailed electroanatomical characterization of arrhythmia substrate with endocardial and epicardial mapping may better define the potential targets for catheter ablation.
- Newer mapping strategies, technologies, and indications for catheter ablation also improve the procedural outcome.

INTRODUCTION

Ventricular tachycardia (VT) and ventricular fibrillation (VF) are important and significant causes of morbidity and sudden cardiac death (SCD) in patients with structural and ischemic heart disease. Implantable cardioverter defibrillators (ICD) have been able to reduce mortality and morbidity from VT or VF[1]; however, recurrence of VT and ICD therapies are associated with an increase in morbidity,[2] and also in mortality.[3]

Antiarrhythmic drugs (AADs) are used frequently in the treatment of VT, and are often done as initial treatment of VT. However, AADs have relatively narrow therapeutic windows, with significant risks of proarrhythmia and side effects. A recent systematic review and meta-analysis of randomized controlled trials suggested an increased mortality with amiodarone.[4] With continued evolution of ablation technologies and techniques, catheter VT ablation is becoming an increasing standard in the management of VT and VF, especially in patients with prior myocardial infarction (**Fig. 1**).[5,6]

INCIDENCE AND PREVALENCE

The incidence of ventricular tachyarrhythmias and sudden deaths was estimated to account for 5.6% of all mortality, claiming 350,000 to 400,000 lives annually in the United States.[7] The overall incidence of sustained VT or VF during an acute myocardial infarction (MI) is approximately 10.2%.[8] Approximately 85% of VT and VF occurred within the first 48 hours after MI. Patients with VT or VF during acute MI have a high in-hospital mortality rate of up to 27%.[9] Recurrence VT and VF can develop in up to 60% of patients who had prior episodes of spontaneous sustained VT.[10] In patients with an ischemic cardiomyopathy and nonsustained VT, sudden death mortality is 28% at 2 years and up to 32% at 5 years.[11] In patients with a depressed ejection fraction (EF) post MI on contemporary medical therapy who received an implantable loop recorder, a 3% incidence of sustained VT was seen during an average follow-up of 2 years.[12]

The risk of SCD is highest in patients with structural heart disease, and underlying coronary

[a] Electrophysiology and Arrhythmia Service, Veterans Administration Medical Center, Loma Linda University, Mail Code 111C, 11201 Benton Street, Loma Linda, CA 92357, USA; [b] Department of Cardiology, Royal North Shore Hospital, The University of Sydney, Level 5, Acute Service Building, St Leonards, Sydney, North South Wales 2065, Australia; [c] Arrhythmia Service, Veterans Administration Medical Center–San Francisco, MC 111C-6, 4150 Clement Street, San Francisco, CA 94121, USA
* Corresponding author.
E-mail address: henry.hsia@ucsf.edu

Card Electrophysiol Clin 9 (2017) 25–46
http://dx.doi.org/10.1016/j.ccep.2016.10.013
1877-9182/17/Published by Elsevier Inc.

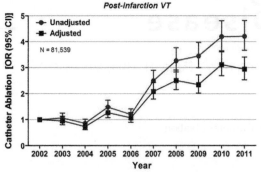

Fig. 1. Trends in catheter VT ablation. The figure illustrates the trends in catheter ablation of postinfarct VT from 2002 to 2011. The data were obtained from the Nationwide Inpatient Sample database to identify all patients ≥18 years of age with a primary diagnosis of VT (International Classification of Diseases, Ninth Edition, Clinical Modification [ICD-9-CM] code 427.1) and who also had a secondary diagnosis of prior history of myocardial infarction (ICD-9-CM412). Of 81,539 patients with postinfarct VT, 4653 (5.7%) underwent catheter ablation. Utilization of catheter ablation increased significantly from 2.8% in 2002 to 10.8% in 2011 (P<.001). CI, confidence interval; OR, odds ratio. (*Adapted from* Palaniswamy C, Kolte D, Harikrishnan P, et al. Catheter ablation of postinfarction ventricular tachycardia: ten-year trends in utilization, in-hospital complications, and in-hospital mortality in the United States. Heart Rhythm 2014;11(11):2060; with permission.)

disease. The risk appears to be highest in patients who have had a prior MI. The overall incidence is estimated to be approximately 2% to 4%.[13] The risk of SCD following MI appears to be greatest in the first 30 days after MI, and declines and plateaus after 12 months. However, the risk of sudden death remains elevated and is significantly higher in those with ventricular dysfunction (left ventricular EF <30%) (**Fig. 2**).[14]

ARRHYTHMOGENIC SUBSTRATE

The majority of VT in ischemic cardiomyopathy is due to reentry associated with areas of scar. The arrhythmogenic substrate appears to develop within weeks after the initial infarction and persists afterward. The development of arrhythmogenic substrate is also influenced by reperfusion status, whether by primary percutaneous coronary intervention or by thrombolytic therapy. Early reperfusion allows salvage of myocardium, resulting in smaller and "more patchy" myocardial scar formation, characterized by a larger scar border region, with small areas of dense scar interspersed with areas of relatively healthy tissue (**Table 1**). Patients who underwent reperfusion therapy for MI are less likely to experience spontaneous VT occurrence (**Fig. 3**); however, the recurrent VT tends to have a shorter cycle length, and are not as reliably assessed during the electrophysiology study.[15,16]

ANATOMY AND HISTOLOGY

VT associated with MI often originated from the subendocardial region of the infarcted myocardium. These are located in the scar regions that are immediately adjacent to the coronary vasculature that was infarcted. The myocardial fibers on the endocardial surface may survive due to

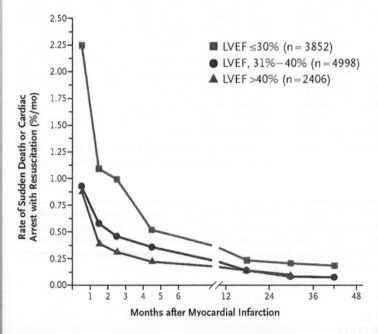

Fig. 2. Sudden death/cardiac arrest after the index MI. The rate of sudden death or cardiac arrest after the index MI over the course of the VALIANT (Valsartan in Acute Myocardial Infarction Trial). The absolute risk is greatest in the early period after myocardial infarction and among patients with the lowest EF and declines over time, reaching a steady state at approximately 2 years. The risk remains increased even though all patients were receiving renin-angiotensin inhibitors and most were receiving beta-blockers and aspirin. LVEF, left ventricular EF. (*Adapted from* Solomon SD, Zelenkofske S, McMurray JJ, et al. Sudden death in patients with myocardial infarction and left ventricular dysfunction, heart failure, or both. N Engl J Med 2005;352(25):2586; with permission.)

Table 1
Effects of reperfusion of ischemic VT substrate

	Reperfused	Nonreperfused	P
No. of spontaneous VT	1.4 ± 1.3	1.7 ± 1.1	.4
Spontaneous VT CL, ms	*299 ± 152*	*378 ± 77*	*.01*
No. of induced VT	2.1 ± 1.7	2.5 ± 1.6	.5
Induced VT CL, ms	*270 ± 58*	*362 ± 74*	*.001*
Scar area, cm²	65 ± 48	85 ± 46	.2
Dense scar area, cm²	*21 ± 25*	*42 ± 21*	*.02*
Border, % of scar	*76 ± 17*	*54 ± 21*	*.002*
Patchy pattern, %	*71*	*14*	*.001*

Abbreviations: CL, cycle length; VT, ventricular tachycardia.

Scar size and pattern defined by electroanatomical maps in patients with VT with and without reperfusion during after an acute MI. There was a nonsignificant difference in the number of spontaneous VTs (P = .4), the number of induced VT at electrophysiology study (P = .5), and also the overall scar area (P = .2). The VT cycle length was significantly shorter in reperfused patients compared with nonreperfused patients (P = .001). The dense scar area was also significantly smaller in the reperfused group compared with the nonreperfused group (P = .02). A patchy scar pattern was significantly noted more frequently in the reperfused group (P = .001). Values in italics symbolizes statistical significance, P <.05.

Adapted from Wijnmaalen AP, Schalij MJ, von der Thusen JH, et al. Early reperfusion during acute myocardial infarction affects ventricular tachycardia characteristics and the chronic electroanatomic and histological substrate. Circulation 2010;121(17):1892; with permission.

perfusion of blood from the ventricular cavity. These areas of viable tissue become interspersed in fibrotic scar that is characterized by slowed and nonuniform anisotropic conduction.[17]

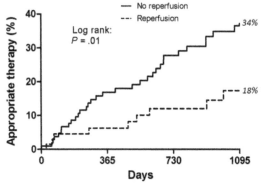

Fig. 3. Occurrence of appropriate ICD therapy in primary prevention, relationship to reperfusion status. The development of arrhythmogenic substrate may be influenced by reperfusion status. Early reperfusion during acute ischemia results in myocardial salvage with smaller, less confluent myocardial scar formation. The reperfused patients were less likely to have spontaneous VT during follow-up, but such events manifested as faster VTs and were less reliably assessed by EP study. (*Adapted from* Piers SR, Wijnmaalen AP, Borleffs CJ, et al. Early reperfusion therapy affects inducibility, cycle length, and occurrence of ventricular tachycardia late after myocardial infarction. Circ Arrhythm Electrophysiol 2011;4(2):199; with permission.)

Histologic studies have shown that the slow conduction areas appear in the infarcted tissue with a "zigzag" course through the myocardium (**Fig. 4**).[18,19] Reentry through these surviving myocardial fibers is primarily on the subendocardium, but can occur in the midmyocardium and also the epicardium. Activation of the abnormal myocardium results in nonuniform anisotropic conduction and gives rise to the long-fractioned electrograms commonly recorded at the border zones of infarcted tissue.[20,21] Subendocardial resection of infarcted myocardium for successful surgical ablation of postinfarction VTs have confirmed the endocardial locations as the substrate for VT after MI.[22] Purkinje fibers have also been shown to participate in the reentry in scar-based VT. The arborization along the border zone of the scar may serve as specialized localized reentry networks for VT, as well as triggers for polymorphic arrhythmias/VF.[23] These also account for the relatively narrow QRS (<145 ms) complexes seen in Purkinje-related VT.[24]

Most patients with VT after MI (60%–80%) often have multiple and distinct morphologies of VT. The reentrant circuits associated with different VT morphologies are commonly within the same region, less likely (16%–18%) originated from disparate sites or different regions of the infarct as demonstrated by animal studies and surgical ablation data.[25,26] For postinfarction VTs of multiple morphologies, a "shared" isthmus may be present in approximately 43% of arrhythmias. Such VTs may rotate in different directions along the

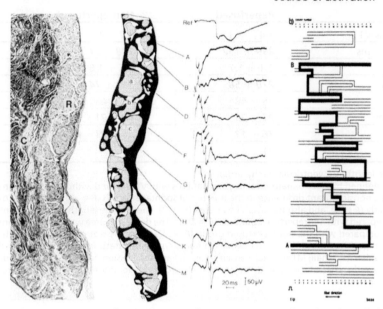

Slow conduction in the
infarcted tissue, with 'zigzag'
course of activation

Fig. 4. Electrical "zigzag" course of activation. In a human specimen of a subendocardial resection with viable myocardial cells, some myocardial bundles (R) are tightly spaced, and others were widely separated with areas of dense connective tissue (C). Electrograms recorded from A-M demonstrate the varying degrees of fractionation and conduction delay. The right panel demonstrates a 3-dimensional reconstruction of the border zone with a "zigzag" course of activation. (*From* de Bakker JM, van Capelle FJ, Janse MJ, et al. Slow conduction in the infarcted human heart. 'Zigzag' course of activation. Circulation 1993;88(3):923; with permission; and de Bakker JM, van Capelle FJ, Janse MJ, et al. Reentry as a cause of ventricular tachycardia in patients with chronic ischemic heart disease: electrophysiologic and anatomic correlation. Circulation 1988;77(3):599; with permission.)

isthmus, with variable extent of central line of block, or exiting the circuit at different sites/directions.[27,28]

PREPROCEDURE PLANNING

Defining the severity of the underlying structural heart disease and the extent of myocardial ischemia is an important part of the clinical evaluation of patients with VT with ischemic heart disease. Multiple preprocedural tests, such as 12-lead electrocardiograms (ECGs), echocardiography, nuclear stress test imaging, ventriculography, MRI, and computed tomography (CT) imaging may be considered.

The ECG provides noninvasive clues for localization of the potential VT "site-of-origin" to a generalized area of the heart. The initial presence of Q waves on the 12-lead ECG reveals general locations of prior MI and potential arrhythmia substrates. In patients with a single prior infarction, the ECG is likely to contain the VT site-of-origin with analysis of the VT morphology. A useful ECG

algorithm developed by Miller and colleagues[22] based on 12-lead ECG allows localization of "site-of-origin" for ischemic VTs with a reasonable (>70%) predictive accuracy to guide further mapping efforts. In the absence of monomorphic VT, premature ventricular contraction (PVC) morphologies during sinus rhythm also can be useful to locate the generalized regions of the macro-reentrant circuit or ascertain the possibility of Purkinje involvement. Furthermore, various QRS morphologic criteria based on a surface ECG have been used to distinguish endocardial from possible epicardial or nonendocardial sites of origins.[29–31]

However, the 12-lead ECGs of the spontaneous presenting VTs are often unavailable. Utilization of the stored electrograms from patients' ICDs can be helpful in providing additional data. Comparison of cycle lengths and the intracardiac "far-field" or "near-field" electrogram morphologies during induced VTs can be used to distinguish "clinical" VT from "nonclinical" arrhythmias. This may focus mapping efforts, streamline workflow, and improve ablation outcomes.[32]

Echocardiography is useful to identify regions of wall motion abnormalities consistent with prior infarcts, areas of myocardial thinning, or aneurysm, suggesting potential locations of arrhythmogenic substrate. Echocardiography also allows identification of mobile/friable intracardiac thrombus, which would preclude an endocardial approach. The presence of aortic or mitral valve stenosis or calcification may influence and guide retrograde aortic versus transseptal ablation approach. Patients with both mechanical aortic and mitral valves may require an epicardial approach, or alternative endocardial access, such as a transapical approach or a transventricular septal approach.[33]

MRI with gadolinium delayed enhancement (DE) to identify scar areas has increasingly been used for localization of myocardial scar.[34] In addition, infarct tissue heterogeneity assessed using MRI is also a strong predictor of spontaneous ventricular arrhythmia occurrence (**Fig. 5**).[35,36] The structural substrate, defined by DE on MRI, as well as wall thinning on CT scan, have been correlated with abnormal electrical substrate with low-voltage areas and critical sites of ischemic VT when combined with electroanatomical maps.[37,38] The integration of merged DE on MRI data and multi-slice CT allows combining substrate assessment with high spatial resolution to define structure-function relationship in scar-related VT. Such integrated images demonstrated that 95% of low-voltage/scar regions were inside MRI DE areas.

Regional wall motion abnormalities and wall thinning (WT) detected on multislice CT were also correlated to significant local conduction delay defined by late potentials or local abnormal ventricular activities (LAVA), with 93% of the very late low-voltage signals present within 3 mm of the thinnest region.[38] The integration of CT imaging and electroanatomical maps can be used to focus mapping on the arrhythmogenic substrate in patients who are unable to have MRI due to implanted cardiac devices.[39]

ENDOCARDIAL ABLATION STRATEGIES

With high-density electroanatomical mapping, Nakahara and colleagues[40] demonstrated the low-voltage (<1.5 mV) area and the dense scar

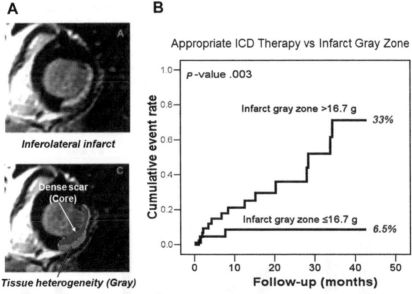

A

Inferolateral infarct

Dense scar (Core)

Tissue heterogeneity (Gray)

B

Appropriate ICD Therapy vs Infarct Gray Zone

p-value .003

Infarct gray zone >16.7 g — 33%

Infarct gray zone ≤16.7 g — 6.5%

Cumulative event rate

Follow-up (months)

Fig. 5. Cardiac MRI in ischemic VT substrate characterization. (*A*) Tissue heterogeneity within human infarcts was quantitatively analyzed by MRI. The image showed an inferolateral infarct that is located mostly near the subendocardium. High signal intensity representing the core (dense scar) with the gray zone representing the border zone with tissue heterogeneity. More extensive tissue heterogeneity correlates with increased ventricular irritability by programmed electrical stimulation. (*B*) Kaplan-Meier curve showing difference in appropriate ICD therapy stratified according to infarct gray zone. More patients (33%) with a large extent of infarct gray zone (infarct gray zone >16.7 g) received appropriate therapy compared with only 6.5% of the patients with a small extent of infarct gray zone (infarct gray zone ≤16.7 g) (*P* = .003). (*From* Roes SD, Borleffs CJ, van der Geest RJ, et al. Infarct tissue heterogeneity assessed with contrast-enhanced MRI predicts spontaneous ventricular arrhythmia in patients with ischemic cardiomyopathy and implantable cardioverter-defibrillator. Circ Cardiovasc Imaging 2009;2(3):189; with permission; and Schmidt A, Azevedo CF, Cheng A, et al. Infarct tissue heterogeneity by magnetic resonance imaging identifies enhanced cardiac arrhythmia susceptibility in patients with left ventricular dysfunction. Circulation 2007;115:2008; with permission.)

(<0.5 mV) were at least twice as large on the endo-cardium compared with the epicardial surface in patients with ischemic cardiomyopathy. Such endocardial preference of scar location was not observed in patients with nonischemic cardiomy-opathy (**Fig. 6**).[40]

Conventional mapping techniques, such as acti-vation and/or entrainment mapping, allow for char-acterization of the functional components of the reentrant VT circuit. Localization of the potential VT circuit based on activation and entrainment mapping is dependent on the hemodynamic toler-ance of the arrhythmia. However, most VTs are poorly tolerated and conventional activation and entrainment mapping strategies have a limited role. A paradigm shift in ablation strategies has focused on a substrate-based approach.

A systematic approach in identification of the VT circuit thereby requires both conventional mapping techniques and also substrate mapping techniques (**Fig. 7**). Mapping is often performed during sinus or paced rhythm to generate a high-density bipolar voltage map of the endocar-dial surface. Areas of the endocardium that are relatively heathy or "normal" generally have endo-cardial bipolar voltages greater than 1.5 mV. Areas in the border zone between healthy and scar regions typically have bipolar voltages from 0.5 mV to 1.5 mV. Areas with lower voltage, less than 0.5 mV, are arbitrarily classified as "dense scar."[41]

Based on detailed entrainment mapping of he-modynamically tolerated VTs, most VT isthmus or entrance sites (84%) were located in the dense scar region of less than 0.5 mV (**Table 2**).[42] Once the low-voltage "scar" area has been identified, pace mapping along the border zone (0.5–1.5 mV) around the scar can then be performed to approx-imate the "exit" site of the VT circuit. This is based on the principle that pacing at the exit site of the VT should yield a similar-paced QRS morphology as that of the spontaneous clinical VT. At the putative "exit," the paced QRS morphology should be similar to the spontaneous arrhythmia with a short stimulus-QRS interval (within 40 ms).[43] Once the approximate exit of the VT is identified, further mapping effort can be focused away from the border zone and into the dense scar region where the critical isthmus is often located.

CHANNELS

Histology of endocardial resection specimen from postinfarction patients with sustained VT revealed isolated bundles of viable myocardial fibers and strands of fibrous tissue interwoven within the infarct tissue, often associated with fractionation of electrograms and slow conduction.[19,44] Electri-cal recordings/signals from these surviving myo-fibers in zones of slow conduction may exhibit a higher signal amplitude/voltage compared with the surrounding nonconducting scar.

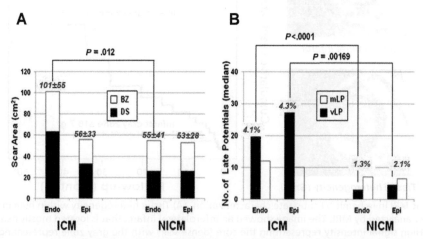

Fig. 6. Differences in scar area and LP between nonischemic cardiomyopathy (NICM) and ischemic cardiomyopa-thy (ICM) substrates. (*A*) With high-density electroanatomical maps of patients with ICM, the dense scar was twice as large on the endocardium as compared with the epicardium. Such predilection for endocardial scar was not as prominent in patients with NICM, with nearly equal extent of scar on the endocardium and epicardium. Less-dense scar (DS) (*solid bars*) was observed in patients with NICM. Open bars indicate border zone (BZ). (*B*) Patients with ICM had more LP and evidence of slow conduction than did patients with NICM. This difference was driven by a greater number of very LPs (vLP) (*solid bars*) in ICM. mLP, moderate late potentials. (*Adapted from* Nakahara S, Tung R, Ramirez RJ, et al. Characterization of the arrhythmogenic substrate in ischemic and nonischemic car-diomyopathy implications for catheter ablation of hemodynamically unstable ventricular tachycardia. J Am Coll Cardiol 2010;55(21):2360; with permission.)

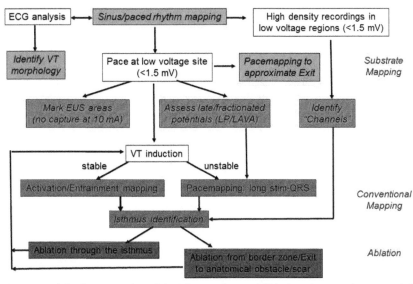

Fig. 7. Systemic approach in the strategies of the VT mapping and ablation. A systemic approach in the identification of the VT circuit requires both conventional mapping techniques and also substrate mapping techniques. (*Adapted from* Al-Ahmad AA, Callans DJ, Hsia HH, et al, editors. Hands-on ablation: the experts' approach. Minneapolis (MN): Cardiotext Publishing, LLC; 2013; with permission.)

These channels are often characterized by a passage demonstrating (1) contiguous electrogram recordings with higher amplitudes/voltages compared with the surrounding tissue; (2) local capture with a long stimulus-QRS interval; and (3) multicomponent, fractionated recordings within the channels. Such channels may be identified in 75% to 88% of patients using high-density electroanatomical mapping focusing on low-voltage areas (<1.5 mV), especially near the dense scar (<0.5 mV). Small adjustments of the bipolar voltage map and the color gradient during the sinus/paced rhythm are made. A single cutoff voltage threshold may not be feasible in all cases, and constant adjustment of the voltage color thresholds is needed to visualize the potential channels, depicted by a passageway of relatively higher

bipolar voltage surrounded by an area of lower-voltage scar.

Channels have been correlated to the zone of slow conduction and critical isthmuses of the VT circuit by entrainment mapping.[42] However, the mere presence of channels within myocardial scar has a low specificity in predicting the location of the VT isthmus site and additional mapping criteria are needed to confirm its functional significance (**Fig. 8**). The presence of isolated late potentials (LPs) inside the voltage channel significantly increase the specificity for identifying the clinical VT isthmus.[45] Most such "VT-related" channels are located in scar areas with bipolar voltages between 0.2 and 0.3 mV,[46] and can be identified noninvasively by contrast-enhanced MRI.[47]

Table 2
Anatomic characterization of substrate for hemodynamically stable ventricular tachycardia

	Entrance	Central Isthmus	Exit	Outer Loop
Dense scar, <0.5 mV	17	30	18	6
Border zone, 0.5–1.5 mV	2	7	26	18
Normal, >1.5 mV	—	—	4	8
Total	19	37	48	32

Most ventricular tachycardia critical isthmus sites or entrance sites were located in the dense scar region of less than 0.5 mV, whereas most exit sites are located in the border zone region.

Adapted from Hsia HH, Lin D, Sauer WH, et al. Anatomic characterization of endocardial substrate for hemodynamically stable reentrant ventricular tachycardia: identification of endocardial conducting channels. Heart Rhythm 2006;3(5):507; with permission.

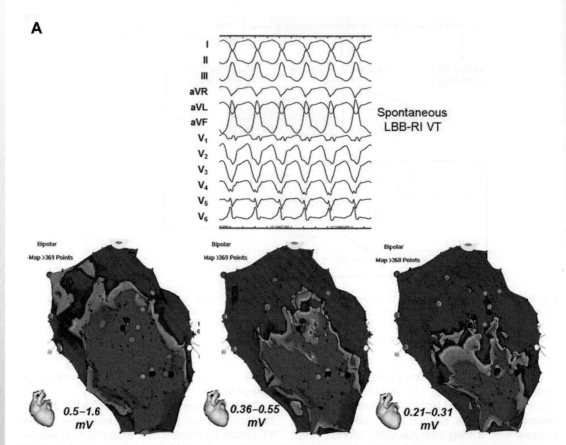

Fig. 8. Catheter mapping and ablation in a patient with a large anterior MI and spontaneous VT. (*A*) The spontaneous VT has a left bundle branch block-right-inferior (LBB-RI) QRS morphology. The exit site of the LBB-RI VT can be located to the left ventricular anterior wall, near the basal septum. The endocardial bipolar voltage map showed a large anterior scar. The color gradient adjustments of the bipolar voltage correspond to 0.5 to 1.6 mV, 0.35 to 0.55 mV, and 0.21 to 0.31 mV. A potential VT-related conduction channel can be identified at a color threshold of 0.21 to 0.31 mV. (*B*) With right ventricular pacing at different rates, delayed and fractionated signals were noted with decremental prolongation of the pacing stimuli-to-potential intervals with increasing pacing rates. (*C*) With right ventricular premature stimulation, decremental multicomponent and fractionated local electrograms were also noted, suggesting slow conduction into a potential channel. (*D*) Voltage map inside this channel demonstrate progressively late LP recordings from the border zone into the scar area. Perfect pacemapping was found to be in the conducting channel of the scar region. (*Adapted from* Al-Ahmad AA, Callans DJ, Hsia HH, et al, editors. Hands-on ablation: the experts' approach. Minneapolis (MN): Cardiotext Publishing, LLC; 2013; with permission.)

ELECTRICALLY UNEXCITABLE SCAR

Electrically unexcitable scar (EUS) mapping also has been used to identify potential borders and channels of viable myocardium and dense scar. High-output unipolar pacing (>10 mA at 2-ms pulse width) in scar regions that failed to capture myocardium were marked as EUS, and has been correlated to areas of dense scar with a local bipolar voltage of less than 0.25 mV. Potential isthmuses or channels often can be located between areas of EUS[48] with EUS commonly located in proximity to VT isthmus and potential conducting channels.

LATE POTENTIALS AND LOCAL ABNORMAL VENTRICULAR ACTIVITIES

The presence of late or fractionated potentials as a marker of local abnormal slow conduction was much more prevalent and a potential-guided ablation strategy was more effective in patients with ischemic heart disease compared with those with nonischemic cardiomyopathy.[40]

LAVA is a general term that incorporates all abnormal ventricular electrograms that represent near-field signals recorded from nonuniform anisotropic slow conduction from the surviving viable myocardial fibers within the potential VT

B

Decremental Late Potentials During RV Paced Rhythm

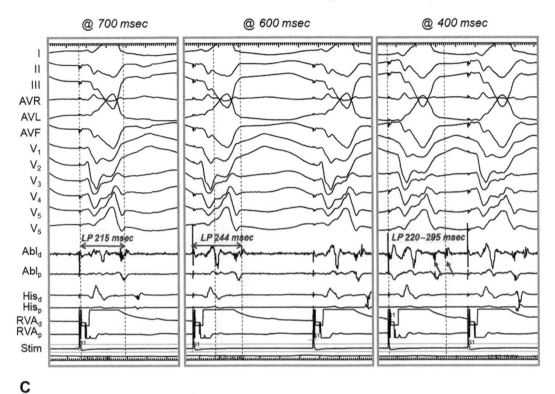

C

Late Potential Recordings:
Decremental Conduction Delay During RVA Extrastimulation @600 msec

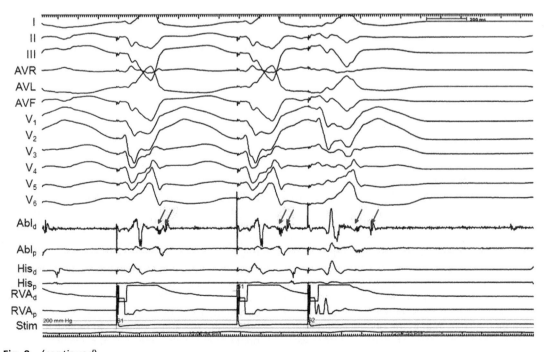

Fig. 8. *(continued)*

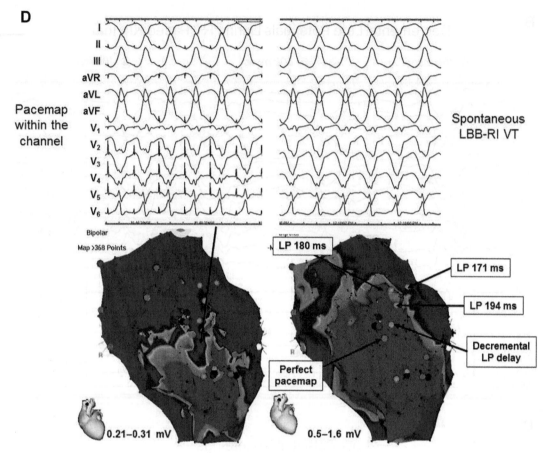

Fig. 8. (*continued*)

isthmus (**Fig. 9**).[21,49] Most LAVAs reside in scar or border-zone tissue and may appear as LPs or electrograms with isolated delayed components (E-IDC) recorded after the ventricular activation/surface QRS.[50,51] Using contrast-enhanced CT, LAVAs were located within regional WT (<5 mm thickness) or at its border. Very late LAVAs (LP > 100 ms after QRS complex) with the latest electrical activation were almost exclusively (93%) detected within the thinnest scar area (<3 mm thickness), demonstrating a structure-function relationship.[38] Pacing at these locations often results in good pace maps suggesting LAVAs represent areas that are likely critical isthmus of VT circuits.[52]

However, the latency and the ability to detect LAVA/LP is determined by the activation wave-fronts with variable fusion of near-field versus far-field signals, and thus affected to a large extent by their locations (see **Fig. 9**). LAVAs were more frequently detected after the QRS complex in the epicardium (91%) than in the endocardium (66%, P<.001), and only 3% of septal LAVAs were detectable and separated from far-field ventricular

electrograms.[53] Ventricular pacing or differential pacing at different rates may provide a different wavefront that may unmask areas of slow conduction.[46,54] Delivery of ventricular extrastimuli also can reveal decremental impulse propagation in areas with slow conduction demonstrating increased fractionation of LAVA/LP signals (see **Fig. 8C**).

The primary goal of catheter ablation of scar-related VT is the interruption of critical areas of slow conduction responsible for the development and maintenance of the reentrant circuit. Most patients with scar-related VT present with unstable arrhythmias that are not amenable to point-by-point conventional mapping techniques based on intracardiac activation sequence and the response to entrainment mapping. Ablation strategies targeting the abnormal electroanatomical substrate, guided by low bipolar voltage recordings, pacemapping, EUS, presence of conduction channels, and LAVA, allow focusing additional mapping efforts, formulating appropriate lesion sets, and perhaps limiting number of ablations.[6,55,56]

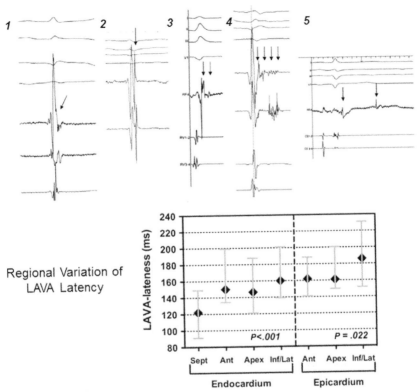

Fig. 9. Electrogram recordings showing various characteristics of local abnormal ventricular activities (LAVAs; *arrows*). (1) The potential may fused with the terminal portion of the far-field ventricular signal, making it difficult to identify. (2) LAVA potential occurs just after the far-field ventricular potential, within the QRS complex. (3) A double-component LAVA potential that closely follows the far-field ventricular signal. (4) LAVAs are represented by multi-component signals without isoelectric intervals. These signals can be visualized distinctly from the preceding far-field ventricular signal. (5) LAVA presenting as late potentials. The late component is recorded after the inscription of the T wave on the surface ECG. The figure also depicts regional variation of LAVA latency. A significant difference in LAVA lateness was found between regions (*P*<.001 for endocardial regions, *P* = .022 for epicardial regions). Due to simultaneous wave front of activation, only 43% of endocardial septal LAVA were clearly separated by an isoelectric line from far-field ventricular potential. (*From* Jaïs P, Maury P, Khairy P, et al. Elimination of local abnormal ventricular activities: a new end point for substrate modification in patients with scar-related ventricular tachycardia. Circulation 2012;125(18):2186; with permission; and Komatsu Y, Daly M, Sacher F, et al. Electrophysiologic characterization of local abnormal ventricular activities in postinfarction ventricular tachycardia with respect to their anatomic location. Heart Rhythm 2013;10(11):1635; with permission.)

Various substrate modification techniques have been described for unmappable or hemodynamically intolerable VT. Linear radiofrequency (RF) lesions are usually created to transect the potential isthmuses or to connect the VT exit sites to anatomic barriers such as the EUS or the valvular annuli. Noninducibility has been the most frequently used end point of VT ablation. However, programmed stimulation is associated with significant limitations with day-to-day variability and limited reproducibility.[57,58]

LAVAs are present in most patients with ischemic VTs. Abolition and elimination of LAVAs during sinus rhythm or ventricular pacing may be achieved in approximately 70% of patients and represent a useful and effective end point for substrate-based VT ablation. Complete LAVA elimination is associated with a better outcome when compared with persistence of LAVAs, and represents a simple procedural end point (**Fig. 10**).[49,59,60]

The conducting channels identified within the scar substrate are often interconnected. Tung and colleagues[61] demonstrated that most (80%) ablations targeting locations with earlier LPs, near the entrance of the channels, resulted in delay, or partial or complete eliminations of neighboring and remote LPs. "Scar dechanneling" represents an alternative method to LAVA abolition, with focal ablation of the earliest LPs recorded at the entrance sites of the channels, aiming toward the end point of eliminating a consecutive series

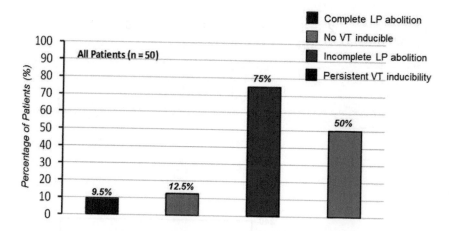

Fig. 10. VT recurrence rate versus ablation strategies. In patients with postinfarction VT, successful LP abolition and postprocedural VT noninducibility constitute significant endpoints after catheter ablation. Complete LP abolition or elimination reduces VT recurrence to exceptionally low rate and compared favorably with postprocedural noninducibility of VT. Persistence of LP/LAVA or persistent inducibility predicts a poor outcome. (*Modified from* Silberbauer J, Oloriz T, Maccabelli G, et al. Noninducibility and late potential abolition: a novel combined prognostic procedural end point for catheter ablation of postinfarction ventricular tachycardia. Circ Arrhythm Electrophysiol 2014;7(3):424–35; with permission.)

of late potentials/LAVA (**Fig. 11**).[62] Scar dechanneling alone results in a lower VT recurrence and mortality rates in more than half of patients. Higher event-free survival rates were observed in patients who were noninducible after scar dechanneling and those with complete elimination of electrograms within the conducting channel. Arrhythmia recurrences are mainly related to incomplete conducting channel-electrogram elimination.[62]

Furthermore, a "core isolation" approach to limit the number of lesions required to eliminate all critical areas for VT maintenance has been developed by Tzou and colleagues.[63] After identification of the area of interest within dense scar, including areas of voltage channels, LPs, isthmus sites identified by conventional criteria, contiguous ablation lesions to either completely surround the region or to anchor it to nearby anatomic anchors are delivered with the end point of exit block or inexcitability within the core area. The "core isolation" approach was achievable in 84% of the patients and was associated with a better VT-free survival.

PROCEDURAL OUTCOMES

Despite the advent of electroanatomical mapping systems, new substrate mapping strategies, and irrigated RF ablation technologies, the long-term efficacy of catheter ablation of postinfarction VT is only modest (**Table 3**).[27,60,64–68] The factors that predict VT recurrences after catheter ablation

have been examined in several multicenter studies. VT recurrences were associated with a history of multiple MIs, the presence of larger scar as assessed by electroanatomical mapping, more numbers of induced VTs, and persistent VT induction after the ablation procedures (**Table 4**).[27,65,69]

Although noninducibility predicts favorably the risk of VT recurrence and perhaps mortality, a combined procedural endpoint of LP/LAVA elimination and noninducibility after VT ablation is associated with a lower VT recurrence rate (16%) compared with noninducibility alone.[60] Such substrate-based ablation approach may be particularly useful because a significant minority of patients were noninducible at baseline. Taken together, these findings suggest that a substrate-based, more extensive ablation approach, targeting all abnormal local potentials within the scar in patients with ischemic heart disease, may be effective to control recurrent ventricular arrhythmia at long-term follow-up (**Fig. 12**). Pooled data from multiple studies showed a 38% risk reduction in VT recurrence using extensive substrate modification compared with limited substrate ablation (**Fig. 13**).

EPICARDIAL ABLATION

In contrast to other substrates like Chagas cardiomyopathy, nonischemic cardiomyopathies

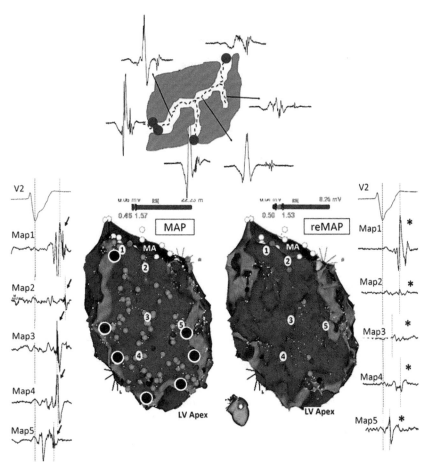

Fig. 11. Scar dechanneling. Inferior view of bipolar voltage electroanatomical substrate maps during sinus rhythm before (MAP) and after (reMAP) scar dechanneling. Electrograms recorded as conducting channel entrances are labeled with black dots and inner sites within the channel are labeled as blue dots. The left MAP demonstrates bipolar electrograms before ablation, and the reMAP demonstrates elimination of the delayed components of the LAVA in the same sites after scar dechanneling (*asterisk*). (*Adapted from* Berruezo A, Fernandez-Armenta J, Andreu D, et al. Scar dechanneling: new method for scar-related left ventricular tachycardia substrate ablation. Circ Arrhythm Electrophysiol 2015;8(2):329; with permission.)

or arrhythmogenic right ventricular cardiomyopathy where epicardial VT substrates are more commonly seen, most postinfarct VT can be ablated endocardially. However, circuits may exist in a midmyocardial or epicardial location, and the epicardium has been targeted for mapping and ablation in selected patients.[70] Although the true incidence of epicardial VTs in ischemic cardiomyopathy is unknown, epicardial VT circuits do appear to be more prevalent in patients with old inferior MIs.[71]

The ECG criteria for differentiation of epicardial versus endocardial VT site-of-origin for nonischemic cardiomyopathy did not reliably identify VTs that require ablation from the epicardium in patients with ischemic heart disease.[72] Thus, an epicardial approach is usually performed after previous failed endocardial ablations. A combined endocardial-epicardial ablation strategy has demonstrated improved outcomes in patients who have failed a prior ablation[73] and when a "homogenization" strategy was used (see **Fig. 12**).[74]

NEW TECHNOLOGIES

Catheter contact force (CF) is an important determinant in RF lesion formation and has been correlated with thrombus formation, steam pops, and risk of perforation. In the absence of CF feedback, up to 20% of endocardial RF applications that are thought to have good contact did not result in lesion formation.[75] Good myocardial contact increases the bipolar and unipolar electrogram amplitudes and improves identification of late,

Table 3
A summary of trials of catheter ablation in postinfarction VT

	n	Indications	LVEF, %	Acute Success, %	Follow-up, mo	Recurrent VT/ICD Rx, %	Adverse Events, %
Reddy et al,[64] 2007; (SMASH-VT)	64	Recur/induc VT/VF	31 ± 10	—	24	13	4.6
Stevenson et al,[65] 2008; ThermoCool VT Ablation	231	MMVT	25	49.0	6	47	7.3
Kuck et al,[66] 2010; VTACH	52	Stable VT	34 ± 9.6	—	21.9 ± 8.3	53	3.8
Tanner et al,[67] 2010; Euro-VT	63	Recur VT	30 ± 13	81.0	12 ± 3	49	5.0
Yokokawa et al,[27] 2013	98	Recur VT ICD Rx	27 ± 13	63.0	35 ± 23	34	7.1
Silberbauer et al,[60] 2014	155	Drug refractory VT	31 ± 9.4	—	~19	32	7.0
Dinov et al,[68] 2014	164	Recur VT	32 ± 11	77.4	27	43	11.1

Abbreviations: ICD, implantable cardioverter defibrillator; induc, inducible; LVEF, left ventricular ejection fraction; MMVT, Monomorphic ventricular tachycardia; Recur, recurrent; Rx, therapies; VF, ventricular fibrillation; VT, ventricular tachycardia; VTACH, Ventricular Tachycardia Ablation in Coronary Heart Disease Study.

fractionated potentials.[76] RF lesion size and depth are also significantly increased with increasing CF, and a CF threshold of usually 9 to 10 g is required for effective lesion formation in ischemic VT.[77]

BIPOLAR RADIOFREQUENCY

RF current delivered during endocardial and epicardial ablations are typically applied in a "unipolar" fashion between the distal electrode and a large grounding pad far away from the catheter. Bipolar RF is performed between the distal electrodes of 2 ablation catheters in close proximity, often on opposite sides of the myocardium, either across the interventricular septum or between the lateral left ventricular wall and the epicardium. Bipolar RF ablation was found to be more likely to achieve transmural lesions (82% vs 33%) in animal models and was more effective in targeting of VT located deep in the midmyocardium.[78]

INTRAMURAL NEEDLE ABLATION

A retractable needle–tipped ablation catheter has been developed for ablation of deep myocardial lesions. In vitro studies have demonstrated that saline-infused needle ablation achieved significantly deeper lesion depths and volume as compared with the conventional irrigated catheters.[79] Direct intramural ethanol injection into the myocardium also has shown feasibility in creating deep intramural lesions.[80] Infusion needle catheter ablation has been shown to be feasible for control of refractory VT in initial human experience.[81] Formal investigation is under way to assess the effectiveness and safety of such ablation device.

AUTONOMIC MODULATION

The autonomic nervous system has been implicated in the pathogenesis of ventricular arrhythmias and SCD.[82,83] Unilateral or bilateral cardiac sympathetic denervation, either surgically or via thoracic epidural anesthesia, have been shown to reduce the burden of ICD shocks and VT in patients with VT storm and refractory ventricular arrhythmias.[84,85] Alternatively, renal sympathetic denervation also has shown promise in control of incessant VT in a case report.[86] Autonomic modulation therefore should be considered as an adjunctive therapy in the management of selected patients with incessant, refractory ventricular arrhythmias.

RECENT STUDIES

There is increasing evidence that VT ablation in ischemic cardiomyopathy is becoming more mainstream, and not limited to a "last-resort" strategy. Previous randomized controlled trials of catheter ablation in ICD patients with ischemic cardiomyopathy and VT, such as Substrate Mapping and

Table 4
VT recurrences after ablation procedure

Stevenson et al,[65] 2008; Thermocool VT Ablation			
	Success (123)	Failure (108)	P
Age	65 (58–70)	69 (62–73)	*.012*
Heart failure, %	52	73	*.002*
LVEF (%)	25 (20–35)	25 (15–35)	.387
Multiple MIs, %	5	14	*.016*
VT events in preceding 6 mo	10 (4–30)	14 (6–38)	.37
No. induced VT/patient	3 (2–4)	4 (3–6)	*.002*
Longest VT CL	440 (370–500)	450 (380–538)	.251
Shortest VT CL	330 (271–400)	305 (272–350)	*.029*
Total no. RF lesions	24 (11–32)	26 (16–39)	*.029*
Postop VT induction	30	58	*<.001*
Yokokawa et al,[27] 2013			
	No Recurrent VT (65)	Recurrent VT (33)	P
LVEF, %	29 ± 14	25 ± 12	.26
Anterior MI	18 (28%)	14 (42%)	.14
Scar area, cm³	69 ± 30	93 ± 40	*.002*
No. clinical VT	4 ± 5	3 ± 3	.29
Clinical VT CL	359 ± 73	350 ± 77	.34
No. induced VT	13 (20%)	9 (27%)	.41
Identified critical sites	3 ± 2	4 ± 3	.49
RF duration, min	63 ± 44	73 ± 48	.35
Postop VT, nonclinical	24/63 (38%)	11/32 (34%)	.72
Postop VT, clinical	0/63 (0%)	0/63 (0%)	1.0

Abbreviations: CL, cycle length; LVEF, left ventricular ejection fraction; MI, myocardial infarction; Postop, postoperative; RF, radiofrequency; VT, ventricular tachycardia.

These studies examined the patient factors that predicted VT recurrence. Patients who had VT recurrences after ablation were older, had more heart failure, a history of multiple MIs, and presence of a larger scar as assessed by electroanatomical mapping. The number of inducible VT, faster VTs, and persistent VT induction were also predictors of worse outcomes. Values in italics symbolizes statistical significance, P <.05.

Ablation in Sinus Rhythm to Halt Ventricular Tachycardia (SMASH-VT) or Ventricular Tachycardia Ablation in Coronary Heart Disease (VTACH) study, have shown a significant benefit of catheter ablation over no ablation in control.[64,66] The recently published multicenter Ventricular Tachycardia Ablation versus Escalated Antiarrhythmic Drug Therapy in Ischemic Heart Disease (VANISH) trial prospectively compared escalating doses of antiarrhythmic drugs with amiodarone and/or mexiletine with catheter ablation. VANISH showed a significantly lower rate of the composite primary outcome of death, VT storm, or appropriate ICD shock in patients undergoing catheter ablation than those receiving an escalation in antiarrhythmic drug therapy.[87]

The International VT Ablation Center Collaborative group study included 2061 patients with structural heart disease undergoing catheter ablation. It was the largest retrospective multicenter study to date that examined the relationship between VT recurrence and mortality. For the first time, the data showed that freedom from VT recurrence after catheter ablation was strongly associated with improved transplant-free survival, independent of EF and heart failure severity, in patients with ischemic and nonischemic cardiomyopathies.[88] In the subset of patients with postinfarction VT and severe ventricular dysfunction (EF <30%), catheter ablation resulted in significant improvement in transplant-free mortality (83% vs 59%) in those without VT recurrence across all New York Heart Association (NYHA) classes (**Fig. 14**). These findings support the use of catheter ablation earlier in a more preemptive strategy in the

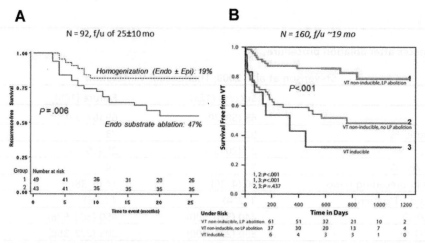

Fig. 12. Ventricular arrhythmia/ICD therapy-free survival by the ablation approach. (*A*) The Kaplan-Meier curve shows a significant difference in VT-free survival rate between a standard endocardial ablation approach and a "homogenization" approach with extensive endocardial and epicardial substrate–guided ablation. A homogenization approach resulted in a decreased VT recurrence rate (47% vs 19%; *P* = .006) compared with endocardial substrate ablation alone at 25 ± 10 months' follow-up. ICD implantable. (*B*) Achieving the combined procedural endpoint of VT noninducibility and LP abolition (Group 1: *green*) significantly reduces VT recurrence rate compared with noninducible patients at the end of the procedure without additional LP abolition (Group 2: *orange*) (16.4% vs 46.0%, *P*<.01) and those with persistent VT inducibility (Group 3: *red*) (16.4% vs 47.4%, *P*<.001). (*Adapted from* [A] Di Biase L, Santangeli P, Burkhardt DJ, et al. Endo-epicardial homogenization of the scar versus limited substrate ablation for the treatment of electrical storms in patients with ischemic cardiomyopathy. J Am Coll Cardiol 2012;60(2):139; with permission; and [B] Silberbauer J, Oloriz T, Maccabelli G, et al. Noninducibility and late potential abolition: a novel combined prognostic procedural end point for catheter ablation of postinfarction ventricular tachycardia. Circ Arrhythm Electrophysiol 2014;7(3):432; with permission.)

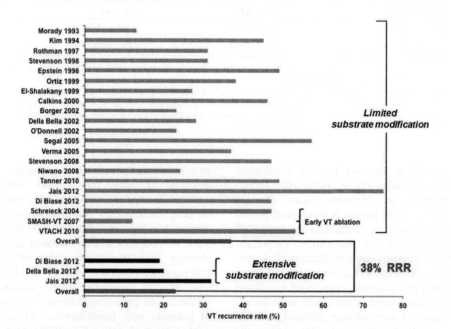

Fig. 13. Recurrence rate after catheter ablation of postinfarct VT. Blue bars represent studies using a limited substrate ablation approach. Green bars represent studies evaluating early intervention with a limited substrate ablation. Black bars represent studies using an extensive substrate-based modification ablation approach. The pooled data are depicted as red bars. RRR, relative risk reduction. [a] Studies included a subgroup of patients with nonischemic cardiomyopathy. (*Adapted from* Santangeli, DiBiase L, Hsia H, et al. Current and future indications for ventricular tachycardia ablation: the evidence from clinical trials. In: Mahapatra S, Marchlinski F, Natale A, et al, editors. VT ablation: a practical guide. Minneapolis (MN): CardioText Publishing; 2014. p. 44; with permission.)

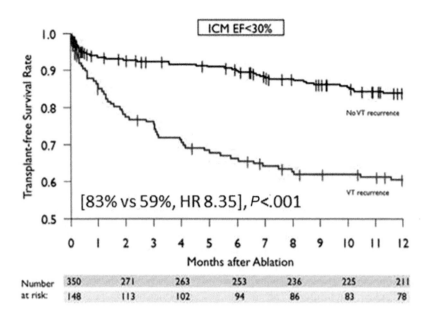

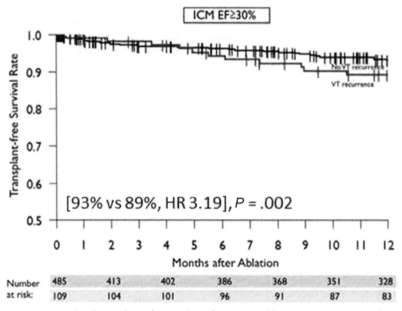

Fig. 14. Kaplan-Meier survival: relationship of transplant-free survival by VT recurrence. Kaplan-Meier curves of transplant-free survival by VT recurrence in patients with EF ≥30% and less than 30%. In patients with EF less than 30% and across all NYHA classes, improved transplant-free survival in those without VT recurrence. (*Adapted from* Tung R, Vaseghi M, Frankel DS, et al. Freedom from recurrent ventricular tachycardia after catheter ablation is associated with improved survival in patients with structural heart disease: an International VT Ablation Center Collaborative Group study. Heart Rhythm 2015;12(9):2004; with permission.)

management of patients with structural heart disease and VT.

Future Developments

Catheter ablation of VT is generally seen as an alternative of adjunct to antiarrhythmic therapy.

However, in contrast to VT in nonischemic structural heart disease, catheter ablation can now be considered as a first-line therapy in patients with ischemic heart disease and sustained monomorphic VT.[89] Catheter ablation has been shown to be superior to antiarrhythmic drugs in reduction of VT recurrences. Retrospective study also showed that freedom from VT recurrence after catheter ablation was associated with improved mortality. Prospective clinical trials are necessary and ongoing to examine the potential mortality impact of catheter ablation. Decrease in death as part of a composite endpoint that includes other important morbidity indicators, such as ICD shocks, has been observed. The impact on quality of life and severity of heart failure is also important to consider. This will hopefully be addressed with the ongoing PARTITA (Does Timing of VT Ablation Affect Prognosis in Patients With an Implantable Cardioverter-defibrillator?) trial.

Recent improvement in electroanatomical mapping technology and software development allowing for better identification of potential targets for catheter ablation such as conduction channels within the scar substrate. Ripple mapping is performed with electroanatomical mapping with postprocessing to display electrograms as a bar changing in length to its voltage and time relationship to identify conducting channels. Ablation of conducting channels using a ripple mapping algorithm has been shown to be promising with no VT recurrence during a mean 480 days of follow-up.[90]

SUMMARY

Ventricular arrhythmias arise from a complex substrate and remain a significant cause of morbidity and mortality in patients with ischemic heart disease. A systematic approach with detailed substrate characterization has been shown to improve VT ablation outcomes in recent trials. There have been continued advancements in mapping technologies and techniques allowing for better definition of potential targets for catheter ablation. Targeting LAVA along with a modified homogenization or de-channeling strategy may improve the procedural outcome and minimize complication. Catheter VT ablation has shifted to a potential first-line therapy and for early intervention. Further studies are needed to address outcomes in relation to quality of life, heart failure, and mortality after catheter ablation of VT.

REFERENCES

1. Moss AJ, Greenberg H, Case RB, et al. Long-term clinical course of patients after termination of ventricular tachyarrhythmia by an implanted defibrillator. Circulation 2004;110(25):3760–5.
2. Sears SF Jr, Conti JB. Quality of life and psychological functioning of ICD patients. Heart 2002;87(5): 488–93.
3. Poole JE, Johnson GW, Hellkamp AS, et al. Prognostic importance of defibrillator shocks in patients with heart failure. N Engl J Med 2008;359(10): 1009–17.
4. Santangeli P, Muser D, Maeda S, et al. Comparative effectiveness of antiarrhythmic drugs and catheter ablation for the prevention of recurrent ventricular tachycardia in patients with implantable cardioverter-defibrillators: a systematic review and meta-analysis of randomized controlled trials. Heart Rhythm 2016;13(7):1552–9.
5. Palaniswamy C, Kolte D, Harikrishnan P, et al. Catheter ablation of postinfarction ventricular tachycardia: ten-year trends in utilization, in-hospital complications, and in-hospital mortality in the United States. Heart Rhythm 2014;11(11):2056–63.
6. Aliot EM, Stevenson WG, Almendral-Garrote JM, et al. EHRA/HRS expert consensus on catheter ablation of ventricular arrhythmias: developed in a partnership with the European heart rhythm association (EHRA), a registered branch of the European Society of Cardiology (ESC), and the Heart Rhythm Society (HRS); in collaboration with the American College of Cardiology (ACC) and the American Heart Association (AHA). Heart Rhythm 2009;6(6): 886–933.
7. Go AS, Mozaffarian D, Roger VL, et al. Heart disease and stroke statistics–2014 update: a report from the American Heart Association. Circulation 2014;129(3):e28–292.
8. Newby KH, Thompson T, Stebbins A, et al. Sustained ventricular arrhythmias in patients receiving thrombolytic therapy: incidence and outcomes. The GUSTO Investigators. Circulation 1998;98(23):2567–73.
9. Tofler GH, Stone PH, Muller JE, et al. Prognosis after cardiac arrest due to ventricular tachycardia or ventricular fibrillation associated with acute myocardial infarction (the MILIS Study). Multicenter Investigation of the Limitation of Infarct Size. Am J Cardiol 1987;60(10):755–61.
10. Stevenson WG, Soejima K. Catheter ablation for ventricular tachycardia. Circulation 2007;115(21): 2750–60.
11. Buxton AE, Lee KL, Fisher JD, et al. A randomized study of the prevention of sudden death in patients with coronary artery disease. Multicenter Unsustained Tachycardia Trial Investigators. N Engl J Med 1999;341(25):1882–90.
12. Bloch Thomsen PE, Jons C, Raatikainen MJ, et al. Long-term recording of cardiac arrhythmias with an implantable cardiac monitor in patients with reduced ejection fraction after acute myocardial infarction: the Cardiac Arrhythmias and Risk Stratification after Acute Myocardial Infarction (CARISMA) study. Circulation 2010;122(13):1258–64.
13. Berger CJ, Murabito JM, Evans JC, et al. Prognosis after first myocardial infarction. Comparison of

Q-wave and non-Q-wave myocardial infarction in the Framingham Heart Study. JAMA 1992;268(12): 1545–51.

14. Solomon SD, Zelenkofske S, McMurray JJ, et al. Sudden death in patients with myocardial infarction and left ventricular dysfunction, heart failure, or both. N Engl J Med 2005;352(25):2581–8.

15. Wijnmaalen AP, Schalij MJ, von der Thusen JH, et al. Early reperfusion during acute myocardial infarction affects ventricular tachycardia characteristics and the chronic electroanatomic and histological substrate. Circulation 2010;121(17):1887–95.

16. Piers SR, Wijnmaalen AP, Borleffs CJ, et al. Early reperfusion therapy affects inducibility, cycle length, and occurrence of ventricular tachycardia late after myocardial infarction. Circ Arrhythm Electrophysiol 2011;4(2):195–201.

17. Friedman PL, Fenoglio JJ, Wit AL. Time course for reversal of electrophysiological and ultrastructural abnormalities in subendocardial Purkinje fibers surviving extensive myocardial infarction in dogs. Circ Res 1975;36(1):127–44.

18. Fenoglio JJ Jr, Pham TD, Harken AH, et al. Recurrent sustained ventricular tachycardia: structure and ultrastructure of subendocardial regions in which tachycardia originates. Circulation 1983;68(3): 518–33.

19. de Bakker JM, van Capelle FJ, Janse MJ, et al. Slow conduction in the infarcted human heart. 'Zigzag' course of activation. Circulation 1993;88(3):915–26.

20. Rutherford SL, Trew ML, Sands GB, et al. High-resolution 3-dimensional reconstruction of the infarct border zone: impact of structural remodeling on electrical activation. Circ Res 2012;111(3):301–11.

21. Gardner PI, Ursell PC, Fenoglio JJ Jr, et al. Electrophysiologic and anatomic basis for fractionated electrograms recorded from healed myocardial infarcts. Circulation 1985;72(3):596–611.

22. Miller JM, Marchlinski FE, Buxton AE, et al. Relationship between the 12-lead electrocardiogram during ventricular tachycardia and endocardial site of origin in patients with coronary artery disease. Circulation 1988;77(4):759–66.

23. Park KM, Nam GB, Choi KJ, et al. Recurrent polymorphic ventricular tachycardia treated by ablation of Purkinje arborization within an infarct borderzone. Tex Heart Inst J 2011;38(3):291–4.

24. Bogun F, Good E, Reich S, et al. Role of Purkinje fibers in post-infarction ventricular tachycardia. J Am Coll Cardiol 2006;48(12):2500–7.

25. Miller JM, Kienzle MG, Harken AH, et al. Morphologically distinct sustained ventricular tachycardias in coronary artery disease: significance and surgical results. J Am Coll Cardiol 1984;4(6):1073–9.

26. Costeas C, Peters NS, Waldecker B, et al. Mechanisms causing sustained ventricular tachycardia with multiple QRS morphologies: results of mapping studies in the infarcted canine heart. Circulation 1997;96(10):3721–31.

27. Yokokawa M, Desjardins B, Crawford T, et al. Reasons for recurrent ventricular tachycardia after catheter ablation of post-infarction ventricular tachycardia. J Am Coll Cardiol 2013;61(1):66–73.

28. Bogun F, Hohnloser SH, Bender B, et al. Mechanism of ventricular tachycardia termination by pacing at left ventricular sites in patients with coronary artery disease. J Interv Card Electrophysiol 2002; 6(1):35–41.

29. Valles E, Bazan V, Marchlinski FE. ECG criteria to identify epicardial ventricular tachycardia in nonischemic cardiomyopathy. Circ Arrhythm Electrophysiol 2010;3(1):63–71.

30. Berruezo A, Mont L, Nava S, et al. Electrocardiographic recognition of the epicardial origin of ventricular tachycardias. Circulation 2004;109(15): 1842–7.

31. Daniels DV, Lu YY, Morton JB, et al. Idiopathic epicardial left ventricular tachycardia originating remote from the sinus of Valsalva: electrophysiological characteristics, catheter ablation, and identification from the 12-lead electrocardiogram. Circulation 2006;113(13):1659–66.

32. Yoshida K, Liu TY, Scott C, et al. The value of defibrillator electrograms for recognition of clinical ventricular tachycardias and for pace mapping of post-infarction ventricular tachycardia. J Am Coll Cardiol 2010;56(12):969–79.

33. Vaseghi M, Macias C, Tung R, et al. Percutaneous interventricular septal access in a patient with aortic and mitral mechanical valves: a novel technique for catheter ablation of ventricular tachycardia. Heart Rhythm 2013;10(7):1069–73.

34. McCrohon JA, Moon JC, Prasad SK, et al. Differentiation of heart failure related to dilated cardiomyopathy and coronary artery disease using gadolinium-enhanced cardiovascular magnetic resonance. Circulation 2003;108(1):54–9.

35. Roes SD, Borleffs CJ, van der Geest RJ, et al. Infarct tissue heterogeneity assessed with contrast-enhanced MRI predicts spontaneous ventricular arrhythmia in patients with ischemic cardiomyopathy and implantable cardioverter-defibrillator. Circ Cardiovasc Imaging 2009;2(3):183–90.

36. Estner HL, Zviman MM, Herzka D, et al. The critical isthmus sites of ischemic ventricular tachycardia are in zones of tissue heterogeneity, visualized by magnetic resonance imaging. Heart Rhythm 2011;8(12): 1942–9.

37. Cochet H, Komatsu Y, Sacher F, et al. Integration of merged delayed-enhanced magnetic resonance imaging and multidetector computed tomography for the guidance of ventricular tachycardia ablation: a pilot study. J Cardiovasc Electrophysiol 2013;24(4): 419–26.

38. Komatsu Y, Cochet H, Jadidi A, et al. Regional myocardial wall thinning at multidetector computed tomography correlates to arrhythmogenic substrate in postinfarction ventricular tachycardia: assessment of structural and electrical substrate. Circ Arrhythm Electrophysiol 2013;6(2):342–50.

39. Zeppenfeld K, Tops LF, Bax JJ, et al. Images in cardiovascular medicine. Epicardial radiofrequency catheter ablation of ventricular tachycardia in the vicinity of coronary arteries is facilitated by fusion of 3-dimensional electroanatomical mapping with multislice computed tomography. Circulation 2006;114(3):e51–2.

40. Nakahara S, Tung R, Ramirez RJ, et al. Characterization of the arrhythmogenic substrate in ischemic and nonischemic cardiomyopathy implications for catheter ablation of hemodynamically unstable ventricular tachycardia. J Am Coll Cardiol 2010;55(21):2355–65.

41. Marchlinski FE, Callans DJ, Gottlieb CD, et al. Linear ablation lesions for control of unmappable ventricular tachycardia in patients with ischemic and nonischemic cardiomyopathy. Circulation 2000;101(11):1288–96.

42. Hsia HH, Lin D, Sauer WH, et al. Anatomic characterization of endocardial substrate for hemodynamically stable reentrant ventricular tachycardia: identification of endocardial conducting channels. Heart Rhythm 2006;3(5):503–12.

43. Josephson ME, Waxman HL, Cain ME, et al. Ventricular activation during ventricular endocardial pacing. II. Role of pace-mapping to localize origin of ventricular tachycardia. Am J Cardiol 1982;50(1):11–22.

44. de Bakker JM, van Capelle FJ, Janse MJ, et al. Reentry as a cause of ventricular tachycardia in patients with chronic ischemic heart disease: electrophysiologic and anatomic correlation. Circulation 1988;77(3):589–606.

45. Mountantonakis SE, Park RE, Frankel DS, et al. Relationship between voltage map "channels" and the location of critical isthmus sites in patients with post-infarction cardiomyopathy and ventricular tachycardia. J Am Coll Cardiol 2013;61(20):2088–95.

46. Arenal A, del Castillo S, Gonzalez-Torrecilla E, et al. Tachycardia-related channel in the scar tissue in patients with sustained monomorphic ventricular tachycardias: influence of the voltage scar definition. Circulation 2004;110(17):2568–74.

47. Perez-David E, Arenal A, Rubio-Guivernau JL, et al. Noninvasive identification of ventricular tachycardia-related conducting channels using contrast-enhanced magnetic resonance imaging in patients with chronic myocardial infarction: comparison of signal intensity scar mapping and endocardial voltage mapping. J Am Coll Cardiol 2011;57(2):184–94.

48. Soejima K, Stevenson WG, Maisel WH, et al. Electrically unexcitable scar mapping based on pacing threshold for identification of the reentry circuit isthmus: feasibility for guiding ventricular tachycardia ablation. Circulation 2002;106(13):1678–83.

49. Jais P, Maury P, Khairy P, et al. Elimination of local abnormal ventricular activities: a new end point for substrate modification in patients with scar-related ventricular tachycardia. Circulation 2012;125(18):2184–96.

50. Arenal A, Glez-Torrecilla E, Ortiz M, et al. Ablation of electrograms with an isolated, delayed component as treatment of unmappable monomorphic ventricular tachycardias in patients with structural heart disease. J Am Coll Cardiol 2003;41(1):81–92.

51. Hsia HH, Lin D, Sauer WH, et al. Relationship of late potentials to the ventricular tachycardia circuit defined by entrainment. J Interv Card Electrophysiol 2009;26(1):21–9.

52. Bogun F, Good E, Reich S, et al. Isolated potentials during sinus rhythm and pace-mapping within scars as guides for ablation of post-infarction ventricular tachycardia. J Am Coll Cardiol 2006;47(10):2013–9.

53. Komatsu Y, Daly M, Sacher F, et al. Electrophysiologic characterization of local abnormal ventricular activities in postinfarction ventricular tachycardia with respect to their anatomic location. Heart Rhythm 2013;10(11):1630–7.

54. Brunckhorst CB, Delacretaz E, Soejima K, et al. Ventricular mapping during atrial and right ventricular pacing: relation of electrogram parameters to ventricular tachycardia reentry circuits after myocardial infarction. J Interv Card Electrophysiol 2004;11(3):183–91.

55. Priori SG, Blomstrom-Lundqvist C, Mazzanti A, et al. 2015 ESC guidelines for the management of patients with ventricular arrhythmias and the prevention of sudden cardiac death: the task force for the management of patients with ventricular arrhythmias and the prevention of sudden cardiac death of the European Society of Cardiology (ESC). Endorsed by: Association for European Paediatric and Congenital Cardiology (AEPC). Eur Heart J 2015;36(41):2793–867.

56. Santangeli P, Marchlinski FE. Substrate mapping for unstable ventricular tachycardia. Heart Rhythm 2016;13(2):569–83.

57. Cooper MJ, Hunt LJ, Palmer KJ, et al. Quantitation of day to day variability in mode of induction of ventricular tachyarrhythmias by programmed stimulation. J Am Coll Cardiol 1988;11(1):101–8.

58. McPherson CA, Rosenfeld LE, Batsford WP. Day-to-day reproducibility of responses to right ventricular programmed electrical stimulation: implications for serial drug testing. Am J Cardiol 1985;55(6):689–95.

59. Sacher F, Lim HS, Derval N, et al. Substrate mapping and ablation for ventricular tachycardia: the LAVA approach. J Cardiovasc Electrophysiol 2015; 26(4):464–71.

60. Silberbauer J, Oloriz T, Maccabelli G, et al. Noninducibility and late potential abolition: a novel combined prognostic procedural end point for catheter ablation of postinfarction ventricular tachycardia. Circ Arrhythm Electrophysiol 2014;7(3):424–35.

61. Tung R, Mathuria NS, Nagel R, et al. Impact of local ablation on interconnected channels within ventricular scar: mechanistic implications for substrate modification. Circ Arrhythm Electrophysiol 2013; 6(6):1131–8.

62. Berruezo A, Fernandez-Armenta J, Andreu D, et al. Scar dechanneling: new method for scar-related left ventricular tachycardia substrate ablation. Circ Arrhythm Electrophysiol 2015;8(2):326–36.

63. Tzou WS, Frankel DS, Hegeman T, et al. Core isolation of critical arrhythmia elements for treatment of multiple scar-based ventricular tachycardias. Circ Arrhythm Electrophysiol 2015;8(2):353–61.

64. Reddy VY, Reynolds MR, Neuzil P, et al. Prophylactic catheter ablation for the prevention of defibrillator therapy. N Engl J Med 2007;357(26):2657–65.

65. Stevenson WG, Wilber DJ, Natale A, et al. Irrigated radiofrequency catheter ablation guided by electroanatomic mapping for recurrent ventricular tachycardia after myocardial infarction: the multicenter thermocool ventricular tachycardia ablation trial. Circulation 2008;118(25):2773–82.

66. Kuck KH, Schaumann A, Eckardt L, et al. Catheter ablation of stable ventricular tachycardia before defibrillator implantation in patients with coronary heart disease (VTACH): a multicentre randomised controlled trial. Lancet 2010;375(9708):31–40.

67. Tanner H, Hindricks G, Volkmer M, et al. Catheter ablation of recurrent scar-related ventricular tachycardia using electroanatomical mapping and irrigated ablation technology: results of the prospective multicenter Euro-VT-study. J Cardiovasc Electrophysiol 2010;21(1):47–53.

68. Dinov B, Fiedler L, Schonbauer R, et al. Outcomes in catheter ablation of ventricular tachycardia in dilated nonischemic cardiomyopathy compared with ischemic cardiomyopathy: results from the Prospective Heart Centre of Leipzig VT (HELP-VT) Study. Circulation 2014;129(7):728–36.

69. Tung R, Josephson ME, Reddy V, et al. Influence of clinical and procedural predictors on ventricular tachycardia ablation outcomes: an analysis from the substrate mapping and ablation in Sinus Rhythm to Halt Ventricular Tachycardia Trial (SMASH-VT). J Cardiovasc Electrophysiol 2010; 21(7):799–803.

70. Sosa E, Scanavacca M, D'Avila A, et al. Endocardial and epicardial ablation guided by nonsurgical transthoracic epicardial mapping to treat recurrent ventricular tachycardia. J Cardiovasc Electrophysiol 1998;9(3):229–39.

71. Sosa E, Scanavacca M, d'Avila A, et al. Nonsurgical transthoracic epicardial catheter ablation to treat recurrent ventricular tachycardia occurring late after myocardial infarction. J Am Coll Cardiol 2000;35(6): 1442–9.

72. Martinek M, Stevenson WG, Inada K, et al. QRS characteristics fail to reliably identify ventricular tachycardias that require epicardial ablation in ischemic heart disease. J Cardiovasc Electrophysiol 2012;23(2):188–93.

73. Tung R, Michowitz Y, Yu R, et al. Epicardial ablation of ventricular tachycardia: an institutional experience of safety and efficacy. Heart Rhythm 2013; 10(4):490–8.

74. Di Biase L, Santangeli P, Burkhardt DJ, et al. Endoepicardial homogenization of the scar versus limited substrate ablation for the treatment of electrical storms in patients with ischemic cardiomyopathy. J Am Coll Cardiol 2012;60(2):132–41.

75. Sacher F, Wright M, Derval N, et al. Endocardial versus epicardial ventricular radiofrequency ablation: utility of in vivo contact force assessment. Circ Arrhythm Electrophysiol 2013;6(1):144–50.

76. Mizuno H, Vergara P, Maccabelli G, et al. Contact force monitoring for cardiac mapping in patients with ventricular tachycardia. J Cardiovasc Electrophysiol 2013;24(5):519–24.

77. Thiagalingam A, D'Avila A, Foley L, et al. Importance of catheter contact force during irrigated radiofrequency ablation: evaluation in a porcine ex vivo model using a force-sensing catheter. J Cardiovasc Electrophysiol 2010;21(7):806–11.

78. Koruth JS, Dukkipati S, Miller MA, et al. Bipolar irrigated radiofrequency ablation: a therapeutic option for refractory intramural atrial and ventricular tachycardia circuits. Heart Rhythm 2012;9(12):1932–41.

79. Sapp JL, Cooper JM, Soejima K, et al. Deep myocardial ablation lesions can be created with a retractable needle-tipped catheter. Pacing Clin Electrophysiol 2004;27(5):594–9.

80. Callans DJ, Ren JF, Narula N, et al. Left ventricular catheter ablation using direct, intramural ethanol injection in swine. J Interv Card Electrophysiol 2002; 6(3):225–31.

81. Sapp JL, Beeckler C, Pike R, et al. Initial human feasibility of infusion needle catheter ablation for refractory ventricular tachycardia. Circulation 2013; 128(21):2289–95.

82. Vaseghi M, Shivkumar K. The role of the autonomic nervous system in sudden cardiac death. Prog Cardiovasc Dis 2008;50(6):404–19.

83. Shen MJ, Zipes DP. Role of the autonomic nervous system in modulating cardiac arrhythmias. Circ Res 2014;114(6):1004–21.

84. Bourke T, Vaseghi M, Michowitz Y, et al. Neuraxial modulation for refractory ventricular arrhythmias: value of thoracic epidural anesthesia and surgical left cardiac sympathetic denervation. Circulation 2010;121(21):2255–62.

85. Vaseghi M, Gima J, Kanaan C, et al. Cardiac sympathetic denervation in patients with refractory ventricular arrhythmias or electrical storm: intermediate and long-term follow-up. Heart Rhythm 2014;11(3): 360–6.

86. Ukena C, Bauer A, Mahfoud F, et al. Renal sympathetic denervation for treatment of electrical storm: first-in-man experience. Clin Res Cardiol 2012; 101(1):63–7.

87. Sapp JL, Wells GA, Parkash R, et al. Ventricular tachycardia ablation versus escalation of antiarrhythmic drugs. N Engl J Med 2016; 375(2):111–21.

88. Tung R, Vaseghi M, Frankel DS, et al. Freedom from recurrent ventricular tachycardia after catheter ablation is associated with improved survival in patients with structural heart disease: an International VT Ablation Center Collaborative Group study. Heart Rhythm 2015;12(9):1997–2007.

89. Pedersen CT, Kay GN, Kalman J, et al. EHRA/HRS/ APHRS expert consensus on ventricular arrhythmias. Heart Rhythm 2014;11(10):e166–96.

90. Jamil-Copley S, Vergara P, Carbucicchio C, et al. Application of ripple mapping to visualize slow conduction channels within the infarct-related left ventricular scar. Circ Arrhythm Electrophysiol 2015; 8(1):76–86.

Catheter Ablation for Ventricular Tachycardia in Patients with Nonischemic Cardiomyopathy

Nathaniel Thompson, MD*, Antonio Frontera, MD,
Masateru Takigawa, MD, Ghassen Cheniti, MD,
Gregoire Massoullie, MD, Hubert Cochet, MD, PhD,
Arnaud Denis, MD, Arnaud Chaumeil, MD,
Nicolas Derval, MD, Meleze Hocini, MD,
Michel Haissaguerre, MD, Pierre Jais, MD,
Frederic Sacher, MD, PhD

KEYWORDS

• Ventricular tachycardia • Ablation • Nonischemic cardiomyopathy

KEY POINTS

- Nonischemic cardiomyopathy (NICM) is an umbrella term for a mixed group of disease processes that often involve the intramyocardium and epicardium.
- Cardiac MRI is a powerful tool that can identify substrate involvement (and sites critical to the maintenance of ventricular tachycardia [VT]), which is sometimes not possible with conventional mapping.
- Clinicians should consider cardiac MRI in all patients with NICM before an implantable cardioverter-defibrillator or device implant in anticipation of future VT.
- Alternative technologies can create deeper lesions than conventional catheter ablation techniques and are valuable options for clinicians, particularly when targeting the interventricular septum or the midmyocardium.

Catheter ablation of ventricular tachycardia (VT) has become an increasingly performed procedure. Studies have shown that ablation can reduce episodes of VT in patients with ischemic heart disease (and likely scar-mediated tachycardia).[1,2]

The number of patients with nonischemic cardiomyopathy (NICM) requiring VT ablation has increased in proportion.[3] However, in those patients with NICM, the results have been more mixed,[4] and generally inferior when compared

Disclosures: Dr A. Denis received speaking honoraria from Medtronic and Boston Scientific. Dr N. Derval received speaking honoraria from Medtronic, Boston Scientific, and Biosense Webster. Dr M. Haissaguerre received consulting fees from Biosense Webster and is a stock holder of Cardio Insight. Dr M. Hocini received consulting fees from Medtronic and Biosense Webster and is a stock holder of Cardio Insight. Dr P. Jais received consulting fees from Biosense Webster, Boston Scientific, St. Jude Medical and is a stock holder of Cardio Insight. Dr F. Sacher received speaking honoraria from Biosense Webster, Medtronic, St. Jude Medical, Sorin Group, Boehringer Ingelheim, Bayer HealthCare, Pfizer, and Buchang Pharma; consulting fees from St. Jude Medical, Bayer Healthcare, and the Sorin Group; and a research grant from Medtronic.
Bordeaux University Hospital, LIRYC Institute, INSERM 1045, Bordeaux University, France
* Corresponding author. Hopital Haut-Leveque, Av. Magellan, Pessac 33600, France.
E-mail address: n.clark.thompson@gmail.com

with patients with ischemic cardiomyopathy (ICM). That patients with NICM fared worse may be explained by the variety and extent of the disease processes (including epicardial and intramural involvement) as well as the ablation strategies used.[5] What is required for the best chance of procedural success is a careful diagnosis of the arrhythmia mechanism and the substrate necessary for its maintenance.

PREPROCEDURE ASSESSMENT

Before the procedure it is important to try to localize the VT and identify regions of substrate involvement (septal vs lateral, periannular, endocardial vs epicardial and intramural). The electrocardiogram can identify epicardial tachycardias[6,7] and can provide other clues during a normal rhythm (eg, arrhythmogenic right ventricular cardiomyopathy [ARVC], sarcoidosis, laminopathy). Acquiring an echocardiogram is standard and provides information on valvular function and overall ventricular function, and can rule out thrombus (a contraindication to endocardial mapping). Preprocedural imaging with computed tomography (CT) and cardiac MRI is particularly helpful. Cardiac MRI with delayed enhancement can help diagnose infiltrative processes such as ARVC and sarcoidosis, and can more generally localize regions of fibrosis or scar (**Fig. 1**).[8] This ability is useful in crafting an ablation strategy (whether to approach epicardially or endocardially) or if other techniques, such as septal or transcoronary alcohol ablation techniques, should be considered. Reconstructed images of both CT

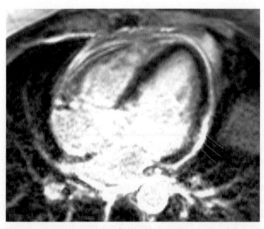

Fig. 1. An example of cardiac MRI with delayed enhancement identifying subepicardial scar in the lateral left ventricle (*red arrows*) in a patient with postmyocarditis VT. Endocardium is preserved without wall thinning. Endocardial ablation in this patient has little chance to be successful.

and MRI can be imported into three-dimensional mapping systems; overlaid images can guide mapping and ablation of critical regions and also avoid important structures (eg, coronary arteries) (**Fig. 2**). In anticipation of future requirements for VT ablation, the authors perform cardiac MRI in all patients with NICM referred for implantable cardioverter-defibrillator or device implantation.

PROCEDURE AND MAPPING STRATEGIES

Initial choice of catheter access is guided by the preablation work-up. The left ventricle (LV) can be accessed retrograde across the aortic valve, antegrade with a transseptal puncture, and from an epicardial approach. Similarly, the right ventricle (RV) can be accessed from the endocardium or from the epicardium. The transseptal approach is effective to reach most of the left ventricular endocardium, although it requires the use of a large, curved, steerable sheath to maneuver easily. It is more difficult to access the basal septum and aortic outflow tract. The retrograde aortic approach is more effective in these scenarios.

The authors recommend diagnostic catheters placed in the His position (useful to diagnose bundle branch reentry and as a landmark during the transseptal puncture) and another to make electrogram recordings from the RV, or from the LV via the coronary sinus. Ventricular capture thresholds should be tested at the beginning of the procedure to be ready for entrainment or pace termination of the clinical tachycardia. High-resolution mapping catheters with multiple electrodes, such as the Livewire (St. Jude Medical, Saint Paul, MN), Orion mapping catheter (Boston Scientific, Marlborough, MA), and the Pentaray mapping catheter (Biosense Webster, Diamond Bar, CA), can rapidly acquire points and are better able to resolve near-field from far-field ventricular signals than more conventional mapping catheters. Their maneuverability in the pericardial space is generally not a problem. However, it may be more challenging to map the endocardium and negotiate the left ventricular space, particularly when the ventricles are not dilated.

To safely arrive at the proper diagnosis and treatment plan, the authors try to be systematic in the use of maneuvers (**Table 1**). After gaining arterial and venous access and diagnostic catheters are in place (and before full anticoagulation), we proceed with pericardial access if there is evidence of epicardial involvement.[9] We then create a map of the epicardial substrate and tag local abnormal ventricular activity potentials. Afterward, we access the left ventricular endocardium via a

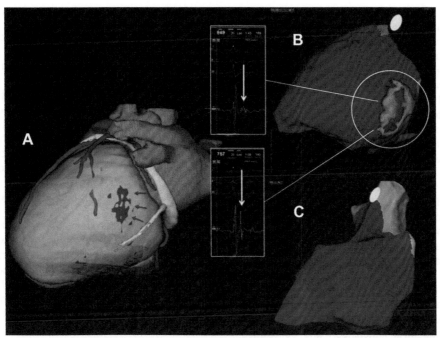

Fig. 2. (*A*) MRI scan integration with a three-dimensional mapping system (Carto, Biosense Webster) for the same patient as in **Fig. 1**. Important structures such as the coronary arteries are shown, with substrate involvement (*red arrows*) of the lateral wall of the LV. (*B*) An epicardial bipolar voltage map shows an area of scar (*circle*) with local abnormal ventricular activity potentials (*white arrows*) recorded at its margins. (*C*) An endocardial bipolar voltage map did not show scar.

Table 1
Work flow for ablation of ventricular tachycardia in patients with nonischemic cardiomyopathy

NICM VT Workflow		
Arterial and venous access	His and RV recording catheters placed	Decision to access the pericardium based on preprocedure work-up and imaging
Epicardial access	Epicardial voltage map	LAVA potentials are tagged and scar identified with the help of 3D image integration
Endocardial access (anticoagulation is given)	Endocardial voltage map	LAVA potentials and scar identified with a 3D voltage map
	VT induction and mapping	If hemodynamically stable, mapping of VT with recording catheters initially at sites of interest
Ablation	Conventional catheter ablation	Endocardial and epicardial targets
	RF needle, bipolar RF and transcoronary alcohol ablation	Intramural and intraseptal targets not amenable to conventional techniques

Stepwise approach

Abbreviations: 3D, three dimensional; LAVA, local abnormal ventricular activity; RF, radiofrequency.

transseptal or a retrograde aortic approach (full anticoagulation is then given) and construct a concurrent endocardial substrate map.

After substrate mapping, we attempt to induce VT with a multipolar catheter already positioned in the area of potential interest (either on the epicardial or endocardial surface). If the patient is able to tolerate a stable tachycardia, we can exclude bundle branch reentry with a recording catheter in the His position. Although mapping of the VT mechanisms follows conventional methods, rhythm and hemodynamic instability can limit the ability to make a diagnosis during tachycardia. In addition, fibrosis (and presumed sites critical to VT maintenance) can involve only the intramyocardium with relatively healthy epicardial and endocardial tissue, limiting the ability to make an accurate map (**Fig. 3**). Haqqani and colleagues[10] showed isolated septal intramural substrate in patients with NICM. A significant number of patients had no identifiable bipolar low-voltage substrate with substantial scar identified with cardiac MRI. Hutchinson and colleagues[11] showed that unipolar endocardial voltage with thresholds less than 8.3 mV for the LV and less than 5.5 mV for the RV can identify intramural or epicardial scar in patients with normal bipolar endocardial voltage.

CONSIDERATIONS BY SUBSTRATE DISORDER

It is not possible here to make a comprehensive review of the NICM types. However, there are practical considerations for clinicians when creating an ablation strategy.

Chagas cardiomyopathy, an infection by a protozoan parasite, is a chronic infection with reparative fibrosis and typically affects the epicardium. Most tachycardias originate from the base of the LV,[12] and require epicardial access and ablation. This procedure was pioneered by Sosa and colleagues[13,14] with success and should be considered an initial strategy in those patients diagnosed with the disease.

Cardiac sarcoidosis, a multisystem inflammatory disease, starts within the myocardium with extension to the epicardium and endocardium and most often involves the basal septum and conduction system.[15] Fibrosis of the LV is patchy and the mechanism of VT is most often scar mediated. Patients can present with multiple different tachycardias requiring extensive ablation. Combined with antiarrhythmic medications, ablation has yielded a reduction in VT reoccurrences.[16] Imaging can be very helpful during preprocedure evaluation; both PET-CT and cardiac MRI can identify pulmonary and extrapulmonary sarcoidosis.[17]

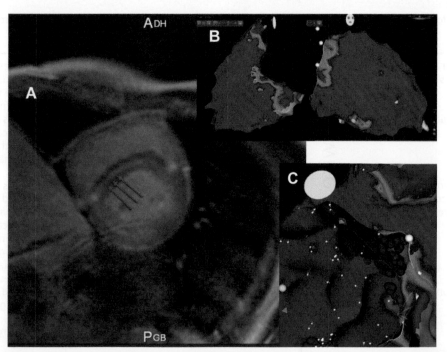

Fig. 3. (*A*) Cardiac MRI of a patient with laminopathy. Note the typical intraseptal scar (*red arrows*). (*B*) Endocardial voltage maps of the left (*left*) and right (*right*) ventricles with limited regions of scar. (*C*) A cutout view of the left side of the interventricular septum. Radiofrequency ablation effectively targeted a region of abnormal substrate guided by initial cardiac MRI.

ARVC is an inherited disease process with fibro-fatty infiltration of subepicardial/midmyocardial tissue of the RV near the annulus with extension to the endocardium, including the LV.[18,19] There is generally greater fibrotic involvement of the epicardium than the endocardium.[19] There is significant overlap in the anatomic distribution of ARVC and cardiac sarcoidosis, and it sometimes is difficult to make a clear distinction. Cardiac MRI can help differentiate between the two; the presence of mediastinal lymphadenopathy and left ventricular septal scar favors a diagnosis of cardiac sarcoidosis.[20] Recent work has shown the need for more extensive ablation in patients with ARVC, particularly at the index procedure.[21,22]

Lamin A/C (LMNA) cardiomyopathy is a group of inherited disease disorders with cardiac involvement, including conduction disease and infiltration of the ventricular septum.[23] In a recent multicenter study, Kumar and colleagues[24] reported poor outcomes with a high rate of recurrence in 25 patients with mutations in the LMNA gene. Multiple VTs (median of 3) were induced in each patient, with most being consistent with origin from scar in the basal LV and septum. Acute success with noninducibility was only achieved in 25% of patients. Partial success (noninducibility of a nonclinical tachycardia) and failure (persistent inducibility of the clinical tachycardia) was attributed to intramyocardial septal substrate in 72% of patients. Bipolar ablation as well as transcoronary alcohol ablation, both described later, may be an option in such patients.

Postsurgical VT can occur after mitral and aortic repair. Eckart and colleagues[25] reported VT occurring either early after surgery or years later in patients without known myocardial infarction. Most tachycardias in this population were related to periannular scar. Often access to the ventricles is limited because of mechanical prosthetic valves. Recently, Soejima and colleagues[26] reported successful epicardial ablation aortic and mitral valve mechanical repair in 6 patients with rheumatic heart disease. Although the endocardium could not be mapped with endocardial catheters, microscopic evaluation in 2 patients revealed dense fibrosis in the epicardium compared with the endocardium. The investigators reported scarring of the anteroapical LV in all patients, with relative sparing of the annulus. The investigators conjectured that anteroapical scarring might be related to surgery-related scar formation or underlying disease.

Chronic or healed myocarditis is a known cause of epicardial scarring that can mimic ARVC,[27] and often requires an epicardial approach.[28] In a retrospective study of 189 patients with NICM, Berte and colleagues[29] reported 12 postmyocarditis patients (6.3%) with epicardial-only scar. Endocardial substrate maps did not identify scarred substrate and epicardial substrate maps required careful manual annotation to delineate scar area. Cardiac MRI was helpful to identify fibrosis and areas to target for ablation. There was 17% recurrence at 24 months after epicardial ablation.

Idiopathic dilated cardiomyopathy (IDCM) is a group of conditions with multiple mechanisms that lead to impaired systolic function. Similar to other types of NICM, a significant percentage of patients have epicardial and intramural fibrosis.[30] Hsia and colleagues[31] described confluent regions of abnormal electrograms confined to the basal and lateral aspects of the LV, adjacent to the annulus. These low-voltage areas involved less than 25% of the total surface area of the endocardial LV. Most mapped VTs originated at the base of the LV in areas with abnormal substrate.

In a significant percentage of patients with IDCM, cardiac MRI is not able to identify fibrosis.[32,33] This may be because of a limitation of the technology to adequately identify abnormal and arrhythmogenic tissue. In general, it is a challenge for clinicians when electrical or anatomic substrate abnormalities cannot be identified. Other tools, including noninvasive panoramic mapping (preprocedure and periprocedure), may be helpful in the future for ablation planning and guidance.[33,34]

SEPTAL AND INTRAMYOCARDIAL MAPPING AND ABLATION

As mentioned earlier, fibrosis and sites critical to the tachycardia can involve only the intramyocardium and septum.[10] Although it is possible to identify endocardial and epicardial breakthrough of the tachycardia, these may be bystander sites that are not part of the circuit. In these situations, advanced imaging is crucial to help identify deep myocardial substrate (see **Figs. 1** and **3**). Ablation of the endocardial and epicardial breakthrough sites can change the surface morphology of the tachycardia without affecting the circuit necessary for its maintenance; this is potentially misleading for operators.

Because patients with NICM often have ventricular substrate that involves the intramyocardium and septum, different strategies may be required to create deeper ablation lesion sets.[35] Transcoronary ethanol ablation is an option after failed endocardial and epicardial ablation, particularly in cases of septal scar.[36] Tokuda and colleagues[37] reported that transcoronary ethanol ablation could prevent recurrences in 36% of the population. The investigators pointed out that patients with inadequate target vessels limited its broader efficacy.

Bipolar radiofrequency ablation is a technique in which 2 catheters oppose each other on both sides of the tissue to create a transmural lesion. In animal studies, this technique was more effective than unipolar radiofrequency ablation to create a lesion across the interventricular septum.[38,39] There also have been human studies, with success creating transmural lesions with good clinical outcomes.[40,41] Recent work has also shown the utility of contrast-enhanced MRI to assess scar formation after unipolar and bipolar ablation across the septum.[42]

Although transcoronary ethanol injection and bipolar radiofrequency ablation have shown promise, neither has been widely adopted. A promising technology to target intramural VT circuits is radiofrequency irrigated needle ablation. Studies have shown that this technique may be useful in patients with VT resistant to conventional ablation.[43–45] In a recent animal study, needle ablation was associated with more frequent, larger, and more often transmural lesions compared with conventional irrigated ablation.[46] MRI in this study was able to assess lesion formation and transmurality in the acute postablation setting. Future work is required to delineate the risks and benefits of needle ablation.

OUTCOMES

In a large retrospective study of 226 patients with NICM treated with VT ablation, Tokuda and colleagues[4] reported freedom from death, heart transplant, and readmission for VT recurrence in 77% of patients. Outcomes varied with the underlying disease process. Patients with ARVC had better outcomes than a dilated cardiomyopathy, whereas patients with sarcoidosis did not do as well.

In a prospective comparison with patients with an ischemic cardiomyopathy, patients with an NICM had 40% compared with 57% freedom from VT at 1-year follow-up.[47] Prioietti and colleagues[48] recently reported similar results comparing outcomes in patients with NICM and ICM with a substrate-based approach; there were significantly lower rates of freedom from VT in patients with NICM compared with ICM (49% vs 74%) over a 21-month period.

Taken as a whole, catheter ablation of VT in the setting of structural heart disease (both NICM and ICM) has proved successful.[49] That patients with NICM have done worse is not surprising given the frequent involvement of the intramural and epicardial substrate. Further studies, including prospective randomized controlled trials describing outcomes of VT ablation in patients with NICM, are necessary.

SUMMARY

VT in patients with a NICM carries significant morbidity and mortality, and remains a challenge for clinicians to adequately treat with catheter ablation. However, with careful preprocedure assessment, particularly with new imaging modalities, and consideration of the differential of pathophysiologic causes, it is possible to create an effective ablation and treatment strategy. Alternative ablation technologies also offer promise to target areas that have until now been recalcitrant to conventional techniques.

REFERENCES

1. Calkins H, Kuck KH, Cappato R, et al. 2012 HRS/EHRA/ECAS expert consensus statement on catheter and surgical ablation of atrial fibrillation: recommendations for patient selection, procedural techniques, patient management and follow-up, definitions, endpoints, and research trial design: a report of the Heart Rhythm Society (HRS) Task Force on Catheter and Surgical Ablation of Atrial Fibrillation. Developed in partnership with the European Heart Rhythm Association (EHRA), a registered branch of the European Society of Cardiology (ESC) and the European Cardiac Arrhythmia Society (ECAS); and in collaboration with the American College of Cardiology (ACC), American Heart Association (AHA), the Asia Pacific Heart Rhythm Society (APHRS), and the Society of Thoracic Surgeons (STS). Endorsed by the governing bodies of the American College of Cardiology Foundation, the American Heart Association, the European Cardiac Arrhythmia Society, the European Heart Rhythm Association, the Society of Thoracic Surgeons, the Asia Pacific Heart Rhythm Society, and the Heart Rhythm Society. Heart Rhythm 2012;9(4):632–96.e21.
2. Sapp JL, Wells GA, Parkash R, et al. Ventricular tachycardia ablation versus escalation of antiarrhythmic drugs. N Engl J Med 2016;375(2):111–21.
3. Sacher F, Tedrow UB, Field ME, et al. Ventricular tachycardia ablation: evolution of patients and procedures over 8 years. Circ Arrhythm Electrophysiol 2008;1(3):153–61.
4. Tokuda M, Tedrow UB, Kojodjojo P, et al. Catheter ablation of ventricular tachycardia in nonischemic heart disease. Circ Arrhythm Electrophysiol 2012; 5(5):992–1000.
5. Liang JJ, Santangeli P, Callans DJ. Long-term outcomes of ventricular tachycardia ablation in different types of structural heart disease. Arrhythm Electrophysiol Rev 2015;4(3):177–83.
6. Valles E, Bazan V, Marchlinski FE. ECG criteria to identify epicardial ventricular tachycardia in

nonischemic cardiomyopathy. Circ Arrhythm Electrophysiol 2010;3(1):63–71.

7. Berruezo A, Mont L, Nava S, et al. Electrocardiographic recognition of the epicardial origin of ventricular tachycardias. Circulation 2004;109(15): 1842–7.

8. Bogun FM, Desjardins B, Good E, et al. Delayed-enhanced magnetic resonance imaging in nonischemic cardiomyopathy: utility for identifying the ventricular arrhythmia substrate. J Am Coll Cardiol 2009;53(13):1138–45.

9. Sacher F, Roberts-Thomson K, Maury P, et al. Epicardial ventricular tachycardia ablation a multicenter safety study. J Am Coll Cardiol 2010;55(21): 2366–72.

10. Haqqani HM, Tschabrunn CM, Tzou WS, et al. Isolated septal substrate for ventricular tachycardia in nonischemic dilated cardiomyopathy: incidence, characterization, and implications. Heart Rhythm 2011;8(8):1169–76.

11. Hutchinson DMD, Gerstenfeld EP, Desjardins B, et al. Endocardial unipolar voltage mapping to detect epicardial ventricular tachycardia substrate in patients with nonischemic left ventricular cardiomyopathy. Circ Arrhythm Electrophysiol 2011;4(1): 49–55.

12. Sarabanda AV, Sosa E, Simões MV, et al. Ventricular tachycardia in Chagas' disease: a comparison of clinical, angiographic, electrophysiologic and myocardial perfusion disturbances between patients presenting with either sustained or nonsustained forms. Int J Cardiol 2005;102(1):9–19.

13. Sosa E, Scanavacca M, d'Avila A, et al. A new technique to perform epicardial mapping in the electrophysiology laboratory. J Cardiovasc Electrophysiol 1996;7(6):531–6.

14. Sosa E, Scanavacca M, D'Avila A, et al. Radiofrequency catheter ablation of ventricular tachycardia guided by nonsurgical epicardial mapping in chronic chagasic heart disease. Pacing Clin Electrophysiol 1999;22(1):128–30.

15. Sekhri V, Sanal S, Delorenzo LJ, et al. Cardiac sarcoidosis: a comprehensive review. Arch Med Sci 2011;7(4):546–54.

16. Kumar S, Barbhaiya C, Nagashima K, et al. Ventricular tachycardia in cardiac sarcoidosis: characterization of ventricular substrate and outcomes of catheter ablation. Circ Arrhythm Electrophysiol 2015;8(1):87–93.

17. Dubrey SW, Falk RH. Diagnosis and management of cardiac sarcoidosis. Prog Cardiovasc Dis 2010; 52(4):336–46.

18. Nasir K, Bomma C, Tandri H, et al. Electrocardiographic features of arrhythmogenic right ventricular dysplasia/cardiomyopathy according to disease severity: a need to broaden diagnostic criteria. Circulation 2004;110(12):1527–34.

19. Kiès P, Bootsma M, Bax J, et al. Arrhythmogenic right ventricular dysplasia/cardiomyopathy: screening, diagnosis, and treatment. Heart Rhythm 2006;3(2): 225–34.

20. Steckman DA, Schneider PM, Schuller JL, et al. Utility of cardiac magnetic resonance imaging to differentiate cardiac sarcoidosis from arrhythmogenic right ventricular cardiomyopathy. Am J Cardiol 2012;110(4):575–9.

21. Berte B, Sacher F, Venlet J, et al. VT recurrence after ablation: incomplete ablation or disease progression? A multicentric European study. J Cardiovasc Electrophysiol 2016;27(1):80–7.

22. Santangeli P, Zado ES, Supple GE, et al. Long-term outcome with catheter ablation of ventricular tachycardia in patients with arrhythmogenic right ventricular cardiomyopathy. Circ Arrhythm Electrophysiol 2015;8(6):1413–21.

23. Rankin J, Ellard S. The laminopathies: a clinical review. Clin Genet 2006;70(4):261–74.

24. Kumar S, Androulakis AF, Sellal JM, et al. Multi-center experience with catheter ablation for ventricular tachycardia in lamin A/C cardiomyopathy. Circ Arrhythm Electrophysiol 2016;9(8):e004357.

25. Eckart RE, Hruczkowski TW, Tedrow UB, et al. Sustained ventricular tachycardia associated with corrective valve surgery. Circulation 2007;116(18): 2005–11.

26. Soejima K, Nogami A, Sekiguchi Y, et al. Epicardial catheter ablation of ventricular tachycardia in no entry left ventricle: mechanical aortic and mitral valves. Circ Arrhythm Electrophysiol 2015;8(2):381–9.

27. Hofmann R, Trappe HJ, Klein H, et al. Chronic (or healed) myocarditis mimicking arrhythmogenic right ventricular dysplasia. Eur Heart J 1993;14(5):717–20.

28. Maccabelli G, Tsiachris D, Silberbauer J, et al. Imaging and epicardial substrate ablation of ventricular tachycardia in patients late after myocarditis. Europace 2014;16(9):1363–72.

29. Berte B, Sacher F, Cochet H, et al. Postmyocarditis ventricular tachycardia in patients with epicardial-only scar: a specific entity requiring a specific approach. J Cardiovasc Electrophysiol 2015;26(1): 42–50.

30. Liuba I, Marchlinski FE. The substrate and ablation of ventricular tachycardia in patients with nonischemic cardiomyopathy. Circ J 2013;77(8):1957–66.

31. Hsia HH, Callans DJ, Marchlinski FE. Characterization of endocardial electrophysiological substrate in patients with nonischemic cardiomyopathy and monomorphic ventricular tachycardia. Circulation 2003;108(6):704–10.

32. McCrohon JA, Moon JC, Prasad SK, et al. Differentiation of heart failure related to dilated cardiomyopathy and coronary artery disease using gadolinium-enhanced cardiovascular magnetic resonance. Circulation 2003;108(1):54–9.

33. Masci PG, Barison A, Aquaro GD, et al. Myocardial delayed enhancement in paucisymptomatic nonischemic dilated cardiomyopathy. Int J Cardiol 2012;157(1):43–7.

34. Shah A, Hocini M, Haissaguerre M, et al. Non-invasive mapping of cardiac arrhythmias. Curr Cardiol Rep 2015;17(8):1–11.

35. Baldinger SH, Kumar S, Barbhaiya CR, et al. Epicardial radiofrequency ablation failure during ablation procedures for ventricular arrhythmias: reasons and implications for outcomes. Circ Arrhythm Electrophysiol 2015;8(6):1422–32.

36. Sacher F, Sobieszczyk P, Tedrow U, et al. Transcoronary ethanol ventricular tachycardia ablation in the modern electrophysiology era. Heart Rhythm 2008; 5(1):62–8.

37. Tokuda M, Sobieszczyk P, Eisenhauer AC, et al. Transcoronary ethanol ablation for recurrent ventricular tachycardia after failed catheter ablation: an update. Circ Arrhythm Electrophysiol 2011;4(6): 889–96.

38. Sivagangabalan G, Barry MA, Huang K, et al. Bipolar ablation of the interventricular septum is more efficient at creating a transmural line than sequential unipolar ablation. Pacing Clin Electrophysiol 2010; 33(1):16–26.

39. Nagashima K, Watanabe I, Okumura Y, et al. Lesion formation by ventricular septal ablation with irrigated electrodes. Circ J 2011;75(3):565–70.

40. Koruth JS, Dukkipati S, Miller MA, et al. Bipolar irrigated radiofrequency ablation: a therapeutic option for refractory intramural atrial and ventricular tachycardia circuits. Heart Rhythm 2012;9(12):1932–41.

41. Gizurarson S, Spears D, Sivagangabalan G, et al. Bipolar ablation for deep intra-myocardial circuits: human ex vivo development and in vivo experience. Europace 2014;16(11):1684–8.

42. Berte B, Sacher F, Mahida S, et al. Impact of septal radiofrequency ventricular tachycardia ablation: insights from magnetic resonance imaging. Circulation 2014;130(8):716–8.

43. Reddy VY, Neuzil P, Taborsky M, et al. Short-term results of substrate mapping and radiofrequency ablation of ischemic ventricular tachycardia using a saline-irrigated catheter. J Am Coll Cardiol 2003; 41(12):2228–36.

44. Sapp JL, Cooper JM, Zei P, et al. Large radiofrequency ablation lesions can be created with a retractable infusion-needle catheter. J Cardiovasc Electrophysiol 2006;17(6):657–61.

45. Sapp JL, Cooper JM, Soejima K, et al. Deep myocardial ablation lesions can be created with a retractable needle-tipped catheter. Pacing Clin Electrophysiol 2004;27(5):594–9.

46. Berte B, Cochet H, Magat J, et al. Irrigated needle ablation creates larger and more transmural ventricular lesions compared with standard unipolar ablation in an ovine model. Circ Arrhythm Electrophysiol 2015;8(6):1498–506.

47. Dinov B, Fiedler L, Schönbauer R, et al. Outcomes in catheter ablation of ventricular tachycardia in dilated nonischemic cardiomyopathy compared with ischemic cardiomyopathy: results from the Prospective Heart Centre of Leipzig VT (HELP-VT) Study. Circulation 2014;129(7):728–36.

48. Proietti R, Essebag V, Beardsall J, et al. Substrate-guided ablation of haemodynamically tolerated and untolerated ventricular tachycardia in patients with structural heart disease: effect of cardiomyopathy type and acute success on long-term outcome. Europace 2015;17(3):461–7.

49. Betensky BP, Marchlinski FE. Outcomes of catheter ablation of ventricular tachycardia in the setting of structural heart disease. Curr Cardiol Rep 2016; 18(7):1–10.

Entrainment Mapping

Saurabh Kumar, BSc(Med), MBBS, PhD, Usha B. Tedrow, MD, MSc,
William G. Stevenson, MD*

KEYWORDS

- Entrainment mapping • Ventricular tachycardia • Postinfarction • Resetting • Fusion
- Concealed entrainment • Catheter ablation

KEY POINTS

- A variety of mapping techniques can be used to attempt to identify the origin of a ventricular tachycardia (VT) and select targets for ablation.
- Entrainment mapping is a technique that uses pacing to confirm the reentrant mechanism of VT and identify critical and noncritical areas of a VT circuit.
- Entrainment mapping is applied to organized, monomorphic, reentrant VTs; ideally, it is applied to reproducibly initiate hemodynamically tolerated VTs. However, short periods of entrainment mapping can be combined with other mapping techniques during VT ablation.
- Entrainment mapping uses a combination of factors such as QRS configuration during entrainment, postpacing interval, the relationship of the stimulus to QRS interval during pacing compared with electrogram to QRS interval during VT, and the ratio of the stimulus to QRS interval during pacing to the VT cycle length to help classify pacing sites as isthmus, bystander, and inner or outer loop sites.
- Ablation is most likely to be successful at terminating VTs at isthmus sites.

INTRODUCTION

Cardiac mapping is the process of characterizing electrophysiologic parameters in relation to the heart's anatomy. A variety of mapping techniques can be used to attempt to identify the origin of a ventricular arrhythmia and select targets for ablation. Substrate mapping characterizes regions of abnormal myocardium, usually where some of the myocardium has been replaced by fibrous tissue, creating barriers to conduction that define reentry circuit paths and contribute to slow conduction that fosters the occurrence of reentry. Substrate mapping can be done during any rhythm and allows characterization of potential arrhythmogenic regions without needing to map during ventricular tachycardia (VT). Activation sequence mapping has been used for decades to define the origin of arrhythmias and reentry circuits. However, it can be difficult and misleading when it is applied in clinical circumstances where sampling is limited and recording methods do not allow reliable identification of local activation times, which is particularly a problem in regions of scar. Entrainment mapping determines the relation of the individual pacing site to the reentry circuit, so requires the presence of tachycardia.

Disclosures: Dr S. Kumar is a recipient of the Neil Hamilton Fairley Overseas Research scholarship cofunded by the National Health and Medical Research Council and the National Heart Foundation of Australia, and the Bushell Travelling Fellowship funded by the Royal Australasian College of Physicians. Dr U.B. Tedrow receives consulting fees/honoraria from Boston Scientific Corp and St. Jude Medical and research funding from Biosense Webster and St. Jude Medical. Dr W.G. Stevenson is coholder of a patent for needle ablation that is consigned to Brigham and Women's Hospital.
Arrhythmia Service, Cardiovascular Division, Department of Medicine, Brigham and Women's Hospital, Harvard Medical School, 75 Francis Street, Boston, MA 02115, USA
* Corresponding author. .
E-mail address: wstevenson@partners.org

Card Electrophysiol Clin 9 (2017) 55–69
http://dx.doi.org/10.1016/j.ccep.2016.10.004
1877-9182/17/Crown Copyright © 2016 Published by Elsevier Inc. All rights reserved.

The mapping approach is determined by whether the arrhythmia is due to a focus (usually automatic or a small reentry circuit) or a large reentry circuit. In patients with structural heart disease, most sustained monomorphic VTs are due to macro-reentry involving an area of ventricular scar[1] and are termed scar-related reentry.[2] Less frequently, VTs are due to reentry or automaticity involving the Purkinje system, which are often more easily targeted for ablation.[3] The focus of this review is to describe the principles of entrainment mapping of VT and its use to identify isthmuses of slow conduction where ablation has a high likelihood of VT termination and to differentiate the critical part of the reentry circuit (isthmus) from bystander pathways that are not a critical part of the VT circuit.

Scar Topography in Structural Heart Disease

In structural heart disease, scar-related macro-reentry may involve endocardial, epicardial, or midmyocardial scar. These reentrant circuits can be complex, large, and 3-dimensional and vary according to scar topography and conducting properties of residual surviving myocytes that form "channels" within the scar and support slow conduction (**Fig. 1A–C**).[4] For these VTs, an isthmus is defined as a corridor of conductive myocardial tissue bound by nonconductive tissue barriers through which a depolarization wavefront must propagate to perpetuate the VT. These barriers are often scar or a natural obstacle such as a valve annulus, but they can also be functional, due to conduction block or collision of wavefronts that is present only during VT (**Fig. 1D**).

The characteristics of scar-related reentrant VT have been extensively studied in patients with prior myocardial infarction (MI),[4–7] but findings are likely translatable to scars related to nonischemic heart disease,[8] including nonischemic cardiomyopathies, valvular heart disease, periaortic scar-related VT, and repaired congenital heart disease.

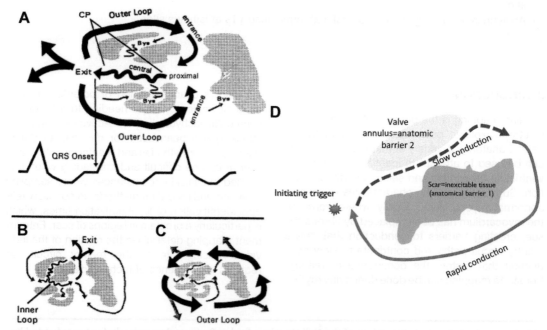

Fig. 1. Anatomic models of reentrant VT. (*A–C*) Three hypothetical reentrant VT circuits. Gray areas are electrically inexcitable scars. The VT circuit is shown in arrows. (*A*) A "figure-of-8" VT circuit with 2 loops through a common pathway (CP). The QRS onset corresponds to the circuit exit. The circuit propagates through the proximal, central, and exit regions, around the border of the scar, and reenters the infarct region through the entrance to reach the proximal portion of the common pathway. Regions that do not participate in the circuit are called bystanders (labeled bys). (*B*) A circuit entirely contained within the infarct. (*C*) A circuit with only an outer loop wavefronts circulating around the margins of the infarct. (*D*) Some of the prerequisites for reentry that include substrate (anatomic boundaries formed by a valve annulus and inexcitable scar), a central area of block (inexcitable scar), an area of slow conduction, and an initiating trigger. (*Adapted from* Stevenson WG, Friedman PL, Sager PT, et al. Exploring postinfarction reentrant ventricular tachycardia with entrainment mapping. J Am Coll Cardiol 1997;29:1181; with permission.)

An Overview of the Authors' Approach to the Use of Entrainment Mapping

Entrainment and activation mapping require that the patient be in VT. It is desirable, however, to limit the duration of time in VT as much as possible. A combination of substrate mapping with activation and entrainment mapping is used with this goal in mind. The authors' approach is to first induce VT with programmed stimulation. Programmed ventricular stimulation is important to confirm the diagnosis,[9] assess the possibility of bundle branch reentry, which requires a different approach, provide a QRS morphology to compare with pace-maps (see later discussion), and inform the use of programmed stimulation as an endpoint for the ablation procedure. Generally, detailed substrate mapping is then performed, including pace-mapping to define the region of interest for the targeted VT. Short episodes of VT are then induced with the ablation catheter placed in this region of interest and entrainment and/or activation mapping then performed to identify the critical region of slow conduction for the targeted VT (**Fig. 2**).[10]

Requirements for Reentry

Entrainment mapping is used for organized, monomorphic, reentrant VTs. Reentry is the continuous repetitive propagation of an activation wavefront, in a circular path, to return to its site of origin to reactivate that site.[11] The prerequisites for reentry are as follows (see **Fig. 1D**)[4,12]:

1. The presence of substrate (myocardial tissue with differences in conduction and refractoriness that are joined proximally and distally);
2. A central area of block (core of inexcitable tissue around which the wavefront circulates);
3. Unidirectional block (facilitates initiation of reentry as it allows an excitation wavefront to travel down one limb of the reentrant circuit, while allowing the other limb to recover conduction);
4. Area of slow conduction (allows excitable tissue to be maintained ahead of the propagating wavefront and recovery in time for the next wavefront, an "excitable gap");
5. Critical mass of tissue that can support reentry;
6. An initiating trigger.[13]

Reentry can be anatomic, when there is a distinct relationship of the reentrant pathway to the underlying tissue structure, and functional when the reentrant circuit occurs at random locations without clearly defined anatomic boundaries. Both conditions likely coexist in reentrant VT circuits. In patients with scar-related VT that is inducible and can be terminated with programmed stimulation, the authors start with the assumption that VT is due to reentry and expect to have that subsequently confirmed during entrainment mapping.

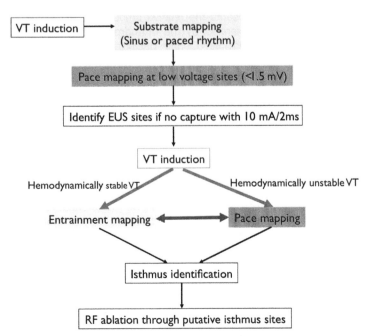

Fig. 2. Schema for mapping of VT in clinical practice, which includes a combination of mapping methods. Note, short periods of VT induction may be performed despite hemodynamic instability to rapidly confirm/refute the location of the pacing site in the putative isthmus of a VT circuit. Pace and entrainment mapping can provide complementary information. EUS, electrically unexcitable scar that does not capture with pacing at 10 mA, 2-ms pulse width. (*Adapted from* Soejima K, Stevenson WG, Maisel WH, et al. Electrically unexcitable scar mapping based on pacing threshold for identification of the reentry circuit isthmus: feasibility for guiding ventricular tachycardia ablation. Circulation 2002;106:1679; with permission.)

Features suggesting reentry (**Fig. 3**A, B)[4] during VT initiation are as follows:

a. Ability to reproducibly initiate and terminate the arrhythmia with programmed ventricular stimulation where a critically timed extrastimulus takes advantage of the excitable gap (**Fig. 3**C, D).[14] The paced wavefront of the extrastimulus finds an area of refractory tissue and conduction is established along the surrounding tissue. This is specific for macro-reentry and is not seen in VT driven by automaticity or triggered rhythms, which are induced with overdrive pacing and/or catecholamines and terminated with vagal maneuvers;

b. Site-specificity for inducibility and termination (**Fig. 3**E).[14] This is based on the principle that the extrastimulus is required to enter the circuit and be blocked unidirectionally. Similar to altering the timing of the extrastimulus, altering the location of the site of extrastimulus may also facilitate entry into the circuit. VTs not driven by macro-reentry do not exhibit this mechanism;

c. An inverse relationship of coupling interval or pacing cycle length (CL) to the CL of the first tachycardia beat during repeated tachycardia initiations (**Fig. 3**F).[14] In macro-reentrant VTs, the shorter the pacing CL, the longer the time is to the first VT beat. Shorter CLs facilitate slow conduction, a major prerequisite for reentry. Shorter pacing CLs often accelerate triggered rhythms.

Entrainment

The demonstration of entrainment proves that the tachycardia is reentrant in nature with rare, theoretic exception. Entrainment is the continuous resetting of a reentry circuit. Resetting is explained in **Fig. 3**.[14] Most VT circuits contain an excitable gap (see **Fig. 3**A).[4] This gap is created by the fact that the time it takes the circulating excitation wave to propagate once around the circuit exceeds the refractory period at each point in the circuit.[4] If a depolarizing stimulus is applied to a site after the site has recovered, but before arrival of the next circulating wavefront, the pacing stimulus captures the myocardium, creating wavefronts that travel in 2 directions in the circuit: the *orthodromic* wavefront that travels in the same direction as the tachycardia wavefronts and the *antidromic* wavefront that travels in the reverse direction and collides with a returning orthodromic wavefront (see **Fig. 3**B).[4] The orthodromic wavefront travels through the circuit, resetting the tachycardia. This sequence can continue until cessation of pacing or development of block somewhere in the circuit. When pacing ceases, the last paced impulse will continue orthodromically at the pacing CL. When pacing at a faster rate than the tachycardia, this manifests as an increase of the tachycardia rate to the pacing rate with resumption of the intrinsic rate back to the baseline rate after pacing.

The demonstration of entrainment can potentially be assessed during the initiation of VT, during pacing in stable VT that continues after pacing, and with VT termination (**Box 1**).[14]

Entrainment proves reentry. The presence of any of the following criteria indicates that entrainment has occurred (**Fig. 4**)[13]:

1. *Fixed fusion* of the paced complexes at a constant pacing rate;
2. *Progressive fusion* at different pacing rates in which the surface electrocardiogram (ECG) looks more like the purely paced configuration and less likely like the tachycardia at progressively shorter pacing CLs; and
3. Conduction block to an orthodromic site that terminates tachycardia followed by activation of that site by a paced wavefront from a different direction (eg, antidromic).[15]

The ability for a pacing train to entrain VT does not require that the pacing site be located with the reentrant circuit. Constant (or fixed) surface ECG fusion during VT occurs when: (a) the paced morphology is of a fixed, hybrid appearance between that of a fully paced complex and a VT complex; and (b) there is a fixed interval between the stimulus artifact and the onset of the surface ECG complex (see **Fig. 4**).[13] The degree of fusion represents the relative amounts of myocardium, depolarized by the orthodromic and antidromic wavefronts. During pacing, fixed (or constant) fusion occurs when there is stability in the collision sites of the antidromic and orthodromic wavefronts. Pacing at the slowest possible CL at sites remote from the circuit exit allows the best opportunity to demonstrate fusion. Progressive fusion is created when at faster pacing rates, there is a progressive increase in the amount of antidromically activated myocardium from the pacing site until a fully paced complex is created (see **Fig. 4**).[13]

Focal VTs (automatic, triggered activity, or micro-reentrant) can be differentiated from macro-reentrant VTs because they do not manifest fixed fusion with overdrive pacing and are frequently suppressed (as with automatic foci) or accelerated (as with triggered activity) with pacing. In the absence of a reentrant mechanism, overdrive pacing frequently reveals only the QRS morphology of the pacing stimulus (or continuously varying degrees of fusion, if exit block out of focus is present).

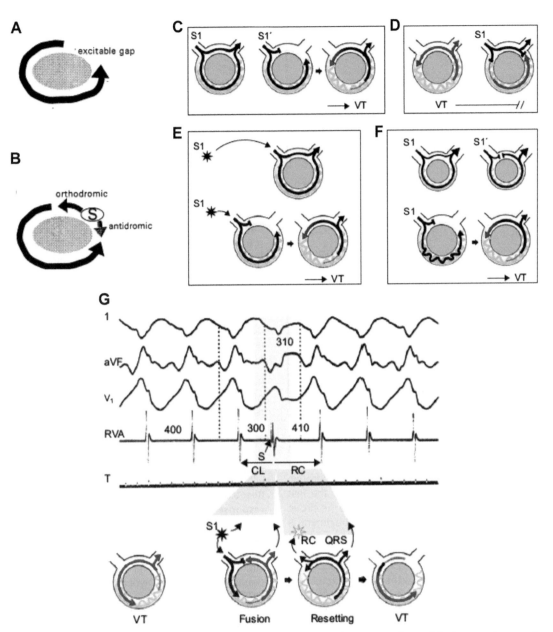

Fig. 3. Features of a reentrant VT circuit. (*A*) VT circuit with a circulating wavefront (*black arrows*) around a central obstacle (*gray area*) and the presence of an excitable gap. (*B*) A premature extrastimulus depolarizes tissue during the excitable gap, producing a stimulated antidromic wavefront that collides with the circulating orthodromic wavefront of the VT. The stimulated orthodromic wavefront then propagates through the circuit resetting the circuit. (*C–E*) Phenomena associated with reentry in VT. (*black and red arrows*) Stimulated and VT beats, respectively. (*C*) A premature extrastimulus enters and exits the circuit (*left*); an even more premature extrastimulus blocks in the region of fast conduction, which is still refractory from the previous beat, conducts antegradely along the slow pathway of the circuit. By the time activation reaches retrogradely the area of fast conduction, this is no longer refractory, and reentry is established (*middle and right*). (*D*) During VT, an extrastimulus is delivered that is blocked in the slow pathway, which is refractory from the previous beat and collides with the VT wavefront in the fast pathway, thus terminating the VT. (*E*) Site specificity of VT initiation is shown wherein an extrastimulus in close proximity is able to penetrate the circuit, whereas pacing from farther away is not. (*F*) Requisite of critical conduction delay for VT initiation. The circuits on the top 2 panels do not have sufficient conduction delay to support reentry. The bottom 2 panels have critical conduction delay to support reentry. (*G*) Resetting with fusion, which is diagnostic of reentry. An extrastimulus (*S*) is delivered at 300 ms from a site far away from the circuit of a VT with CL of 400 ms. The extrastimulus penetrates and interacts

been called a form of concealed entrainment. This form of concealed entrainment can also be shown pacing from the ventricle during AV nodal reentry tachycardia. In contrast, when the pacing site is in or close to the reentry circuit isthmus, proximal to the exit, entrainment may occur without producing QRS fusion, but with the paced QRS maintaining the same configuration as the tachycardia beats known as entrainment with concealed fusion (or a form of concealed entrainment). The presence of entrainment with concealed fusion often indicates that the pacing site is in the reentry circuit isthmus, but exceptions occur when pacing is performed in bystander pathways that connect to the reentry circuit isthmus or exit, or nondominant inner loops that are not critical to the maintenance of reentry. Radiofrequency (RF) ablation is unlikely successfully interrupt VT at these sites as well as at sites that show manifest fusion (discussed in detail later).

Although entrainment is usually assessed during a train of pacing stimuli, single scanning stimuli can also be used, and the effect that is observed is generally referred to as resetting if the stimulus alters the timing of the tachycardia.

Resetting with fusion Resetting is the interaction of a premature wavefront with a tachycardia resulting in either advancement or delay of the subsequent tachycardia beat. Its mechanism is explained earlier (see **Fig. 3**G).[14] Although resetting itself does not prove reentry, resetting with fusion is virtually diagnostic of reentry.[16]

Resetting with an increasing or a mixed response The return CL is the interval from the extrastimulus to the onset of the next beat, corresponding to the time required for the stimulated impulse to reach the circuit, conduct throughout the circuit, emerge from the reentry circuit exit and depolarize sufficient myocardium to produce the QRS onset, or reach the recording site. In contrast to the postpacing interval (PPI), resetting is often assessed from the QRS or activation at a site remote from the pacing site, and many studies of resetting have been done pacing from the RV

Upon cessation of pacing, the last paced wavefront will traverse through the VT isthmus and exit the circuit to produce a nonfused VT complex at the paced CL as there is no longer an antidromic wavefront with which to fuse, and thus, the last paced orthodromic wavefront completes the circuit to maintain the tachycardia. When entrainment is manifest with constant QRS fusion (called manifest fusion), the last captured wavefront is entrained at the pacing CL, but it does not show fusion. When pacing is performed outside the reentry circuit exit, entrainment may occur with no discernible QRS fusion, and the criteria for entrainment may not be demonstrable even though entrainment is occurring within the circuit and may be detectable from recordings within the circuit. This phenomena has

with the VT generating the next beat. The next beat morphology results in QRS morphology that is fused between the paced beat and the VT beat morphology (fusion). The next beat arrives with return cycle length (RCL) of 410 ms, which represents the time required for the stimulated impulse to reach the circuit, conduct throughout the circuit, and return to the stimulation site. RVA, right ventricular apical catheter. ([A, B] from Stevenson WG, Friedman PL, Sager PT, et al. Exploring postinfarction reentrant ventricular tachycardia with entrainment mapping. J Am Coll Cardiol 1997;29:1180–9; with permission. [C–F] from Benito B, Josephson ME. Ventricular tachycardia in coronary artery disease. Rev Esp Cardiol (Engl Ed) 2012;65:939–55. [G] from Almendral JM, Rosenthal ME, Stamato NJ, et al. Analysis of the resetting phenomenon in sustained uniform ventricular tachycardia: incidence and relation to termination. J Am Coll Cardiol 1986;8:294–300 and Benito B, Josephson ME. Ventricular tachycardia in coronary artery disease. Rev Esp Cardiol (Engl Ed) 2012;65:939–55; with permission.)

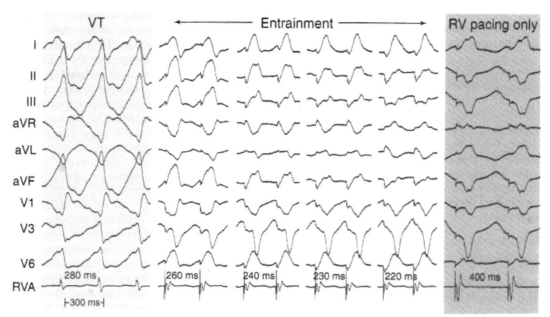

Fig. 4. Examples of QRS fusion during entrainment of VT. QRS morphology of the VT is shown in the left panel. RV pacing QRS morphology is shown in the right panel. During constant pacing, each paced complex is a stable blend of pacing and VT. With increasing pacing CL, progressive ECG fusion is seen, with increasing resemblance to fully paced QRS complexes (*middle panel, left to right*). (*From* Issa ZF, MIller JM, Zipes DP. Clinical arrhythmology and electrophysiology: a companion to Braunwald's heart disease, 2nd ed. Philadelphia: Saunders Elsevier, 2012; with permission.)

apex, remote from the reentry circuit. The relationship between the paced coupling interval and the return CL can show a flat response, increasing response, or a mixed response (combination of the 2). A flat response is when the return CL is stable despite a decreasing extrastimulus coupling interval, suggesting a full excitable gap throughout the circuit. It may also be seen in automatic or triggered VTs. An increasing response is seen when the return CL increases with increasing extrastimulus prematurity. Both increasing and mixed responses suggest reentry but can also be mimicked by slow conduction between an arrhythmia focus and the pacing and recording sites. VT termination with a timed extrastimulus and site specificity of termination are also more consistent with a reentrant mechanism than automaticity.[14]

ANATOMIC MODEL OF THE VENTRICULAR TACHYCARDIA CIRCUIT

Computer models have helped understand likely components of a VT circuit (see **Fig. 1**).[6] Entrainment mapping sites have been related to reentry circuits composed of a central pathway (or isthmus) that has an entry site and an exit site, outer loops, and inner loops. Sites that are not involved in the reentry circuit are designated bystander sites. When 2 loops share a common central region, it is

called "figure-of-8" reentry (see **Fig. 1**A). VT propagates through the common pathway during electrical diastole. This region may be small and bounded by anatomic and functional barriers that prevent the spread of the electrical signals it generates except in the orthodromic direction, making it electrocardiographically silent. The VT wavefront exits the exit site and propagates through any outer loop and the rest of the myocardium. Activation of the exit site corresponds to the onset QRS on surface ECG. The outer loop may be normal tissue along the border of the scar. Outer loops are in the border of the scar. Activation of the outer loop corresponds to electrical systole (QRS). Pacing at an outer loop alters the QRS due to fusion (see later discussion).

An inner loop is a reentry path through the scar region that connects the exit and entrance to the isthmus. It may function as either an integral part of the VT circuit or a bystander. If conduction through the inner loop is slower than the outer loop, then it serves as a bystander (nondominant loop), whereas if conduction is faster than the outer loop, it then serves as a critical part of the circuit (dominant loop). Bystander sites are passively activated during VT and are not essentially part of the circuit. Bystander sites can be remote bystanders (where pacing produces QRS fusion) or adjacent bystanders (where pacing produced concealed fusion). In other types of circuits, the entire circuit may be contained entirely within the scar or the infarct serves as an anatomic obstacle for a single loop along the border of the scar—a single outer loop. Response of pacing at various aforementioned sites was tested in a computer model of reentry; furthermore, the response to RF ablation at these entrainment-identified parts of the VT circuit was also systematically tested in studies with a 4-mm tip nonirrigated catheter.[4,6] Rates of VT termination were highest in isthmus sites (**Table 1**).[4]

As noted above, the simple demonstration of entrainment alone does not indicate the location of the pacing site relative to the reentry circuit. Several other pieces of information can help locate components of the reentry circuit, which include the following:

a. PPI after entrainment,
b. QRS configuration during entrainment, and
c. Stimulus to QRS interval (S-QRS) during entrainment and its relationship to electrogram to QRS (EGM-QRS) during VT and its relationship to the VT CL.

POSTPACING INTERVAL AFTER ENTRAINMENT

The PPI is the interval from the last capturing stimulus to the next activation at the pacing site and a measure of the proximity of a pacing site to the reentry circuit.[6] Pacing sites within a reentry circuit will yield a PPI close to the tachycardia cycle length (TCL) as the stimulated orthodromic wavefront completes the circuit after one revolution around the circuit. Thus, the interval from the last stimulus that captures the next activation at the pacing site

Table 1
Mapping sites and frequency of termination during radiofrequency ablation with a single solid tip radiofrequency ablation lesion

	No. of Sites Terminated	RF-Terminated VT (%)
Isthmus site	85	29
Exit	35	37
Central	22	23
Proximal	28	25
Inner loop	46	9
Adjacent bystander	35	11
Outer loop	116	10
Remote bystander	116	3
Total	398	12

Adapted from Stevenson WG, Friedman PL, Sager PT, et al. Exploring postinfarction reentrant ventricular tachycardia with entrainment mapping. J Am Coll Cardiol 1997;29:1182; with permission.

is equal to the revolution time through the circuit, which is the TCL.[4] When pacing is performed from sites outside the circuit that entrain the time interval from the last pacing stimulus to the subsequent signal indicating activation *at the pacing site* will be a composite of the conduction time from the pacing site to the circuit, then through the circuit, and then back to the pacing site. The aforementioned conduction time yields a PPI longer than the TCL. The farther away the pacing site is located from the circuit, the greater the difference is between the PPI and TCL. In VT related to prior infarction, a PPI minus TCL difference (PPI − TCL) within 30 ms is associated with increased likelihood of VT termination with RF ablation at that site, consistent with close proximity to the reentry circuit.[6]

Accuracy of the PPI requires 3 assumptions be met. First, that pacing is capturing and stably resetting the reentry circuit. Second, that pacing does not slow conduction or alter the reentry path. Pacing rates only slightly faster than the TCL are used to entrain the tachycardia for measurement of the PPI. Rapid pacing may slow conduction velocity or alter the conduction path in the circuit, thus falsely prolonging the TCL.[17] Third, that the EGM selected for measurement of the PPI represents activation at the pacing site. Sometimes, the local activation from the pacing site cannot be deciphered due to long duration, due to fractionated EGMs, or because it is obscured by the stimulus artifact during pacing. Recording from closely adjacent sites (eg, the proximal electrodes of the mapping catheter that are 1–2 mm distant from the distal electrodes) is reasonable with generally good agreement with the measurements made from the distal electrode. One must be cognizant that the difference can be exaggerated in regions of local tissue conduction velocity is severely depressed due to infarction or interelectrode spacing is greater than 2.5 mm.[18] A major source of potential error is the presence of far-field EGMs that are due to activation of sites remote from the pacing sites. Far field EGMs often cause a false PPI that is shorter than the tachycardia CL. Far-field potentials can often be recognized as signals that are present during pacing, indicating that they are generated by a site that is not directly depolarized by the pacing stimulus, but rather is activation by a conducting wavefront that reaches the site after the stimulus.[16]

THE N+1 DIFFERENCE TECHNIQUE

Analysis of the PPI may be difficult if pacing artifact obscures signals. Recording from the proximal electrode may be reasonable; however, errors can occur if low-amplitude EGMs are absent at the proximal recording site or extensive conduction slowing occurs between the proximal and distal electrode in abnormal regions of infarction.[19] If entrainment occurs with concealed fusion, the S-QRS – EGM-QRS difference can be used (see later discussion). However, if fusion is present, or might be present, the N+1 technique can be useful. This technique does not require simultaneous recording of EGMs at the pacing site during entrainment and is not influenced by the presence or absence of QRS fusion.[5]

One can obtain an N+1 difference value by (Fig. 5)

a. Calculating the interval between the last pacing stimulus that entrains tachycardia and the second QRS interval after the stimulus (called the $S\text{-}QRS_{n+1}$); then,
b. Calculating the interval between the QRS and EGM in any of the subsequent beats ($EGM_{n+2}\text{-}QRS_{n+2}$); then
c. Calculating the difference between the 2 (called the N+1 difference).

If the QRS onset is not discernible, another stable, fiducial point such as a right ventricular apical catheter can be used. The N+1 difference is mathematically equal to the PPI – TCL difference and has been shown to have an excellent correlation to PPI-TCL difference in scar-related VT (r = 0.91, P<.0001).[5] An N+1 difference of 30 ms or less has an excellent sensitivity and specificity for predicting a PPI-TCL difference of 30 ms or less, regardless of the presence of absence of QRS fusion.[5]

QRS CONFIGURATION DURING ENTRAINMENT

During scar-related monomorphic VT, the QRS produced is usually determined by the sequence of ventricular myocardial activation that results from propagation of the excitation wavefront away from the exit from the scar. When pacing is performed during VT from a site remote from the circuit, the stimulated wavefronts alter the ventricular activation sequence, thus altering the QRS morphology (see **Fig. 4**; **Figs. 6** and **7**). Stimulated wavefronts collide with VT wavefronts that have traveled orthodromically through the circuit and are now leaving the reentry circuit from its exit. The resultant QRS complex is due to fusion of the wavefronts propagating away directly from the pacing site with those emerging from the VT circuit exit. Constant pacing will produce stable regions of collision between these 2 wavefronts and produce constant fusion with a stable QRS morphology from beat to beat. With increasing pacing rate, the stimulated wavefronts travel further, capturing more of the ventricle resulting in the QRS that morphology more closely resembles that of purely paced QRS complexes in sinus rhythm, and the progressive change with increasing pacing rate is referred to as progressive fusion.

At some sites within the reentry circuit, pacing entrains the VT without changing the QRS configuration (it remains the same as that of the VT), and as such, no fusion is detectable on the EKG (entrainment with concealed fusion, as discussed above). Entrainment with concealed fusion occurs when pacing is performed within the reentry circuit, and collision of the stimulated antidromic wavefronts with the orthodromic wavefronts is occurring very close to the pacing site, in or near the reentry circuit. The pacing-induced wavefronts can only reach the surrounding myocardium by propagating through the circuit and emerging from the exit. In these instances, only a small

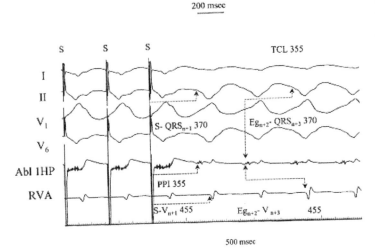

200 msec

TCL 355

S S S

I

II

V_1

V_6

S- QRS_{n-1} 370 $Eg_{n+2} \cdot QRS_{n-3}$ 370

Abl 1HP

PPI 355

RVA

S-V_{n+1} 455 $Eg_{n+2} \cdot V_{n+3}$ 455

500 msec

Fig. 5. Example of the N+1 difference technique. Pacing from an outer loop site. Pacing entrains the VT with QRS fusion. The PPI (355 ms) equals the TCL (355 ms), thus PPI – TCL = 0. The $S\text{-}QRS_{n+1}$ is 370 ms, and the EGM_{n+1} to QRS_{n+3} are both 370 ms, also giving an N+1 difference of 0, which is identical to the PPI-TCL. Similar measurements can be made with the right ventricular apical catheter (RVA) serving as a fiducial point. Abl 1HP, unipolar high pass filtered signal; Eg, electrogram; RVA, right ventricular apical catheter. (*Adapted from* Soejima K, Stevenson WG, Maisel WH, et al. The N + 1 difference: a new measure for entrainment mapping. J Am Coll Cardiol 2001;37: 1390; with permission.)

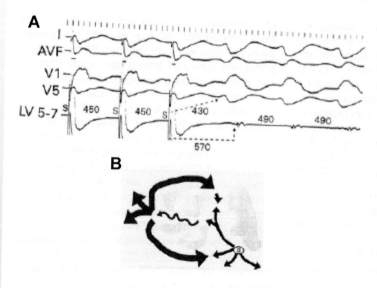

A

I
AVF
V1
V5
LV 5-7   450   450   430   490   490

570

B

Fig. 6. Pacing from a remote bystander site. (*A*) VT of CL 490 ms is entrainment by pacing at a CL of 450 ms with QRS fusion and a PPI – TCL difference of 80 ms (570 ms–490 ms) upon the cessation of pacing; this is consistent with a remote bystander site. (*B*) Pacing from this site creates wavefronts that propagate away from the scar (*gray regions*), thus altering QRS morphology, and also into the circuit within the scar, thus resetting it. The PPI is the conduction time from the pacing site to the circuit, through the circuit and back to the pacing site that exceeds the TCL. (*Adapted from* Stevenson WG, Friedman PL, Sager PT, et al. Exploring postinfarction reentrant ventricular tachycardia with entrainment mapping. J Am Coll Cardiol 1997;29:1184; with permission.)

mass of tissue is depolarized by the antidromic wavefront and is not detectable on the surface ECG. Thus, fusion is occurring at the EGM level and may be detectable by EGM recordings in the scar, but is concealed as regards the surface ECG (**Figs. 8** and **9**).

STIMULUS TO QRS INTERVAL

During entrainment with concealed fusion, the S-QRS interval is an indicator of the conduction time from the pacing site to the reentry circuit exit. For sites within the reentry circuit, the S-QRS interval will equal the EGM-QRS interval and the PPI will approximate the VT CL. When pacing from a bystander site entrains VT with concealed fusion, the S-QRS interval typically exceeds the EGM-QRS interval during VT and the PPI exceeds the VT CL.

Based on the combination of fusion, PPI, and S-QRS during VT, a classification of reentry circuit sites was developed specifying sites in the circuit

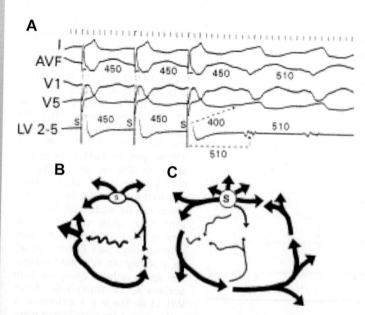

A

I
AVF   450   450   450   510
V1
V5
LV 2-5   450   450   400   510

510

B   **C**

Fig. 7. Pacing from an outer loop site. (*A*) VT of CL 510 ms is entrained by pacing at a CL of 450 ms. There is advancement of all VT complexes to the pacing CL, QRS fusion, and a PPI that approximates the TCL (PPI – TCL = 0). This is consistent with an outer loop site. (*B*) The outer loop site is within the reentry circuit. Pacing creates antidromic wavefronts that propagate away from the infarct border, thereby altering QRS complexes and orthodromic wavefronts that propagate through the circuit, resetting the reentry circuit. Following the last extrastimulus, the pacing site is depolarized by the orthodromic wavefront that has made one revolution through the circuit. The PPI thus equals TCL. (*C*) Similar findings are seen when pacing from a circuit that solely contains an outer loop. (*Adapted from* Stevenson WG, Friedman PL, Sager PT, et al. Exploring postinfarction reentrant ventricular tachycardia with entrainment mapping. J Am Coll Cardiol 1997;29:1185; with permission.)

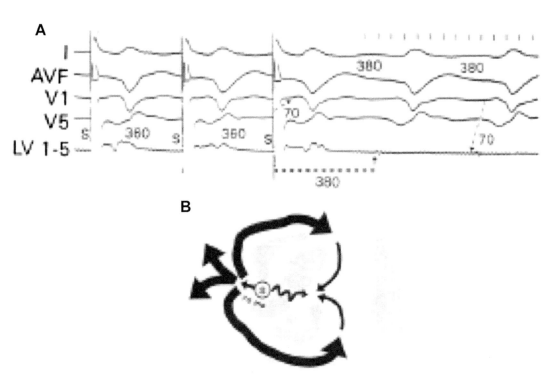

Fig. 8. Pacing from an exit site. (*A*) VT of CL 380 ms is entrained by pacing at a CL of 360 ms with no alteration of QRS morphology (concealed entrainment). At the cessation of pacing, the PPI matches the TCL, consistent with pacing location within a reentry circuit site. The S-QRS (70 ms) also equals the EGM-QRS (70 ms), and the S-QRS is 18% of the VT CL (70 ms/380 ms), consistent with pacing from an exit site in the circuit (see **Figs. 1** and **8**). (*B*) The stimulated antidromic wavefront collides with and is extinguished within the circuit by the returning orthodromic VT wavefront. The stimulated orthodromic wavefront exits the infarct from the same site as the VT wavefront, advancing the QRS complex without altering its configuration (entrainment with concealed fusion). The next depolarized signal at the pacing site has made one complete revolution through the circuit; thus the PPI will match the TCL. The EGM-QRS is equal to the conduction time from the mapping site to the exit site, which approximates the S-QRS during pacing. (*Adapted from* Stevenson WG, Friedman PL, Sager PT, et al. Exploring postinfarction reentrant ventricular tachycardia with entrainment mapping. J Am Coll Cardiol 1997;29:1185; with permission.)

as exit, central, or proximal isthmus sites, and outer or inner loop sites, and sites outside the circuit as adjacent or remote bystander sites. These sites are further discussed later with relevant examples.

FEATURES OF MAPPING SITES
Remote Bystanders

Any site not located within the reentry circuit is a bystander site. Pacing from bystander sites for sufficiently longer periods can usually entrain the tachycardia, but the PPI will exceed the TCL. At most bystanders, the pacing-induced wavefronts also alter the ventricular activation sequence, and thus, the QRS configuration will be fused between a paced QRS and a VT QRS configuration (see **Fig. 6**). RF ablation at remote bystanders will rarely terminate VT (see **Table 1**). It is important to recognize, however, patients with scar-related VTs often have multiple inducible VTs,

and in scar regions, a bystander site for one VT can potentially be involved in the reentry circuit of a different VT.

Outer Loop Sites

Outer loops are likely to be paths along the border of an infarct or scar region and participate in the VT. When pacing from outer loop sites, the antidromic wavefronts are not confined to within the anatomic and functional boundaries of the reentry circuit, and the stimulated wavefronts can propagate away from the scar region to depolarize the remainder of the myocardium, thus altering the QRS configuration (QRS fusion). However, as the site is located within the circuit, the PPI will equal the TCL (see **Fig. 7**). As these sites are in the border of the infarct region in continuity with the rest of the myocardium, they can be broad. Therefore, RF termination occasionally terminates VT during ablation in an outer loop, particularly if

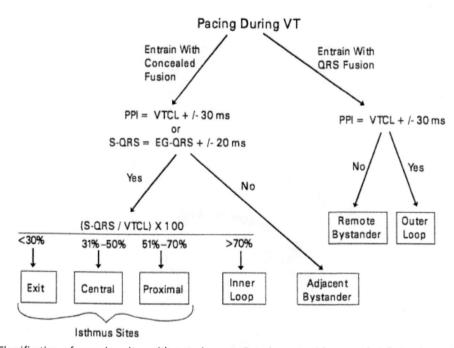

Fig. 9. Classification of mapping sites with entrainment. Entrainment with concealed fusion but without the presence of a PPI to TCL or S-QRS to EGM-QRS approximation suggests pacing from an adjacent bystander. If the latter 2 parameters are approximated, the sites are within the circuit. Further classification is then based on the ratio of S-QRS/VT CL. Sites with a ratio less than 70% are classified as isthmus sites. Pacing with QRS fusion and PPI matching the TCL suggests pacing from an outer loop, whereas if the PPI exceeds the TCL, it suggests pacing from a remote bystander. (*Adapted from* Stevenson WG, Friedman PL, Sager PT, et al. Exploring postinfarction reentrant ventricular tachycardia with entrainment mapping. J Am Coll Cardiol 1997;29:1187; with permission.)

an isolated potential is also present at the site, but this may be due to heating of the adjacent isthmus rather than interruption of conduction through the loop (see **Table 1**). A series of RF lesions may be able to interrupt an outer loop in some reentry circuits.

Exit Sites

When pacing from the circuit exit site, the stimulated antidromic wavefronts collide with the orthodromic wavefronts within the anatomic and functional boundaries of the circuit and are extinguished. The stimulated orthodromic wavefront will propagate away from the circuit exit producing a QRS configuration identical to the VT (concealed entrainment). The PPI will also match the TCL. The S-QRS interval during entrainment will match the EGM-QRS interval during VT (see **Fig. 8**). At such sites, the S-QRS is short (≤30% of the TCL) as the conduction time from the pacing site to the exit (the point at which the QRS onset occurs) is short. Exit sites are one of the preferred sites of RF ablation with a high rate of expected VT termination (see **Table 1**). Exits can, however, be broad or funnel shaped, and ablation may alter the QRS

morphology by altering propagation from the exit without terminating the tachycardia. When the S-QRS is very short (<40 ms), the site may actually be part of the outer loop rather than the exit region and fail to interrupt tachycardia. Pace-mapping in an exit region during sinus rhythm is expected to produce a QRS morphology similar to VT, although this may not always be the case due to areas of functional block that may be present during VT and not during sinus rhythm. In animal models of infarct scar-related VT, the exit regions where the excitation wavefront curves around the region of block contains the slowest conduction in the circuit.[20]

Central, Proximal, and Inner Loop Sites

Entrainment at central and proximal isthmus sites will produce concealed fusion and an S-QRS matching the EGM-QRS. However, as the pacing site is moved further from the exit, to more proximal sites in the circuit, the S-QRS interval increases. The percentage of S-QRS to VT CL (S-QRS/VT CL × 100) has been used to characterize sites as exit, central, or proximal isthmus on the basis of the ratio being less than or equal to 30%, 31% to 50%, 51% to 70%, respectively (see **Fig. 9**). These designations were arrived at empirically, based on the observation that VT was infrequently interrupted at S-QRS greater than 70% of the VT CL sites (inner loops). As the S-QRS indicates conduction time that is determined by distance and conduction velocity, the S-QRS does not necessarily indicate the length of the isthmus distal to the pacing site. RF ablation is frequently effective in interrupting VT at central and proximal sites.[6]

Inner loop sites have a long S-QRS during entrainment (>70% of VT CL) and show concealed fusion (**Fig. 10**). The S-QRS interval is as long as the pacing site is proximal to isthmus. Ablation at inner loops is less effective than isthmus sites (see **Table 1**). Some sites that appear to be inner loops are actually outer loops, or very close to the outer loop, such that increasing the pacing rate slightly will produce QRS fusion.

Adjacent Bystanders

Adjacent bystander sites are those that are connected to the reentry circuit, but are not critical to the reentry circuit (blind loops or alleys). Here, pacing will demonstrate entrainment with concealed fusion, but the PPI exceeds the TCL and the S-QRS is longer than the EGM-QRS (**Fig. 11**). Occasionally, pacing at an isthmus site will falsely appear as an adjacent bystander due to slowing of conduction during pacing that prolongs the PPI and S-QRS an observation that likely occurs with rapid pacing.

These entrainment criteria do offer incremental improvement in the predictive value for successful RF termination of VT. Bogun and colleagues[21] found that the positive predictive value of concealed entrainment for successful ablation was 54%, which increased to 72% in the presence of an S-QRS/VT CL of less than or equal to 70%, to 82% in the presence of an S-QRS = EGM-QRS, and to 89% in the presence of isolated middiastolic potentials that could not be dissociated from VT during entrainment. However, concealed entrainment with the combination of S-QRS = EGM-QRS during VT, in combination with the presence of an isolated diastolic potential, has the best discriminatory value for identifying sites where RF ablation is likely to be successful in patients with prior MI.[22]

LIMITATIONS OF ENTRAINMENT MAPPING

Entrainment mapping has several limitations. VT must be present or inducible and stable for a sufficient amount of time to perform pacing. Entrainment mapping may require only a minute if all that is needed is one pacing run to assess the proximity of the site to the VT, following which VT can be terminated by pacing or cardioversion to restore hemodynamic stability. As noted above, combining entrainment mapping at selected sites first identified by substrate mapping during sinus or paced rhythm can help limit the amount of time spent in VT.

The use of entrainment criteria provides a guide for relating the mapping findings to the likelihood of RF-induced VT termination. Combination of substrate, activation, and entrainment mapping is likely to yield the optimal success.

Rapid pacing may alter conduction in abnormal regions of ventricular myocardium that may be

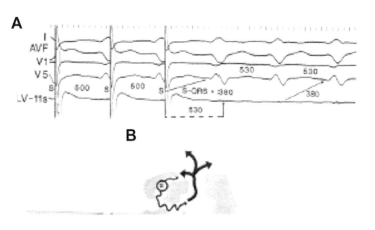

Fig. 10. Pacing from an inner loop site. (A) Pacing at a CL of 500 ms entrains the VT of CL 530 ms with concealed fusion. The PPI approximates the TCL, consistent with a pacing from a reentry circuit site. However, the S-QRS is 71% of the TCL and is thus consistent with an inner loop site (see also **Figs. 1 and 8**). (B) The stimulated antidromic wavefront collides with an orthodromic VT wavefront within the infarct and is contained in the infarct. The stimulated orthodromic wavefront resets the VT with concealed fusion but with a very long S-QRS. This is because of the long conduction time between the pacing site and the exit of the excitation wavefronts from the scar. (*Adapted from* Stevenson WG, Friedman PL, Sager PT, et al. Exploring postinfarction reentrant ventricular tachycardia with entrainment mapping. J Am Coll Cardiol 1997;29:1186; with permission.)

A

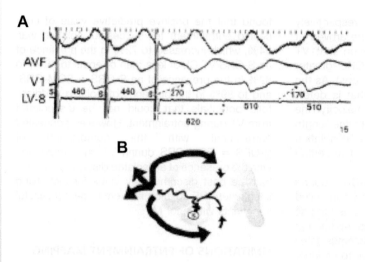

B

Fig. 11. Pacing from an adjacent bystander site. (A) Pacing at a CL of 460 ms entrains the VT of CL 510 ms with concealed fusion. However, PPI exceeds the TCL by 110 ms (PPI 620 ms − TCL 510 ms), consistent with a bystander site. The S-QRS (270 ms) does not approximate the EGM-QRS (170 ms). (B) When pacing from the "dead end" adjacent bystander site, the stimulated wavefronts reach the reentry circuit common pathway and propagate in both directions. The stimulated antidromic wavefront collides with the returning orthodromic VT wavefront and is contained within the infarct. The stimulated orthodromic wavefront entrains the tachycardia with concealed fusion. The PPI is the conduction time from the pacing site to the circuit, through the circuit and back to the pacing site, and exceeds the TCL. (*Adapted from* Stevenson WG, Friedman PL, Sager PT, et al. Exploring postinfarction reentrant ventricular tachycardia with entrainment mapping. J Am Coll Cardiol 1997;29:1186; with permission.)

within reentry circuits falsely increasing PPI and S-QRS intervals.[17] Antiarrhythmic drugs may have the same effect of conduction slowing. Timing of local EGMs and the presence of far-field potentials can make the PPI difficult to decipher. Pacing for entrainment may terminate VT or initiate another VT, complicating mapping attempts. Synchronizing the first beat of the train so that it does not fall at an unduly short interval after the preceding beat and pacing at CLs only 10 to 30 ms shorter than the VT is used to reduce this possibility.

INCORPORATING ENTRAINMENT MAPPING INTO VENTRICULAR TACHYCARDIA ABLATION PROCEDURES

For patients with scar-related VTs, the location of the scar and the QRS morphology of VT usually provide an excellent indication of the likely region of the ventricle containing the reentry circuit exit. The scar location can be further refined with substrate mapping. With this knowledge, initiation of VT and rapid confirmation that a region of interest is in or close to the VT circuit can be used to direct initial ablation lesions. Entrainment mapping can be performed, even if VT is not hemodynamically tolerated. Multiple VTs are often present, and if poorly tolerated, most of the ablation may be performed during sinus rhythm. When a VT is well tolerated hemodynamically, the reentry isthmus can often be found relatively quickly. When initial VT ablation lesions fail to abolish inducible VT, entrainment mapping can clarify whether the target regions are close to the VT circuit. Long PPIs can be very useful in focusing attention

away from bystander regions that have interesting EGMs, but are not involved in the VT. When an extensive substrate-guided ablation approach fails, entrainment mapping can be particularly useful in identifying the region likely to contain the circuit. Whether hemodynamic support to allow entrainment mapping would improve outcomes in some of these patients remains to be determined. When a target site is identified in a high-risk area, as near the conduction system or a branch of a coronary artery in the epicardium, entrainment findings can be useful in assessing the likely impact of ablation before taking the risk of delivering ablation energy to the region. Pacing and capturing at a site during VT provides further evidence that the site has viable myocardium and is not dense, unexcitable fibrous tissue.

SUMMARY

Entrainment mapping forms a critical part of mapping of deciphering VT mechanism and facilitates mapping of macro-reentrant VT circuits such that critical isthmus sites can be identified as targets for ablation. Entrainment mapping incorporates anatomy, functional properties of the scar, and electrophysiologic response from pacing to categorize the role of the pacing site within a VT circuit. Other forms of mapping (substrate, pace, and activation) serve as an incremental role in the catheter ablation of VT. Although limitations exist, entrainment mapping can rapidly identify critical isthmus sites during VT and facilitate efficacious catheter ablation.

REFERENCES

1. Stevenson WG. Current treatment of ventricular arrhythmias: state of the art. Heart Rhythm 2013;10: 1919–26.
2. Aliot EM, Stevenson WG, Almendral-Garrote JM, et al. EHRA/HRS expert consensus on catheter ablation of ventricular arrhythmias: developed in a partnership with the European Heart Rhythm Association (EHRA), a registered branch of the European Society of Cardiology (ESC), and the Heart Rhythm Society (HRS); in collaboration with the American College of Cardiology (ACC) and the American Heart Association (AHA). Heart Rhythm 2009;6:886–933.
3. Lopera G, Stevenson WG, Soejima K, et al. Identification and ablation of three types of ventricular tachycardia involving the his-purkinje system in patients with heart disease. J Cardiovasc Electrophysiol 2004;15:52–8.
4. Stevenson WG, Friedman PL, Sager PT, et al. Exploring postinfarction reentrant ventricular tachycardia with entrainment mapping. J Am Coll Cardiol 1997;29:1180–9.
5. Soejima K, Stevenson WG, Maisel WH, et al. The N + 1 difference: a new measure for entrainment mapping. J Am Coll Cardiol 2001;37:1386–94.
6. Stevenson WG, Khan H, Sager P, et al. Identification of reentry circuit sites during catheter mapping and radiofrequency ablation of ventricular tachycardia late after myocardial infarction. Circulation 1993;88: 1647–70.
7. Tung S, Soejima K, Maisel WH, et al. Recognition of far-field electrograms during entrainment mapping of ventricular tachycardia. J Am Coll Cardiol 2003; 42:110–5.
8. Ellison KE, Friedman PL, Ganz LI, et al. Entrainment mapping and radiofrequency catheter ablation of ventricular tachycardia in right ventricular dysplasia. J Am Coll Cardiol 1998;32:724–8.
9. Nazer B, Woods C, Dewland T, et al. Importance of ventricular tachycardia induction and mapping for patients referred for epicardial ablation. Pacing Clin Electrophysiol 2015;38:1333–42.
10. Soejima K, Stevenson WG, Maisel WH, et al. Electrically unexcitable scar mapping based on pacing threshold for identification of the reentry circuit isthmus: feasibility for guiding ventricular tachycardia ablation. Circulation 2002;106:1678–83.
11. Zipes DP. Mechanisms of clinical arrhythmias. J Cardiovasc Electrophysiol 2003;14:902–12.
12. Mines GR. On dynamic equilibrium in the heart. J Physiol 1913;46:349–83.
13. Issa ZF, MIller JM, Zipes DP. Mapping and navigation modalities. In: Issa ZF, MIller JM, Zipes DP, editors. Clinical arrhythmology and electrophysiology: a companion to Braunwald's heart disease. 1st edition. China: Saunders; 2009. p. 57–99.
14. Benito B, Josephson ME. Ventricular tachycardia in coronary artery disease. Rev Esp Cardiol (Engl Ed) 2012;65:939–55.
15. Almendral JM, Gottlieb CD, Rosenthal ME, et al. Entrainment of ventricular tachycardia: explanation for surface electrocardiographic phenomena by analysis of electrograms recorded within the tachycardia circuit. Circulation 1988;77:569–80.
16. Rosenthal ME, Stamato NJ, Almendral JM, et al. Resetting of ventricular tachycardia with electrocardiographic fusion: incidence and significance. Circulation 1988;77:581–8.
17. el-Sherif N, Gough WB, Restivo M. Reentrant ventricular arrhythmias in the late myocardial infarction period: 14. Mechanisms of resetting, entrainment, acceleration, or termination of reentrant tachycardia by programmed electrical stimulation. Pacing Clin Electrophysiol 1987;10:341–71.
18. de Bakker JM, van Capelle FJ, Janse MJ, et al. Macroreentry in the infarcted human heart: the mechanism of ventricular tachycardias with a "focal" activation pattern. J Am Coll Cardiol 1991;18: 1005–14.
19. Hadjis TA, Harada T, Stevenson WG, et al. Effect of recording site on postpacing interval measurement during catheter mapping and entrainment of postinfarction ventricular tachycardia. J Cardiovasc Electrophysiol 1997;8:398–404.
20. Anter E, Tschabrunn CM, Buxton AE, et al. High-resolution mapping of postinfarction reentrant ventricular tachycardia: electrophysiological characterization of the circuit. Circulation 2016;134: 314–27.
21. Bogun F, Bahu M, Knight BP, et al. Comparison of effective and ineffective target sites that demonstrate concealed entrainment in patients with coronary artery disease undergoing radiofrequency ablation of ventricular tachycardia. Circulation 1997;95:183–90.
22. Bogun F, Kim HM, Han J, et al. Comparison of mapping criteria for hemodynamically tolerated, postinfarction ventricular tachycardia. Heart Rhythm 2006;3:20–6.

Pace Mapping to Localize the Critical Isthmus of Ventricular Tachycardia

Christian de Chillou, MD, PhD[a,b],*, Jean-Marc Sellal, MD[a,b],
Isabelle Magnin-Poull, MD[a,b]

KEYWORDS

- Catheter ablation • Electroanatomical mapping • Ischemic cardiomyopathy • Pace-mapping
- Ventricular tachycardia

KEY POINTS

- The "protected isthmus" of the reentrant circuit is critical for the maintenance of postinfarct ventricular tachycardias (VTs) and the target for catheter ablation.
- In this article, the authors describe the technique of pace-mapping during sinus rhythm to unmask postinfarct VT isthmuses.
- A pace-mapping map should be considered as the surrogate of an activation map during VT, both in patients with a normal heart and in patients with a structural heart disease.
- The color-coded sequence (from the best to the poorest matching sites) on the pace-mapping map reveals a figure-of-8 picture matching the VT activation time map.
- An abrupt change in paced QRS morphology occurs between both sides of the midisthmus line, allowing the identification of a VT isthmus.

INTRODUCTION

In patients with a structural heart disease, in particular, postinfarct patients, ventricular tachycardias (VT) are mostly related to the presence of a ventricular scar in which surviving myocytes are surrounded by a certain amount of fibrous tissue, which favors slow conduction. Because slow conduction is one of the electrophysiological characteristics of such scars, it explains why macroreentry[1–3] is the underlying mechanisms of most scar-related VTs. The so-called protected isthmus of the reentrant circuit is the critical element for the maintenance of these VTs and, therefore, the target for ablation.[4]

Identifying such a protected isthmus may be performed by a conventional electrophysiological approach either based on VT entrainment techniques or by an electroanatomical activation mapping during VT using a 3-dimensional (3D) mapping system.[4–6] In greater than 90% of postinfarct mappable VTs, complete activation maps during VT[6] demonstrate an endocardial macroreentrant circuit, usually with 2 loops rotating around a protected isthmus bounded by 2 approximately parallel conduction barriers, which consist of either a line of double potentials, a scar area, or the mitral annulus. On average, these critical isthmuses are about 31 mm long and 16 mm wide and

Conflict of Interest Disclosures: Dr C. de Chillou has received lecture fees from Biosense Webster, Boston Scientific, and St Jude Medial for less than 10,000 annual USD. Dr J.M. Sellal has received research grants or lectures fees from Biosense Webster and St Jude Medical for less than 10,000 annual USD.
[a] Department of Cardiology, University Hospital Nancy, rue du Morvan, 54511 Vandœuvre lès-Nancy F-54500, France; [b] INSERM-IADI, U947, rue du Morvan, 54511 Vandœuvre lès-Nancy F-54500, France
* Corresponding author. Department of Cardiology, Hôpitaux de Brabois, 1, rue du Morvan, Vandœuvre lès Nancy 54511, France.
E-mail address: c.dechillou@chru-nancy.fr

harbor diastolic electrograms. Activation mapping, however, cannot be used to define the protected VT isthmus in the presence of a poorly tolerated, unmappable VT. Several investigators[7–11] have proposed a substrate-based approach either relying on sinus rhythm (SR) scar definition, using bipolar voltage and pace mapping to create linear lesions, or targeting electrograms showing late potentials (or fractionation). Recently,[12] pace-mapping has also been demonstrated to be a very powerful technique to unmask the isthmuses of postinfarct VT circuits.

GENERAL CONSIDERATIONS ABOUT PACE-MAPPING

Many years ago, pace mapping during SR emerged as one of the most efficacious techniques to localize the site of origin of focal VTs in patients without structural heart disease, especially in patients with right or left ventricular outflow tract VTs. Indeed, most investigators[13–16] report successful ablation at sites with identical or near identical matches in all 12 surface-electrocardiogram (ECG) leads. Comparison of a 12-lead ECG obtained at a given pace-mapping site with the 12-lead ECG recorded during VT can be carried out visually with the result to be expressed according to the number of matching leads using a scale from 0 to 12 (**Fig. 1**).

Nevertheless, this is a qualitative analysis. Furthermore, the reproducibility of this method (both interobserver and intraobserver variability) has not been evaluated, whereas this factor may have a significant impact on the results. However, the use of computerized algorithms for comparison of paced and tachycardia QRS morphologies results in quantifiable and reliable data, which dramatically improve the precision of the pace-mapping (see **Fig. 1**). In addition, computer-assisted comparisons allow the generation of a "pace-mapping map" (**Fig. 2**). In patients with a focal VT (such as outflow tract VTs in the absence of structural heart disease), the probability of obtaining an exact pace-mapping match decreases gradually as the distance of the pacing site from the site of VT origin increases and vice versa. As a consequence, pace-mapping and activation mapping are highly correlated,[17] such that a pace-mapping map should be considered as a surrogate of an activation map in patients with a focal VT and no structural heart disease.

The spatial resolution of pace-mapping maps depends on several factors. Indeed, rapid myocardial conduction velocity, high pacing outputs, bipolar pacing, and large interelectrode distances decrease the precision of pace-mapping. As a consequence, unipolar pacing should be preferred, and the authors recommend using the lowest possible output to minimize the possibility

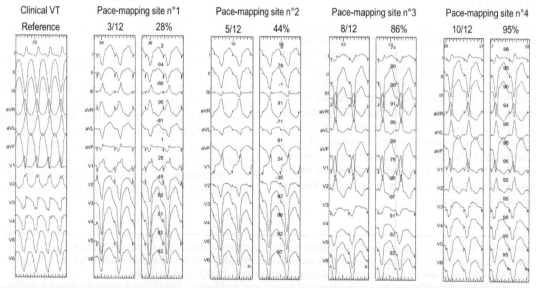

Fig. 1. Example of four 12-lead ECG obtained during pace-mapping at 4 different sites (*1–4*) in the same patient. For each pace-mapping site, both the visual and the automated comparison with the clinical VT are shown. Each visual comparison is given as a number of matching leads out of 12. Each computerized comparison, first calculated lead per lead (*small figures*) is expressed as the global average percentage of correlation with the clinical VT. Computerized comparison allows a higher reproducibility and increases the accuracy as well as the sharpness of the pace-mapping map.

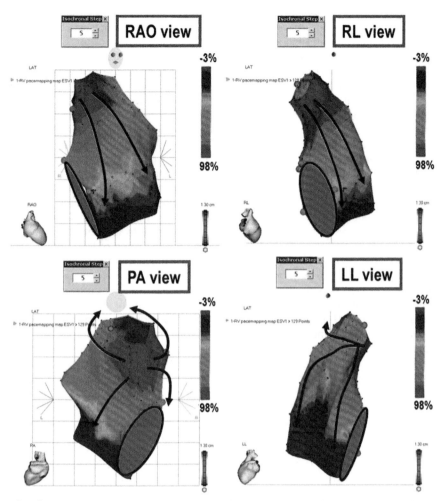

Fig. 2. Example of a pace-mapping map in a patient with an idiopathic right ventricular outflow tract tachycardia. Different views of the right ventricle are shown. The color coding indicates the percentage of matching with the clinical VT for each pacing site, the best matching (98%) being in red and the poorest matching (−3%) in purple. The VT exit corresponds to the site with the best correlation (98%) with the clinical VT and is located at the posterior part of the right ventricular outflow tract. The percentage of correlation with the clinical VT gradually and progressively decreases (5% step isochrones) when moving away from the VT exit site. This pace-mapping map shows a centrifugal pattern, which matches the activation time mapping during VT. LL, left lateral; PA, posteroanterior; RAO, right anterior oblique; RL, right lateral.

of far-field capture. Smaller electrodes certainly lead to more focal myocardial depolarization and should therefore show a better pace-mapping spatial resolution as compared with larger-tip electrodes commonly used for ablation. At the present time, however, there are no data comparing pace-mapping maps using large-tip electrodes as compared with small-tip electrodes.

It has also been suggested that varying the pacing rate may alter the paced-QRS morphology[18] and, to minimize this, pacing at VT cycle length is advised. Based on hundreds of pacing sites with varying pacing rates between 600 and 300 ms, the authors' (unpublished) data do not support, however, the need to pace at VT cycle length. Indeed, they only could observe, and inconsistently, a minimal QRS alteration that did not significantly affect the pace-mapping map.

PACE-MAPPING IN (AND AROUND) POSTINFARCT VENTRICULAR TACHYCARDIA ISTHMUSES

Pace-mapping has also been proposed[19,20] as a technique to identify the exit site of postinfarct macro-reentrant VTs. Typically, VT exit site pacing will yield a matched QRS morphology with a short stimulus-to-QRS (S-QRS) interval. As the pacing site moves away from the exit region to the VT entrance site within the VT isthmus, the S-QRS interval theoretically gets longer and longer with a QRS morphology still perfectly matching the VT. This is, however, partially true because the authors demonstrated recently[12] that an abrupt transition between a paced-QRS that matches the clinical VT (exit site) and a nonmatched paced-QRS (entrance site) identifies the core of a VT isthmus. Importantly, this observation was made in a systematic way in all patients for whom an endocardial macro-reentrant VT circuit was highlighted.

What does this abrupt transition actually mean? Consider a high-density pace-mapping map within a VT isthmus. In all patients and in all identified isthmuses, the authors observed a perfect match with VT morphology when pacing at the isthmus exit but also at all pacing sites located on the exit side of the isthmus, up to the midisthmus zone. Oppositely, when pacing at the isthmus entrance, the authors always noticed a poor 12-lead ECG match with VT morphology. This poor match was found at isthmus entrance but also at all pacing sites placed on the entrance side of a VT isthmus, up to the midisthmus zone (**Fig. 3**). An abrupt change in QRS morphology is

therefore observed when slightly moving the mapping catheter from one side to the other of the (virtual) midisthmus line. The only possible explanation for such a finding is the following: when pacing at the exit side of the midisthmus line, the activation wavefront propagates in both directions with respect to the isthmus orientation, but more rapidly to the exit zone of the isthmus as compared with the entrance zone of the isthmus. As a consequence, the myocardial depolarization outside the isthmus begins at the exit side of the isthmus and spreads away from there to depolarize the ventricles. On the contrary, when pacing at the entrance side of the midisthmus line, the activation wavefront propagates more rapidly to the entrance zone as compared with the exit zone of the isthmus, which leads to a depolarization of the ventricles starting at the entrance zone of the isthmus. Because an isthmus is 31 mm long on average, the resulting ECG are markedly different when pacing at one or the other side of a midisthmus line (**Fig. 4**).

This finding is in contrast to VT entrainment, where concealed fusion can be observed all along the isthmus, including both the entrance and the exit locations, the only remarkable difference being

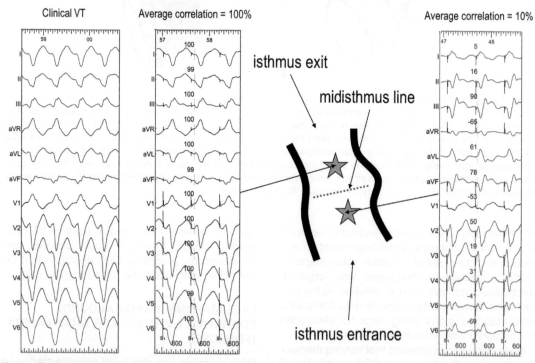

Fig. 3. Illustration of the difference in QRS morphology obtained when pacing on one or the other side of the midisthmus line of a VT isthmus. When pacing at the exit side of the midisthmus line, the 12-lead ECG obtained shows a perfect match with the clinical VT (AC of 100%). On the contrary, pacing on the entrance side of the midisthmus line generates a 12-lead ECG with a poor match (AC of 10%) with the clinical VT. An abrupt difference in paced-QRS is observed within a short distance, the transition being demarcated by the midisthmus line.

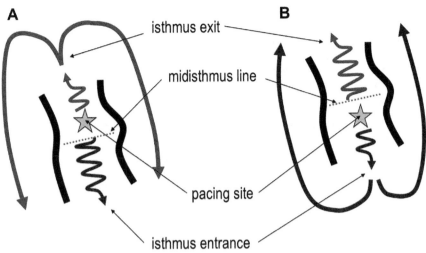

Fig. 4. Schema explaining the difference in QRS morphology shown in **Fig. 3** (see text for details). (*A*) When pacing at the exit side of the midisthmus line, the activation wavefront propagates but more rapidly to the exit zone (*red zigzag-shaped arrow*) and spreads away from there to depolarize the ventricles (*red full arrows*). (*B*) When pacing at the entrance side of the midisthmus line, the activation wavefront propagates but more rapidly to the exit zone (*blue zigzag-shaped arrow*) and spreads away from there to depolarize the ventricles (*blue full arrows*). The resulting ECGs are therefore significantly different when pacing at one or the other side of a midisthmus line.

the value of the S-QRS interval, which is short at isthmus exit and gets longer and longer when moving step by step the pacing site from the exit to the entrance part of the isthmus (**Fig. 5**). Such a long S-QRS interval is due to the slow longitudinal conduction within the isthmus, and it also indicates that myocardial cells depolarized between the pacing site (isthmus entrance) and the onset of the QRS complex (isthmus exit) do not contribute

to the morphology of the QRS complex because they are depolarized before the QRS complex onset. When pacing within the protected isthmus, VT entrainment is explained by 2 opposite (orthodromic and antidromic) wavefronts with respect to the VT activation sequence. During VT entrainment, the collision between the antidromic (N) paced wavefront with the previous (N−1) orthodromic wavefront prevents any change in QRS

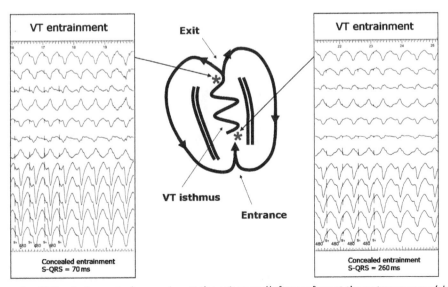

Fig. 5. Example of VT entrainment when pacing at the exit zone (*left panel*) or at the entrance zone (*right panel*) of a VT circuit. In both cases, concealed entrainment is observed with the difference of a longer S-QRS interval (260 ms vs 70 ms) when pacing at the entrance site as compared with the exit site.

morphology whatever the pacing site along the VT isthmus (**Fig. 6**), as opposed to what is observed when pace-mapping is performed during SR.

HOW TO DELINEATE A POSTINFARCT VENTRICULAR TACHYCARDIA ISTHMUS USING PACE-MAPPING?

Since 2007, pace-mapping during SR is the first-choice approach to identify postinfarct VT isthmuses. Indeed, as the authors have shown before, an abrupt change in paced QRS morphology can be used to identify a VT isthmus. In total, there are 4 steps to unmask a VT isthmus.

Step 1: Ventricular Programmed Electrical Stimulation

The aim of this first step is to obtain a 12-lead ECG of the targeted clinical VT in a given patient. This is usually achieved with a bipolar catheter inserted via the femoral vein and positioned at the right ventricular apex (RVA). With this catheter, ventricular programmed electrical stimulation (PES) is used to induce VT, applying up to 3 extrastimuli during spontaneous rhythm and during paced rhythm (600 ms, then 400 ms basic cycle length). The same protocol should be applied at the right ventricular outflow tract and then in the left ventricle (in the vicinity of the scar), when no VT was induced by PES at the RVA. In the authors' experience, absence of VT inducibility is observed in less than 5% of cases after PES has been performed at up to 3 ventricular sites in postinfarct patients with a documented VT.

After VT has been induced, SR is promptly restored by overdrive pacing in order to pass on to the next stage. A template reference of the 12-lead ECG during VT is selected for matching purpose (see step 3).

Step 2: Ventricular 3-Dimensional Reconstruction

Using a 3D mapping system (CARTO, Biosense-Webster, Diamond Bar, CA, USA; Ensite Precision, St Jude Medical, St Paul, MN, USA; and so forth), the second step consists of re-creating the geometry of the ventricles from point-by-point high-density sampling during SR and then to display the resulting bipolar voltage map with a lower and higher cutoff value of 0.5 and 1.5 mV, respectively. The postinfarct scar will hence be roughly delineated, with the so-called dense scar' depicted in red (voltage <0.5 mV) and healthy tissue (voltage >1.5 mV) depicted in purple. Importantly, the low-voltage (voltage <1.5 mV) region contains the reentry circuit.[21]

Step 3: Ventricular Pace-Mapping

Pace-mapping (pacing rate at 600 ms/2-ms pulse width at twice the diastolic threshold) during SR is the third step. Pace-mapping should be performed at many (30–60) sites within, and all around, the infarct area with the resulting 12-lead ECG obtained at each pacing site and then compared

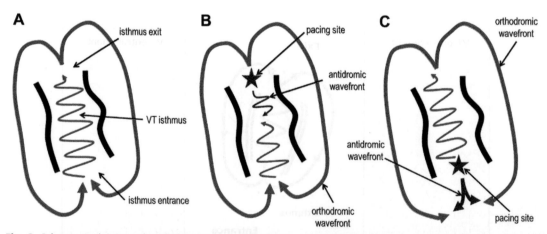

Fig. 6. Schema explaining why identical QRS morphologies are observed when pacing at the entrance or exit zone of a VT circuit during entrainment maneuvers. (*A*) Activation sequence during VT represented by the red arrows. (*B*) Activation sequence during VT entrainment when pacing at the exit site of the VT circuit. (*C*) Activation sequence during VT entrainment when pacing at the entrance site of the VT circuit. The blue arrows represent both the antidromic wavefronts and the amount of myocardial cells depolarized in a different way during VT entrainment as compared with nonentrained VT. During VT entrainment, the main wavefronts activations outside the VT isthmus are identical whatever the pacing site. As a consequence, entrainment with concealed fusion is observed on the corresponding 12-lead ECGs obtained in *A–C*.

with the 12-lead ECG during VT. Each comparison is done automatically by the data-processing template-matching software integrated into the BARD (Boston Scientific, Arden Hills, MN, USA) workstation or integrated into a marketed 3D mapping system (CARTO, Biosense-Webster, Diamond Bar, CA, USA or Ensite Precision, St Jude Medical, St Paul, MN, USA). Briefly, a reference QRS is selected on the 12-lead ECG obtained during the induced clinical VT, and the one to be compared with the reference is selected on a pace-mapping 12-lead ECG. The different available software "slides" the reference over the incoming data until the best local match is found by using a correlation calculation. This calculation is repeated at multiple positions for each of the ECG leads. The position that yields the highest average correlation (AC) across all of the leads is the best local match. This position is marked, and the values for each lead are calculated and displayed along with an AC value for the entire ECG. As a result, an ECG-AC value toward 99% to 100% means a perfect match between two 12-lead ECG morphologies, whereas an ECG-AC value toward zero (or even negative values) identifies a poor match between the two 12-lead ECG morphologies compared beforehand. For each lead-to-lead comparison, both the polarity and the amplitude of the QRS complexes play an important role as to the resulting value of the percentage of correlation calculated by the different software.

Each pacing site is attributed a color representing the value of the ECG-AC, which will be displayed on the 3D shell of the reconstructed ventricle. Zones with the highest ECG-AC values are displayed in red, and those with a lower ECG-AC are color-coded in yellow, then green, then blue, and finally purple for areas showing the lowest ECG-AC values. This newly generated color-coded map is given the name "pace-mapping map."

Although the pace-mapping sites may be relatively scattered, it is important to look for the VT exit zone first. The VT exit zone will correspond to pace-mapping sites, where a good match (>90% of correlation) with the reference VT is observed.

Step 4: Tips and Tricks to Acquire and Interpret the Pace-Mapping Map

Although the pace-mapping sites may be relatively scattered, it is important to look for the VT exit zone first. It is therefore important to perform pace-mapping at many sites until the exit zone has been identified. The VT exit zone corresponds to the myocardial area, where all pace-mapping sites show a good match (>90% of correlation)

with the reference VT. Despite a high-density and homogenous distribution of pace-mapping sites all over the endocardial surface of the ventricle, it may be possible that the exit site of the VT is not identified, that is, there is no pace-mapping site with a good match with the clinical VT. In such a case, it is necessary to apply step 2 and step 3 again in the other ventricle or on the epicardial surface of the ventricles to eventually identify the VT exit site.

Once the VT exit area has been identified, pace-mapping should be performed at adjacent (10–15 mm) sites all around the exit zone to find places where pace-mapping abruptly shows a poor correlation with the clinical VT. In postinfarct VT patients, absence of an abrupt transition at any site all around the exit area is rarely observed (<10% of cases). In such cases, the pace-mapping maps show a centrifugal depolarization pattern, with points at the exit VT zone showing a good QRS match, and the percentages of correlation gradually and homogenously decreasing when moving away in all directions from the best pace-mapping zone, as it is typically observed in normal heart patients with right ventricular outflow tract tachycardia (see **Fig. 2**). In postinfarct VT patients, an endocardial pace-mapping map with a centrifugal pattern is either related to a focal VT or is explained by an endocardial breakthrough of an intramural or epicardial reentrant circuit. Mapping of other side of the ventricular wall is then necessary to understand the underlying mechanism.

However, in the great majority of postinfarct VT patients, a poor paced-QRS correlation is found at some pacing sites around the exit zone and in close vicinity (10–15 mm) of points with a good paced-QRS correlation. Such an abrupt transition between a paced-QRS that matches the clinical VT (exit site) and a nonmatched paced-QRS (entrance site) identifies the core of a VT isthmus. The line demarcating the exit area, on one side, from the entrance area, on the other side, is defined as the midisthmus line (**Fig. 7**). It remains then to identify the lateral boundaries of the isthmus. Looking at the pace-mapping map, a gradual and progressive decrease in the percentage of correlation values is noticed (with the corresponding colors changing from red to orange, yellow, green, and so forth) when moving from the exit zone to the outer part of the isthmus. When following the isochronal color-coded sequence on the pace-mapping map, a figure-of-8 picture, matching the VT activation time mapping (**Fig. 8**), can be observed. Therefore, a pace-mapping map should also be considered as the surrogate of an activation map during VT in postinfarct patients and could be used to define

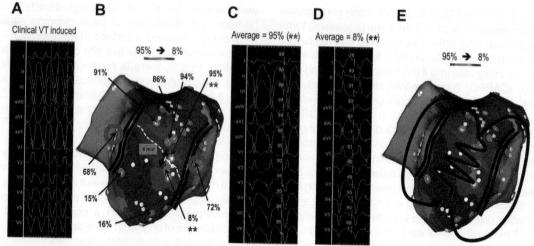

Fig. 7. Example of a deductive reconstruction (only based on pace mapping [PMs]) of a VT reentrant circuit in a patient with a poorly tolerated postmyocardial infarction (MI) VT. (A) 12-lead ECG of the clinical VT induced during the EP study. (B) PM-map (5% step isochrones) of the 3D reconstructed LV (CARTO picture/inferior oblique view), with yellow tags representing PM sites. The percentage of matching between the 12-lead ECG during VT and those obtained during PM ranges from 95% to 8%. The white dotted line represents the midisthmus line. There are 2 pacing sites (red circles) with intermediate QRS matching (68% and 72%, respectively) very close to sites with a good QRS matching, which delineate the lateral borders of the VT isthmus (see text for details). (C, D) 12-lead ECGs obtained during PM at 2 different, 6-mm-apart, LV sites (red and blue asterisks on B). (E) Reconstruction of the VT circuit with isthmus boundaries corresponding to lines of conduction block. EP, electrophysiological; LV, left ventricle.

the lateral boundaries of the isthmus (see **Fig. 8**). A more precise approach consists of acquiring more pace-mapping points all along the "exit side" of the midisthmus line. When doing so, a good match with the clinical VT is observed but, when moving laterally in one direction along the isthmus line, the extremity of the midisthmus line will be encountered where a pace-mapping point will not any longer match the VT morphology (see **Fig. 7**). Such a point is just outside the VT isthmus.

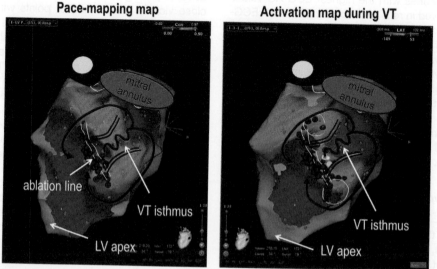

Fig. 8. Example of a 3D reconstruction (CARTO picture/posterosuperior oblique view) showing the PM map and the activation map during VT in the same patient. Arrows following the isochronal color-coded sequence on the PM (left) depict a figure-of-8, which looks like the VT activation time mapping (right). As a consequence, a PM map should be considered as a surrogate of an activation map in post-MI patients. LV, left ventricle.

The corresponding lateral boundary of the isthmus is then defined as a barrier roughly perpendicular to the midisthmus line and passing between this very point found immediately outside the isthmus and an adjacent point located within the isthmus. The second boundary of the isthmus will be found using the same method in getting more pace-mapping points in the other direction of the mid-isthmus line.

After the VT isthmus is identified, point-by-point radiofrequency ablation can be performed with the aim to transect the VT isthmus at any site from its entrance (see **Fig. 8**) to its exit.

SUMMARY

Pace-mapping during SR is a valuable tool to localize the critical isthmus of postinfarct VTs with definition of isthmuses boundaries identified by detailed activation mapping and displayed on electroanatomical mapping system.

Importantly, the orientation of the isthmus of a reentrant postinfarct VT circuit may be recognized using pace mapping with the identification of 2 adjacent zones consistent with the exit (area with pace mapping showing a good correlation with the 12-lead ECG during VT) and the entrance (area with pace mapping showing a poor correlation with the 12-lead ECG during VT) of the VT circuit.

REFERENCES

1. El-Sherif N, Scherlag BJ, Lazzara R, et al. Re-entrant ventricular arrhythmias in the late myocardial infarction period. 1. Conduction characteristics in the infarct zone. Circulation 1977;55:686–702.
2. Klein H, Karp RB, Kouchoukos NT, et al. Intra-operative electrophysiologic mapping of the ventricle during sinus rhythm in patients with a previous myocardial infarction: identification of the electrophysiologic substrate of ventricular arrhythmias. Circulation 1982;66:847–53.
3. de Bakker JMT, van Capelle FJL, Janse MJ, et al. Reentry as a cause of ventricular tachycardia in patients with chronic ischemic heart disease: electrophysiologic and anatomic correlation. Circulation 1988;77:589–606.
4. Stevenson WG, Khan H, Sager P, et al. Identification of reentry circuit sites during catheter mapping and radiofrequency ablation of ventricular tachycardia late after myocardial infarction. Circulation 1993;88: 1647–70.
5. Stevenson WG, Friedman PL, Sager PT, et al. Exploring postinfarction reentrant ventricular tachycardia with entrainment mapping. J Am Coll Cardiol 1997;29:1180–9.
6. de Chillou C, Lacroix D, Klug D, et al. Isthmus characteristics of reentrant ventricular tachycardia after myocardial infarction. Circulation 2002;105:726–31.
7. Marchlinski FE, Callans DJ, Gottlieb CD, et al. Linear ablation lesions for control of unmappable ventricular tachycardia in patients with ischemic and nonischemic cardiomyopathy. Circulation 2000;101: 1288–96.
8. Soejima K, Suzuki M, Maisel WH, et al. Catheter ablation in patients with multiple and unstable ventricular tachycardias after myocardial infarction. Short ablation lines guided by reentry circuit isthmuses and sinus rhythm mapping. Circulation 2001;104:664–9.
9. Kottkamp H, Wetzel U, Schirdewahn P, et al. Catheter ablation of ventricular tachycardia in remote myocardial infarction: substrate description guiding placement of individual linear lesions targeting noninducibility. J Cardiovasc Electrophysiol 2003;14: 675–81.
10. Arenal A, del Castillo S, Gonzalez-Torrecilla E, et al. Tachycardia-related channel in the scar tissue in patients with sustained monomorphic ventricular tachycardias influence of the voltage scar definition. Circulation 2004;110:2568–74.
11. Jaïs P, Maury P, Khairy P, et al. Elimination of local abnormal ventricular activities: a new end point for substrate modification in patients with scar-related ventricular tachycardia. Circulation 2012;125: 2184–96.
12. de Chillou C, Groben L, Magnin-Poull I, et al. Localizing the critical isthmus of post-infarct ventricular tachycardia: the value of pace-mapping during sinus rhythm. Heart Rhythm 2014;11:175–81.
13. Wilber DJ, Baerman J, Olshansky B, et al. Adenosine-sensitive ventricular tachycardia: clinical characteristics and response to catheter ablation. Circulation 1993;87:126–34.
14. Calkins H, Kalbfleisch SJ, El-Atassi R, et al. Relation between efficacy of radiofrequency catheter ablation and site of origin of idiopathic ventricular tachycardia. Am J Cardiol 1993;71:827–33.
15. Coggins DL, Lee RJ, Sweeney J, et al. Radiofrequency catheter ablation as a cure for idiopathic tachycardia of both left and right ventricular origin. J Am Coll Cardiol 1994;23:133–41.
16. Movsowitz C, Schwartzman D, Callans DJ, et al. Idiopathic right ventricular outflow tract tachycardia: narrowing the anatomic location for successful ablation. Am Heart J 1996;131:930–6.
17. Azegami K, Wilber DJ, Arruda M, et al. Spatial resolution of pacemapping and activation mapping in patients with idiopathic right ventricular outflow tract tachycardia. J Cardiovasc Electrophysiol 2005;16: 823–9.
18. Goyal R, Harvey M, Daoud EG, et al. Effect of coupling interval and pacing cycle length on

morphology of paced ventricular complexes. Implications for pace mapping. Circulation 1996;94: 2843–9.

19. Brunckhorst CB, Delacretaz E, Soejima K, et al. Identification of the ventricular tachycardia isthmus after infarction by pace mapping. Circulation 2004; 110:652–9.

20. Stevenson WG, Soejima K. Catheter ablation for ventricular tachycardia. Circulation 2007;115:2750–60.

21. Hsia HH, Lin D, Sauer WH, et al. Anatomic characterization of endocardial substrate for hemodynamically stable re-entrant ventricular tachycardia: identification of endocardial conducting channels. Heart Rhythm 2006;3:503–12.

Substrate Ablation of Ventricular Tachycardia: Late Potentials, Scar Dechanneling, Local Abnormal Ventricular Activities, Core Isolation, and Homogenization

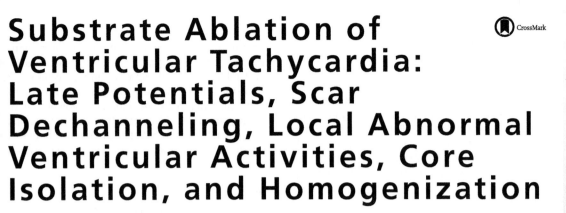

David F. Briceño, MD[a], Jorge Romero, MD[a],
Carola Gianni, MD, PhD[b], Sanghamitra Mohanty, MD, MS[b],
Pedro A. Villablanca, MSc, MD[a], Andrea Natale, MD, FHRS, FESC[b,c],
Luigi Di Biase, MD, PhD[a,b,c,d],*

KEYWORDS

- Ventricular tachycardia • Ventricular arrhythmia • Substrate ablation • Structural heart disease

KEY POINTS

- Ventricular arrhythmias are a frequent cause of mortality in patients with ischemic cardiomyopathy (ICM) and nonischemic cardiomyopathy (NICM).
- Scar-related reentry represents the most common arrhythmia substrate in patients with recurrent episodes of sustained ventricular tachycardia (VT).
- Initial mapping of scar-related VT circuits is focused on identifying arrhythmogenic tissue, which can be based on identification of abnormal electrograms during sinus rhythm or pacing, obviating activation and entrainment mapping during an episode of VT to delineate reentry circuit isthmuses and exits.
- The substrate-based strategies include targeting late potentials (LPs), scar dechanneling, local abnormal ventricular activities (LAVAs), core isolation (CI), and homogenization of the scar.
- Even though substrate-based strategies for VT ablation have shown promising outcomes for patients with structural heart disease (SHD) related to ICM, the data are scarce for patients with nonischemic substrates.

Disclosures: Dr L. Di Biase is a consultant for Stereotaxis, Biosense Webster, Boston Scientific, and St. Jude Medical. Dr L. Di Biase received speaker honoraria/travel from Medtronic, Janssen, Pfizer, EPiEP, and Biotronik. Dr A. Natale has received speaker honoraria from Boston Scientific, Biosense Webster, St. Jude Medical, Biotronik, and Medtronic and is a consultant for Biosense Webster, St. Jude Medical, and Janssen. The remaining authors have no disclosures.

[a] Division of Cardiovascular Disease, Montefiore Medical Center, Albert Einstein College of Medicine, 111 East 210th Street, Bronx, NY 10467, USA; [b] Department of Cardiology, Texas Cardiac Arrhythmia Institute, St. David's Medical Center, 3000 N. IH-35, Austin, TX 78705, USA; [c] Department of Biomedical Engineering, University of Texas, 107 W Dean Keeton Street, Austin, TX 78712, USA; [d] Department of Cardiology, University of Foggia, Via Antonio Gramsci, 71122 Foggia FG, Italy
* Corresponding author. Montefiore Einstein Center for Heart and Vascular Care, Montefiore Medical Center, Albert Einstein College of Medicine, 111 East 210th Street, Bronx, NY 10467.
E-mail address: dibbia@gmail.com

cardiacEP.theclinics.com

INTRODUCTION

Ventricular arrhythmias are a frequent cause of mortality in patients with ischemic cardiomyopathy (ICM).[1] The increased mortality risk that these patients experience can be mitigated by implantation of a cardioverter-defibrillator which still carries significant limitations, because no device is fully protective against life-threatening arrhythmias, such as ventricular tachycardia (VT).[2] Even though implantable cardioverter-defibrillators (ICD) prolong survival, frequent shocks are associated with decreased quality of life, hospital readmissions, and increased mortality.[3,4]

Catheter ablation (CA) and antiarrhythmic drugs (AADs) are used to reduce ICD shocks and potentially improve survival rates in patients with VT.[5] AADs have shown no survival benefit and suboptimal outcomes on ICD shock reduction as well as serious side effects.[3] Recently, the VANISH trial (Ventricular Tachycardia Ablation versus Escalation of Antiarrhythmic Drugs) demonstrated that in patients with ICM, an ICD, and recurrent VT, despite the use of AAD, there was a significantly lower rate of the composite primary outcome of death, VT storm, or appropriate ICD shock among patients undergoing CA than among those receiving an escalation in AAD,[6] highlighting the importance of CA of VT. Despite significant technical advances, however, VT ablation is an evolving treatment modality, which frequently requires more than 1 procedure to achieve high success rates.

Accordingly, with the evolution of advanced cardiac-mapping systems, substrate-based CA has emerged as a useful alternative to more conventional ablation methods.[7] Despite becoming a widespread strategy for VT ablation, however, different clinical studies have adopted heterogeneous characterization of abnormal electrograms resulting in diverse substrates definitions having a major impact on ablation goals.[7] Therefore, this review describes the available evidence from different definitions and approaches for substrate-based ablation of VT.

SUBSTRATE MAPPING FOR VENTRICULAR TACHYCARDIA ABLATION

The mapping techniques used to guide VT ablation depend on the mechanism of VT and the nature of its substrate. Scar-related reentry represents the most common arrhythmia substrate in patients with recurrent episodes of sustained VT,[8] which is commonly caused by a prior myocardial infarction. Causes of non-ischemic cardiomyopathy (NICM) are less common and include arrhythmogenic right ventricular cardiomyopathy (ARVC), sarcoidosis, and dilated cardiomyopathy, among others.[9,10] Scar-related circuits are often large, are complex, and demonstrate variable involvement of the myocardium. CA targets these circuits, which are typically composed of an isthmus with an exit and an entrance (**Fig. 1**).[11] Briefly, initial mapping

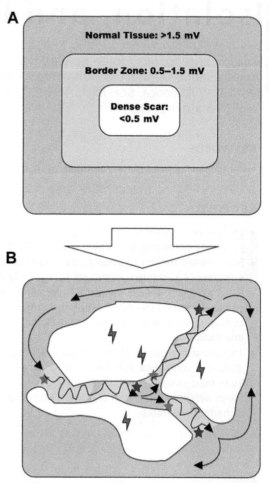

Fig. 1. (A) Tissue voltage definitions. Endocardially, normal voltage is defined as greater than 1.5 mV, whereas dense scar as less than 0.5 mV, and scar border zone as 0.5 mV to 1.5 mV (bipolar electrograms recorded from catheters with a 4-mm tip electrode, 1-mm interelectrode spacing, and filtered at 10–400 Hz). (B) Schematic of scar related circuits: entrance (*green star*), isthmus (*gray zone*), and exit (*red star*). These are often large and complex and demonstrate variable involvement of the myocardium. Additionally, evidence suggests that ablation of scar channels alone does not work as well as extensive ablation because areas between these channels often have electrical activity giving rise to VT substrates (*thunderbolts*). Substrate-based ablation targets abnormal electrical activity.

is focused on recognizing the arrhythmogenic tissue, which can be based on 2 strategies (**Fig. 2**): (1) identification of abnormal electrograms during sinus rhythm or pacing (substrate mapping) and (2) activation and entrainment mapping during an episode of VT to define reentry circuit isthmuses and exits (standard mapping).[8] Substrate mapping is often combined with limited activation and entrainment mapping.[9] Recent evidence suggests, however, that VT induction and mapping before substrate ablation prolong the procedure, radiation exposure, and need for electrical cardioversion without improving acute results and long-term ablation outcomes compared with substrate ablation alone.[12]

Substrate mapping is used to target electroanatomic scar substrates, a term used to quantify myocardial scar based on a specific tissue voltage, initially described by Marchlinski and colleagues[13] in 2000 (see **Fig. 1**). Endocardially, normal voltage is defined as greater than 1.5 mV whereas dense scar as less than 0.5 mV and scar border zone as 0.5 mV to 1.5 mV (bipolar electrograms recorded from catheters with a 4-mm tip electrode and 1-mm interelectrode spacing and and filtered at 10–400 Hz).[9,13] Different parameters are used during epicardial mapping, with the low-voltage area defined as bipolar signal amplitude less than 1.0 mV.[14] Endocardial unipolar voltage mapping can also be useful in specific scenarios, specifically to predict epicardial arrhythmia substrate, as in patients with dilated cardiomyopathy where normal left ventricular (LV) tissue has been reported to be greater than or equal to 8.27 mV and greater

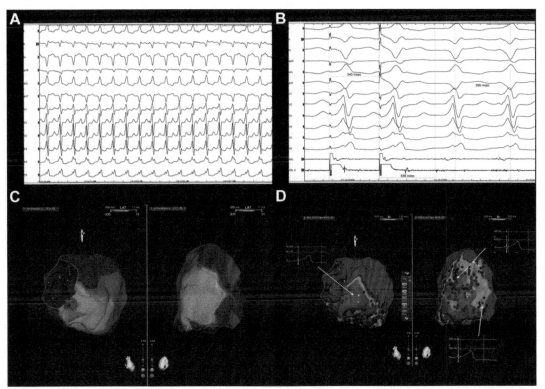

Fig. 2. VT catheter ablation comparing standard ablation versus substrate-based ablation (homogenization) technique in the same patient. Note the difference in ablation points between the 2 strategies to achieve a successful outcome. (*A*) Twelve-lead electrocardiogram of the clinical VT (RS pattern in precordial lead with left superior axis) indicating basal inferoseptal origin. (*B*) Concealed entrainment of the clinical VT with a postpacing interval identical to the tachycardia cycle length (ie, 598 ms). (*C*) Endocardial activation map during VT. Red regions represent earliest endocardial activation and the purple region is activated late during the cardiac cycle. Red dots display ablation point across the VT isthmus where concealed entrainment was obtained. (*D*) Bipolar voltage map of the endocardial LV during sinus rhythm. In the left side, arrow depicts scar area without abnormal potentials, hence no ablation lesions were applied. In the right, arrows show areas with abnormal potentials where lesions were applied. Red regions represent scar (bipolar voltage <0.5 mV), and purple regions represent normal myocardium (bipolar voltage >1.5 mV). Other colored regions represent abnormal myocardial regions probably scar border (bipolar voltage between 0.5 and 1.5 mV). Red dots display ablation points in areas of abnormal electrograms.

than or equal to 5.5 mV for normal right ventricular tissue in patients with ARVC.[10,15]

Substrate-based ablation of VT evolved from initial pioneering studies in the 1970s by Josephson and colleagues,[16–18] where a surgical approach, based on subendocardial resection, achieved more than 80% success in the long-term management of recurrent VT.[19] Subsequently, as stated previously, with the advent of improved technology, substrate-based CA became widespread.[13,20,21] Since then, several studies have suggested that a substrate-based ablation is superior to standard ablation of VT.[22–26]

To further explore this hypothesis of superiority among substrate-based ablation compared with standard ablation of VT, the authors performed an exploratory pooled analysis of studies comparing substrate-based versus standard ablation of VT in patients with SHD. Ventricular arrhythmia recurrence, all-cause mortality and a composite of these outcomes (**Fig. 3**) was assessed; six studies were included (n=396 patients). The mean follow-up was 24+/−15 months. Substrate-based ablation was associated with decreased VA recurrence/all-cause mortality compared to standard ablation of stable VTs (RR 0.57, 95% CI 0.40–0.81). Although there was a trend favoring substrate ablation, there was no difference in VA recurrence or in all-cause mortality between substrate-based ablation versus standard ablation of stable VTs when doing separate analysis (RR 0.68, 95% CI 0.40–1.15; RR 0.56, 95% CI 0.29–1.09, respectively). These preliminary results suggest an advantage of substrate-based ablation strategies compared to standard ablation of VT. The specific strategies available for substrate-based ablation of VT are summarized in **Fig. 4**.

STRATEGIES FOR SUBSTRATE ABLATION OF VENTRICULAR TACHYCARDIA
Late Potentials

Definitions of LPs has been heterogeneous over the years. Early work by Cassidy and colleagues[17] described LPs as any type of electrogram with a duration that extended beyond the end of the surface QRS interval. In this context, they defined a normal electrogram with an amplitude of 3 mV or greater, a duration of 70 ms or less, and/or an amplitude/duration ratio of 0.046 or greater. These investigators showed that ablation strategies based on targeting LPs is effective.[16,17,27] Subsequently, derivations from this definition were used to characterize the different substrate-based techniques. Overall, LPs reveal the location of slow

conducting channels (CCs) (ie, isthmuses) that cause VTs to occur through the ventricular substrate.

Evidence
Arenal and colleagues[21] studied 24 patients with documented monomorphic VT, who underwent CA guided by LPs. Endocardial electroanatomic activation maps during sinus rhythm and right ventricular apex pacing were obtained to define areas for which an electrogram displayed isolated, delayed components. Ablation guided by LPs suppressed all but one clinical VT whose inducibility suppression was tested. During a follow-up period of 9 ± 4 months, five patients had VT recurrences.

More recently, Vergara and colleagues[25] reported in 2012 the efficacy of radiofrequency CA of VT ablation targeting complete LP activity. They evaluated 64 consecutive patients with recurrent VTs and ICM or NICM; 50 patients (47 male; 66.2 ± 10.1 years) had LPs at electroanatomic mapping; 35 patients had at least one VT inducible at basal programmed stimulation. After substrate mapping, radiofrequency ablation was performed with the endpoint of all LPs abolition. LPs could not be abolished in five patients despite extensive ablation, in one patient because of localization near an apical thrombus, and in two patients because of possible phrenic nerve injury. At the end of procedure, VT was still inducible in 5/8 patients with incomplete LP abolition and in five of 42 patients (16.1%) with complete LP abolition (P<.01). After a follow-up of 13.4 ± 4.0 months, 10 patients (20.0%) had VT recurrences and one of them died after surgical VT ablation; VT recurrence was 9.5% in patients with LPs abolition (4/42 patients) and 75.0% (6/8 patients) in those with incomplete abolition. These findings suggested that LPs abolition is an effective endpoint of VT ablation, and its prognostic value compares favorably to that achieved by programmed electrical stimulation (programmed electrical stimulation was repeated when all LP activity was abolished to assess the acute result of ablation).

An area that needs further study is the impact of substrate-based ablation in NICM. Nakahara and colleagues[28] evaluated the impact of LPs target in ICM versus NICM. They showed that an ablation approach incorporating LPs ablation and pace-mapping had limited success in patients with NICM compared with ICM. They evaluated 33 patients with SHD (NICM, n = 16; ICM, n = 17) referred for CA of VT. An LP-targeted ablation strategy was effective in ICM patients (82% nonrecurrence at 12 ± 10 months of follow-up), whereas NICM patients had less favorable outcomes (50%

A

Ventricular Arrhythmia Recurrence / All-Cause Mortality

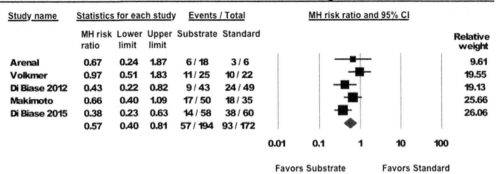

Study name	MH risk ratio	Lower limit	Upper limit	Substrate	Standard		Relative weight
Arenal	0.67	0.24	1.87	6 / 18	3 / 6		9.61
Volkmer	0.97	0.51	1.83	11 / 25	10 / 22		19.55
Di Biase 2012	0.43	0.22	0.82	9 / 43	24 / 49		19.13
Makimoto	0.66	0.40	1.09	17 / 50	18 / 35		25.66
Di Biase 2015	0.38	0.23	0.63	14 / 58	38 / 60		26.06
	0.57	0.40	0.81	57 / 194	93 / 172		

Random effects models
Heterogeneity: Tau2 = 0.06; Chi2 = 6.48; df = 4; P = .17; I2 = 38.3%
Test for overall effect Z = -3.13 (p = .00)

B

Ventricular Arrhythmia Recurrence

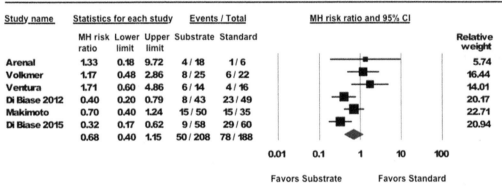

Study name	MH risk ratio	Lower limit	Upper limit	Substrate	Standard		Relative weight
Arenal	1.33	0.18	9.72	4 / 18	1 / 6		5.74
Volkmer	1.17	0.48	2.86	8 / 25	6 / 22		16.44
Ventura	1.71	0.60	4.86	6 / 14	4 / 16		14.01
Di Biase 2012	0.40	0.20	0.79	8 / 43	23 / 49		20.17
Makimoto	0.70	0.40	1.24	15 / 50	15 / 35		22.71
Di Biase 2015	0.32	0.17	0.62	9 / 58	29 / 60		20.94
	0.68	0.40	1.15	50 / 208	78 / 188		

Random effects models
Heterogeneity: Tau2 = 0.23; Chi2 = 12; df = 5; P = .04; I2 = 58.2%
Test for overall effect Z = -1.44 (p = .15)

C

All-Cause Mortality

Study name	MH risk ratio	Lower limit	Upper limit	Substrate	Standard		Relative weight
Arenal	0.33	0.06	1.88	2 / 18	2 / 6		14.59
Volkmer	0.66	0.17	2.63	3 / 25	4 / 22		20.69
Di Biase 2012	1.14	0.07	17.67	1 / 43	1 / 49		4.55
Makimoto	0.47	0.08	2.65	2 / 50	3 / 35		17.16
Di Biase 2015	0.57	0.20	1.61	5 / 58	9 / 60		43.02
	0.56	0.29	1.09	13 / 194	19 / 172		

Fixed effects models
Heterogeneity: Tau2 = 0.00; Chi2 = 0.7; df = 4; P = .95; I2 = 0%
Test for overall effect Z = -1.69 (p = .09)

Fig. 3. Pooled analysis of studies comparing substrate-based versus standard ablation of VT in patients with SHD. (A) Composite VA recurrence/all-cause mortality, (B) VA recurrence, and (C) All-cause mortality. Diamond indicates overall summary estimate for the analysis (width of the diamond represents the 95% CI); width of the shaded square, size of the population. CI, confidence interval; MH, Mantel–Haenszel.

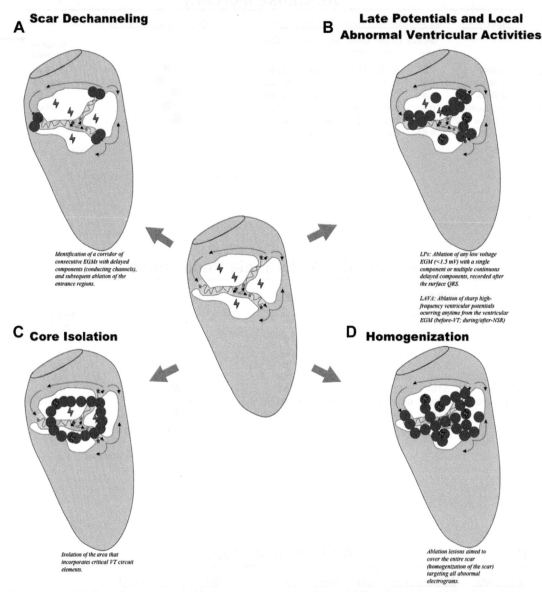

A Scar Dechanneling

Identification of a corridor of consecutive EGMs with delayed components (conducting channels), and subsequent ablation of the entrance regions.

B Late Potentials and Local Abnormal Ventricular Activities

LPs: Ablation of any low voltage EGM (<1.5 mV) with a single component or multiple continuous delayed components, recorded after the surface QRS.

LAVA: Ablation of sharp high-frequency ventricular potentials occurring anytime from the ventricular EGM (before-VT; during/after-NSR)

C Core Isolation

Isolation of the area that incorporates critical VT circuit elements.

D Homogenization

Ablation lesions aimed to cover the entire scar (homogenization of the scar) targeting all abnormal electrograms.

Fig. 4. Strategies for substrate-based ablation. Areas between channels often have electrical activity giving rise to VT substrates (*thunderbolts*); thus, elimination of scar related potentials is a relevant ablation goal and is the basis of different substrate-based ablation strategies. (*A*) Scar dechanneling, (*B*) ablation of LPs and LAVAs, (*C*) CI (core isolation), and (*D*) homogenization of the scar. NSR, normal sinus rhythm.

at 15 ± 13 months of follow-up) using the same ablation technique. These results suggest that the contribution of scar to the electrophysiologic abnormalities targeted for ablation of unstable VT differs between ICM and NICM substrate, when incorporating LPs target. They suggest that patients with NICM have smaller endocardial scar and fewer LPs within endocardial and epicardial scar compared with patients with ICM. The relative paucity of very LPs in patients with NICM may partly account for the challenges in VT ablation

for this population and alternative ablative strategies should be considered. A possible explanation is that because scar in NICM tends to be smaller and less confluent than in ICM, the reentrant circuit may have different anatomic and functional properties that affect propagation.

Scar Dechanneling

Berruezo and colleagues[29] described the scar dechanneling technique.[30,31] They tagged and dichotomously classified electrograms with delayed components as entrance or inner CC points, defined by the presence of a corridor of consecutive electrograms differentiated by higher-voltage amplitude than the surrounding area (which is believed to define the isthmus of the circuit), depending on delayed component precocity during sinus rhythm. The CC entrance is defined as the electrograms with delayed components with the shortest delay between the far-field component of healthy/border zone muscle (low frequency, usually high voltage) and local component (delayed, high frequency, usually fractionated, and low voltage) corresponding to the local activation of myocardial fibers in the scar. To avoid targeting healthy tissue beyond the scar area, CC entrances are tagged in a zone with 0.5 mV to 1.5 mV voltage.

Evidence

This same group published outcomes using scar dechanneling in patients with scar-related VT.[29] They assessed 101 consecutive patients with LV scar–related VT (75 ischemic patients; LV ejection fraction, $36 \pm 13\%$). Procedural endpoint was the elimination of all identified CCs by ablation at the CC entrance followed by abolition of residual inducible VTs. Patients needing only scar dechanneling had a shorter procedure (213 ± 64 vs 244 ± 71 minutes; $P = .027$), fewer radiofrequency applications ($19 \pm 11\%$ vs $27 \pm 18\%$; $P = .01$), and external cardioversion/defibrillation shocks (20% vs 65.2%; $P<.001$). At two years, patients needing scar dechanneling alone had better event-free survival (80% vs 62%) and lower mortality (5% vs 11%). Incomplete CC electrogram elimination was the only independent predictor (hazard ratio, 2.54 [1.06–6.10]) for the primary endpoint.

Contrary to the negative results targeting LPs in NICM, ablation using scar dechanneling has shown promising outcomes in this setting.[31,32] Ferndandez-Armenta and colleagues[32] assessed the link between CC and VT isthmuses in patients with ARVC, finding that CCs more frequently act as the VT substrate in this cardiomyopathy and, therefore, should also be considered to guide substrate-guided ablation. Berruezo and colleagues[31] showed that combined endocardial and epicardial VT ablation incorporating scar dechanneling achieves very good short-term and midterm success rates in patients with ARVC. Using this approach, during a median follow-up of 11 months (6–24 months), only one (9%) patient had a VT recurrence.

Local Abnormal Ventricular Activities

Jais and colleagues[24] described local abnormal ventricular activities (LAVA) in their original study as sharp high-frequency ventricular potentials. These potentials may be of low amplitude, distinct from the far-field ventricular electrogram occurring anytime during or after the far-field ventricular electrogram in sinus rhythm or before the far-field ventricular electrogram during VT. Additionally, potentials can sometime display fractionation or multiple components separated by very low-amplitude signals or an isoelectric interval, and are not well coupled to the rest of the myocardium. These high-frequency sharp signals are considered indicative of local electric activity arising from pathologic tissue. To confirm the nature of LAVAs and to distinguish them from far-field ventricular electrograms in the presence of ambiguity, they used different pacing maneuvers. This strategy uses a high-density catheter to identify the LAVAs.

Evidence

In 2012, Jais and colleagues[24] showed that LAVAs could be identified in most patients with scar-related VT. They revealed that elimination of LAVAs is feasible and safe and is associated with superior survival free from recurrent VT compared with standard ablation (ie, activation and entrainment). They prospectively enrolled 70 patients (67 ± 11 years; 7 female) with VT and structurally abnormal ventricles. Conventional mapping was performed in sinus rhythm, and a high-density PentaRay mapping catheter was used in the endocardium (n = 35) and epicardially. LAVAs were recorded in 67 patients (95.7%). LAVAs were successfully abolished or dissociated in 47 of 67 patients (70.1%). In multivariate analysis, LAVA elimination was independently associated with a reduction in recurrent VT or death (hazard ratio, 0.49; 95% confidence interval, 0.26–0.95; $P<.035$) during long-term follow-up (median, 22 months).

Core Isolation

Tzou and colleagues[33] described core isolation (CI) in their original study. They illustrated that the CI area incorporates critical VT circuit elements confirmed by electrophysiologic data or dense but electrically excitable scar. Practically, to obtain CI, the first step in the ablation procedure is to isolate the dense scar (<0.5 mV) by circumferentially surrounding the putative isthmus or entrance and early exit site(s), which are identified based on pace mapping or entrainment mapping. Sites with ablation termination are uniformly incorporated within CI regions. Regions with electrogram voltage less than 1.0 mV are also targeted if there are features consistent with isthmus, entrance, or early exit sites, as defined previously. If VT is non-inducible at the outset and 12-lead VT ECGs are unavailable, circumferential ablation around dense scar (<0.5 mV) should be performed.

Successful CI was defined by failure to capture the ventricle with pacing from inside the lesion set (exit block) using a pacing output of 20 mA and pulse width of 2 ms from multiple (≥3) discrete sites that had previously demonstrated capture. CI assessment should be done at multiple sites within the isolated region to confirm isolation within the lesion set and not just a segmental effect. CI efficacy is typically assessed after a circumferential lesion set is completed around the region of interest.

Evidence

In 2015, Tzou and colleagues[33] reported CI as a novel strategy with a discrete and measurable endpoint beyond VT inducibility to treat patients with multiple or unmappable VTs. They evaluated patients with SHD presenting for VT radiofrequency ablation at two centers. Strategy involved entrainment/activation mapping if VT was hemodynamically stable and voltage mapping with electrogram analysis and pace mapping in patients with unstable VT. CI was performed incorporating putative isthmus and early exit site(s) based on standard criteria. If VT was noninducible, the dense scar (<0.5 mV) region was isolated. VT inducibility was assessed as procedural endpoint besides testing for successful CI; 44 patients were included (mean age 63; 95% male; 73% ICM; mean LV ejection fraction 31%; 68% with multiple unstable VTs [mean 3 + 2]). CI area was 11 + 12 versus 55 + 40 cm² total scar area. Additional substrate modification was performed in 27 (61%), and epicardial radiofrequency ablation was performed in four (9%) patients. CI was achieved in 37 (84%) and led to better VT-free survival (approximately 89 vs 57%) (log rank P = .013).

These results show that CI is a strategy with a measurable end point beyond VT inducibility, and that the CI region can be selected based on standard characterization of suspected VT isthmus surrogates, thus limiting ablation target size.

Homogenization

Homogenization was described by the authors' group as an empiric extension of ablation throughout the entire scar.[22] In addition to voltage criteria, abnormal electrograms both in the endocardium and the epicardium, including delayed and fragmented recordings, are targeted (eg, LAVA and LP). This strategy involves ablating areas of abnormal electrograms within the dense scar and border zone to homogenize it, preventing isthmuses from forming. Homogenization has the advantage over other substrate-based strategies to target all abnormal signals eliminating all of the scar related potentials, avoiding triggers from "active" zones from different scar areas presumed to be inert. In particular, it may offer advantages over strategies such as CI, where the isolated area may be jeopardized if a lesion fails, reconnecting the circuit. When using an epicardial approach, the areas presenting abnormal recordings are targeted when it contains at least three abnormal electrograms. After endocardial ablation, the epicardial scar is remapped, and if areas of abnormal recordings are still present, then ablation is performed. In this regard, normal electrograms are defined as electrograms with three or fewer sharp and discrete deflections from baseline, amplitude greater than 1.5 mV, and duration less than 70 ms (and/or ratio amplitude/duration >0.046). Any electrogram not fitting this definition is categorized as abnormal and targeted for ablation. Epicardial homogenization is performed only in patients showing large areas of epicardial delayed or fractionated potentials. The goal of this ablation strategy is to cover the entire scar with ablation lesions targeting abnormal electrograms. After substrate ablation, high output pacing at 20 mA from within the scar is performed to confirm that no tissue is captured.

Evidence

The authors reported in 2012[22] the impact on recurrences of two different substrate approaches for the treatment of ventricular arrhythmias; 92 consecutive patients (81% male, age 62 ± 13 years) with ICM and electrical storm underwent CA. Patients were treated either by confining the radiofrequency lesions to the endocardial surface with limited substrate ablation (group 1, n = 49) or underwent endocardial and epicardial ablation of abnormal potentials within the scar (homogenization of the scar, group 2, n = 43). Epicardial access was obtained in all group 2 patients, whereas epicardial ablation was performed in 33% (n = 14) of these patients. Mean ejection fraction was 27 ± 5%. During a mean follow-up of 25 ± 10 months, the ventricular arrhythmias recurrence rate of any VTs was 47% (23 of 49 patients) in group 1 and 19% 8/43 patients) in group 2 (log-rank P = .006); one patient in group 1 and one patient in group 2 died at follow-up for noncardiac reasons. The study demonstrated that ablation using endoepicardial homogenization of the scar significantly increases freedom from ventricular arrhythmias in ICM patients.

Subsequently, in 2015, the authors published the VISTA randomized controlled trial,[23] which evaluated the rates of VT recurrence in patients undergoing ablation limited to clinical VT along with mappable VTs (clinical ablation) versus substrate-based ablation, which consisted of homogenization of the scar. Subjects with ICM and hemodynamically tolerated VT were randomized to clinical ablation (n = 60) versus substrate-based ablation that targeted all abnormal electrograms in the scar (n = 58). Primary endpoint was recurrence of VT. Secondary endpoints included periprocedural complications, 12-month mortality, and rehospitalizations. At 12-month follow-up, 9 (15.5%) and 29 (48.3%) patients had VT recurrence in substrate-based and clinical VT ablation groups, respectively (log-rank $P<.001$). More patients undergoing clinical VT ablation (58%) were on AADs after ablation versus substrate-based ablation (12%; $P<.001$); 7 (12%) patients with substrate ablation and 19 (32%) with clinical ablation required rehospitalization ($P = .014$). Overall 12-month mortality was 11.9%, 8.6% in substrate ablation and 15.0% in clinical ablation groups, respectively (log rank $P = .21$). Combined incidence of rehospitalization and mortality was significantly lower with substrate ablation ($P = .003$). Periprocedural complications were similar in both groups ($P = .61$). These results support that an extensive substrate-based ablation approach is superior to ablation targeting only clinical and stable VTs in patients with ICM presenting with tolerated VT.

SUMMARY

Ventricular arrhythmias are a frequent cause of mortality in patients with ICM and NICM. Scar-related reentry represents the most common arrhythmia substrate in patients with recurrent episodes of sustained VT. Initial mapping of scar-related VT circuits is focused on identifying arrhythmogenic tissue, which can be based on identification of abnormal electrograms during sinus rhythm or pacing (substrate mapping), obviating activation and entrainment mapping during an episode of VT to delineate reentry circuit isthmuses and exits (standard mapping). The substrate-based strategies include targeting LPs, scar dechanneling, LAVAs, CI, and homogenization of the scar. Despite each having a different ablation goal, all have a common endpoint and are performed in sinus rhythm. Evidence suggests that ablation of scar channels alone does not work as well as extensive ablation, in view of areas between these channels often having electrical activity giving rise to VT substrates. Thus, elimination of scar-related potentials is a relevant ablation goal and is the basis of different substrate-based ablation strategies. These strategies have been defined as

- LP: ablation of any type of electrogram with a duration that extends beyond the end of the surface QRS interval, taking into consideration that a normal electrogram has an amplitude of 3 mV or greater, a duration of 70 ms or less, and/or an amplitude/duration ratio of 0.046 or greater
- Scar dechanneling: identification of a corridor of consecutive electrograms with delayed components (CCs) and subsequent ablation of the entrance regions
- LAVA: ablation of sharp high-frequency ventricular potentials occurring anytime during or after the far-field ventricular electrogram in sinus rhythm or before the far-field ventricular electrogram during VT that sometimes displays fractionation or double or multiple components separated by very-low-amplitude signals or an isoelectric interval and are not well coupled to the rest of the myocardium
- CI: ablation lesions creating an isolation area that incorporates critical VT circuit elements confirmed by electrophysiologic data or dense but electrically excitable scar
- Homogenization of the scar: extension of ablation throughout the entire scar with lesions targeting all abnormal electrograms

These ablation strategies have been all associated with higher arrhythmia-free survival, and exploratory analysis of pooled data of studies comparing substrate-based versus standard ablation of VT in patients with SHD not only confirms these studies but also suggests that at long-term follow-up, substrate-based ablation is associated with better outcomes compared with standard ablation. It may be anticipated that future studies will include comparison and combination of substrate-based ablation strategies to continue improving outcomes.[7,34]

Finally, even though substrate-based strategies for VT ablation have shown promising outcomes for patients with SHD, specifically related to myocardial infarction, the data are scarce for patients with nonischemic substrates; hence, further clinical trials are needed to determine the best approach for those patients.

REFERENCES

1. Huikuri HV, Castellanos A, Myerburg RJ. Sudden death due to cardiac arrhythmias. N Engl J Med 2001;345:1473–82.
2. Connolly SJ, Hallstrom AP, Cappato R, et al. Meta-analysis of the implantable cardioverter defibrillator secondary prevention trials. AVID, CASH and CIDS studies.

Antiarrhythmics vs Implantable Defibrillator study. Cardiac Arrest Study Hamburg. Canadian Implantable Defibrillator Study. Eur Heart J 2000;21:2071–8.

3. Bardy GH, Lee KL, Mark DB, et al, Sudden Cardiac Death in Heart Failure Trial I. Amiodarone or an implantable cardioverter-defibrillator for congestive heart failure. N Engl J Med 2005;352:225–37.

4. Poole JE, Johnson GW, Hellkamp AS, et al. Prognostic importance of defibrillator shocks in patients with heart failure. N Engl J Med 2008;359:1009–17.

5. Tung R, Vaseghi M, Frankel DS, et al. Freedom from recurrent ventricular tachycardia after catheter ablation is associated with improved survival in patients with structural heart disease: an International VT Ablation Center Collaborative Group study. Heart Rhythm 2015;12:1997–2007.

6. Sapp JL, Wells GA, Parkash R, et al. Ventricular tachycardia ablation versus escalation of antiarrhythmic drugs. N Engl J Med 2016;375(2):111–21.

7. Santangeli P, Marchlinski FE. Substrate mapping for unstable ventricular tachycardia. Heart Rhythm 2016;13:569–83.

8. Wissner E, Stevenson WG, Kuck KH. Catheter ablation of ventricular tachycardia in ischaemic and nonischaemic cardiomyopathy: where are we today? A clinical review. Eur Heart J 2012;33:1440–50.

9. Natale A, Raviele A, Al-Ahmad A, et al, Venice Chart members. Venice Chart International Consensus document on ventricular tachycardia/ventricular fibrillation ablation. J Cardiovasc Electrophysiol 2010;21:339–79.

10. Tanawuttiwat T, Nazarian S, Calkins H. The role of catheter ablation in the management of ventricular tachycardia. Eur Heart J 2016;37:594–609.

11. Stevenson WG, Khan H, Sager P, et al. Identification of reentry circuit sites during catheter mapping and radiofrequency ablation of ventricular tachycardia late after myocardial infarction. Circulation 1993;88:1647–70.

12. Fernandez-Armenta J, Penela D, Acosta J, et al. Substrate modification or ventricular tachycardia induction, mapping, and ablation as the first step?: A randomized study. Heart Rhythm 2016;13(8):1589–95.

13. Marchlinski FE, Callans DJ, Gottlieb CD, et al. Linear ablation lesions for control of unmappable ventricular tachycardia in patients with ischemic and nonischemic cardiomyopathy. Circulation 2000;101:1288–96.

14. Cano O, Hutchinson M, Lin D, et al. Electroanatomic substrate and ablation outcome for suspected epicardial ventricular tachycardia in left ventricular nonischemic cardiomyopathy. J Am Coll Cardiol 2009;54:799–808.

15. Hutchinson MD, Gerstenfeld EP, Desjardins B, et al. Endocardial unipolar voltage mapping to detect epicardial ventricular tachycardia substrate in patients with nonischemic left ventricular cardiomyopathy. Circ Arrhythm Electrophysiol 2011;4:49–55.

16. Cassidy DM, Vassallo JA, Buxton AE, et al. The value of catheter mapping during sinus rhythm to localize site of origin of ventricular tachycardia. Circulation 1984;69:1103–10.

17. Cassidy DM, Vassallo JA, Miller JM, et al. Endocardial catheter mapping in patients in sinus rhythm: relationship to underlying heart disease and ventricular arrhythmias. Circulation 1986;73:645–52.

18. Kienzle MG, Miller J, Falcone RA, et al. Intraoperative endocardial mapping during sinus rhythm: relationship to site of origin of ventricular tachycardia. Circulation 1984;70:957–65.

19. Betensky BP, Marchlinski FE. Outcomes of catheter ablation of ventricular tachycardia in the setting of structural heart disease. Curr Cardiol Rep 2016;18:68.

20. Reddy VY, Neuzil P, Taborsky M, et al. Short-term results of substrate mapping and radiofrequency ablation of ischemic ventricular tachycardia using a saline-irrigated catheter. J Am Coll Cardiol 2003;41:2228–36.

21. Arenal A, Glez-Torrecilla E, Ortiz M, et al. Ablation of electrograms with an isolated, delayed component as treatment of unmappable monomorphic ventricular tachycardias in patients with structural heart disease. J Am Coll Cardiol 2003;41:81–92.

22. Di Biase L, Santangeli P, Burkhardt DJ, et al. Endo-epicardial homogenization of the scar versus limited substrate ablation for the treatment of electrical storms in patients with ischemic cardiomyopathy. J Am Coll Cardiol 2012;60:132–41.

23. Di Biase L, Burkhardt JD, Lakkireddy D, et al. Ablation of stable VTs versus substrate ablation in ischemic cardiomyopathy: the VISTA randomized multicenter trial. J Am Coll Cardiol 2015;66:2872–82.

24. Jais P, Maury P, Khairy P, et al. Elimination of local abnormal ventricular activities: a new end point for substrate modification in patients with scar-related ventricular tachycardia. Circulation 2012;125:2184–96.

25. Vergara P, Trevisi N, Ricco A, et al. Late potentials abolition as an additional technique for reduction of arrhythmia recurrence in scar related ventricular tachycardia ablation. J Cardiovasc Electrophysiol 2012;23:621–7.

26. Tung R, Mathuria NS, Nagel R, et al. Impact of local ablation on interconnected channels within ventricular scar: mechanistic implications for substrate modification. Circ Arrhythm Electrophysiol 2013;6:1131–8.

27. Miller JM, Tyson GS, Hargrove WC 3rd, et al. Effect of subendocardial resection on sinus rhythm endocardial electrogram abnormalities. Circulation 1995;91:2385–91.

28. Nakahara S, Tung R, Ramirez RJ, et al. Characterization of the arrhythmogenic substrate in ischemic and nonischemic cardiomyopathy implications for

catheter ablation of hemodynamically unstable ventricular tachycardia. J Am Coll Cardiol 2010;55: 2355–65.

29. Berruezo A, Fernandez-Armenta J, Andreu D, et al. Scar dechanneling: new method for scar-related left ventricular tachycardia substrate ablation. Circ Arrhythm Electrophysiol 2015;8:326–36.

30. Fernandez-Armenta J, Berruezo A, Ortiz-Perez JT, et al. Improving safety of epicardial ventricular tachycardia ablation using the scar dechanneling technique and the integration of anatomy, scar components, and coronary arteries into the navigation system. Circulation 2012;125:e466–8.

31. Berruezo A, Fernandez-Armenta J, Mont L, et al. Combined endocardial and epicardial catheter ablation in arrhythmogenic right ventricular dysplasia incorporating scar dechanneling technique. Circ Arrhythm Electrophysiol 2012;5:111–21.

32. Fernandez-Armenta J, Andreu D, Penela D, et al. Sinus rhythm detection of conducting channels and ventricular tachycardia isthmus in arrhythmogenic right ventricular cardiomyopathy. Heart Rhythm 2014;11:747–54.

33. Tzou WS, Frankel DS, Hegeman T, et al. Core isolation of critical arrhythmia elements for treatment of multiple scar-based ventricular tachycardias. Circ Arrhythm Electrophysiol 2015;8:353–61.

34. Santangeli P, Frankel DS, Marchlinski FE. End points for ablation of scar-related ventricular tachycardia. Circ Arrhythm Electrophysiol 2014;7:949–60.

Alternative Approaches for Ablation of Resistant Ventricular Tachycardia

Carola Gianni, MD, PhD[a,b],
Sanghamitra Mohanty, MD, MS[a,c],
Chintan Trivedi, MD, MPH[a], Luigi Di Biase, MD, PhD[a,d,e,f],
Amin Al-Ahmad, MD[a], Andrea Natale, MD, FHRS, FESC[a,c,d,g,h,i,j],
J. David Burkhardt, MD[a,*]

KEYWORDS

- Ventricular tachycardia • Alcohol ablation • Coil embolization • Simultaneous unipolar RF ablation
- Bipolar RF ablation • Surgical ablation • Stereotactic ablative radiosurgery

KEY POINTS

- Unipolar radiofrequency (RF) ablation can be ineffective for ventricular tachycardias (VTs) with a deep intramural origin or cases in which epicardial access is not attainable due to prior cardiac surgery.
- Alternative approaches include alcohol ablation or coil embolization, simultaneous unipolar or bipolar RF ablation, surgical ablation, or noninvasive ablation with stereotactic radiosurgery.
- Alcohol ablation is commonly used to treat resistant VT with good acute and long-term results, although it is limited to the territories vascularized by the target vessel.

INTRODUCTION

Ventricular tachycardia (VT) ablation is usually performed with an ablation catheter that delivers unipolar radiofrequency (RF) energy to eliminate the re-entry circuit responsible for VT. However, there are some instances when unipolar RF ablation fails, notably in VTs with a deep intramural origin or cases in which epicardial access is not attainable due to prior cardiac surgery. To overcome these limitations, several alternative approaches have been used in clinical practice, including alcohol ablation, coil embolization, simultaneous unipolar or bipolar RF ablation, surgical ablation, or noninvasive ablation with stereotactic radiosurgery. This review article describes some of these alternative techniques.

The authors have nothing to disclose.
[a] Texas Cardiac Arrhythmia Institute, St. David's Medical Center, 3000 N. IH-35, Suite 720, Austin, TX 78705, USA; [b] Department of Clinical Sciences and Community Health, University of Milan, Milan, Italy; [c] Department of Internal Medicine, Dell Medical School, University of Texas, Austin, TX, USA; [d] Department of Biomedical Engineering, Cockrell School of Engineering, University of Texas, Austin, TX, USA; [e] Arrhythmia Services, Department of Medicine, Montefiore Medical Center, Albert Einstein College of Medicine, Bronx, NY, USA; [f] Department of Clinical and Experimental Medicine, University of Foggia, Foggia, Italy; [g] Interventional Electrophysiology, Scripps Clinic, La Jolla, CA, USA; [h] Department of Cardiology, MetroHealth Medical Center, Case Western Reserve University School of Medicine, Cleveland, OH, USA; [i] Division of Cardiology, Stanford University, Stanford, CA, USA; [j] Atrial Fibrillation and Arrhythmia Center, California Pacific Medical Center, San Francisco, CA, USA
* Corresponding author.
E-mail address: jdavidburkhardt@gmail.com

ALCOHOL ABLATION

Transcoronary ethanol ablation (TCEA) is performed by intracoronary injection of ethanol. Via direct chemical injury and ischemic injury secondary to vascular damage, ethanol causes coagulative necrosis of the myocardium, which is later replaced by a permanent scar, thereby affecting the circuit that sustains VT.[1]

TCEA can be performed either anterogradely via a coronary artery or retrogradely via the coronary venous system. In anterograde TCEA, selective coronary angiography allows identification of the arterial branches that supply the tachycardia-related region. The target artery is engaged with an angioplasty wire and occluded with an over-the-wire balloon. It is important to exclude vessels with a pronounced collateral circulation to avoid unnecessary damage to distant areas. The angioplasty wire can also be used to record a unipolar electrogram from within the myocardium and select the vessels in close proximity to the area of VT origin with more precision.[2] To do so, only the distal end of the guidewire should be exposed, using either an uninflated angioplasty balloon or a subselector catheter. Once the target vessel is identified, confirmation of the potentially successful site is achieved by inducing the VT and observing its termination after injecting iced saline (2–3 mL). To follow, slow ethanol injection (95%–100%, 1 mL at 1 mL/min up to 5 mL per vessel) is then performed and the balloon remains inflated for approximately 10 minutes after the infusion to prevent backflow of ethanol and ensure good tissue penetration. An alternative approach to TCAE is retrograde intracoronary venous infusion of ethanol.[3] A selective coronary venogram can show the target venous branches that drains the area of VT origin, as determined with activation mapping. As with anterograde TCAE, the target vessel can be cannulated with an angioplasty wire and occluded with an over-the-wire balloon to infuse ethanol (95%–100%, 1 mL at 0.5 mL/min with the balloon inflated for 2 minutes).

Compared with unipolar RF ablation, TCEA allows creation of deeper myocardial lesions; however, it is limited to the territories vascularized by the target vessel. Moreover, the target vessel itself might be inadequate (too small, stenotic, occluded, or with prominent collaterals) and complications are not negligible. In addition to the complications inherent to coronary artery instrumentation (eg, coronary arterial dissection and thrombosis), the reflux of ethanol to nontargeted areas can cause complete heart block (septal alcohol ablation) and myocardial infarction of distant unwanted regions. Additionally, a case of

fatal free wall rupture secondary to intramyocardial dissection has been described.[4]

Several case reports and a few case series (**Table 1**) have demonstrated the feasibility of TCAE for VT ablation; however, both the acute and long-term success rates, as well as the complication rates, remain suboptimal.[2–16] Most of these studies were performed in the setting of ischemic cardiomyopathy, although cases of successful TCAE have been reported for valvular,[4] Chagas',[13] hypertrophic,[17] and dilated idiopathic cardiomyopathies.[2,9–11,15,16]

CORONARY COIL EMBOLIZATION

A recently described approach is transcoronary coil embolization. After selecting the target vessel, coils can be deployed, resulting in coronary occlusion and subsequent myocardial infarction.[18] This might be an alternative in cases with severely reduced systolic dysfunction, given the unpredictable amount of injury when performing TCAE.

SIMULTANEOUS UNIPOLAR OR BIPOLAR RADIOFREQUENCY ABLATION

In conventional unipolar RF, current is delivered from the ablation catheter tip to a grounding patch positioned on the patient's skin: this results in larger current density at the catheter tip (given the smaller surface area) with resistive tissue heating at the catheter-myocardium interface, as well as conductive heating of deeper tissues. To increase efficacy, it is possible to deliver RF current between 2 electrodes positioned on opposing sides of the target deep myocardial tissue. This can be done simultaneously both in a unipolar or bipolar RF fashion. In simultaneous unipolar RF ablation, 2 ablation catheters are connected to 2 RF generators each with their own return electrode, whereas in true bipolar RF ablation, RF current flows between the 2 ablation catheters using 1 as the active electrode and the other as the return electrode. Bipolar RF has been shown to improve lesion transmurality in animal studies compared with both sequential and simultaneous unipolar RF ablation, probably because it depends less on catheter contact and alignment.[19] However, to deliver bipolar RF energy, noncommercially available custom-engineered cable and switch box are necessary to attach the return catheter record and display the temperature from the tip of both catheters, as well as their location on the electroanatomic system. In contrast, simultaneous unipolar RF ablation can be more easily applied, provided 2 RF generators are available.

Table 1
Cases series on ventricular tachycardia alcohol ablation

Author, Year	N	Age (y)	ICM	Acute Success	Complications	Follow-up	Recurrence
Brugada et al,[5] 1989	3	56 ± 10	100%	100%	33% (CHB)	1–6 mo	33%
Dailey et al,[6] 1992	4	NA	100%	100%	25% (CHB)	4–25 mo	50%
Kay et al,[7] 1992	10	62 ± 12	100%	90% any VT	40% (CHB)	372 d	50%
Nellens et al,[8] 1992	10	NA	100%	100%	NA	2–44 mo	14%
Segal et al,[2] 2007	5	70 ± 4	80%	100%	0%	19 ± 17 mo	0%
Sacher et al,[9] 2008	9	55 ± 9	67%	56% any VT 89% clinical VT	33% (1 severe hypotension; 2 groin hematoma)	29 ± 23 mo	33%
Steven et al,[10] 2009[a]	3	NA	NA	100%	0%	NA	NA
Tokuda et al,[11] 2011	22	63 ± 13	52%	46% any VT 82% clinical VT	38% (CHB)	16 d	64%
Baher et al,[3] 2012[b]	2	~67	0%	100% clinical VT	50% (pericarditis)	5 mo	0%

Abbreviations: CHB, complete heart block; ICM, ischemic cardiomyopathy; N, number; NA, not available.
[a] Part of a case series on VT originating from the aortomitral continuity in structural heart disease.
[b] Retrograde TCEA.

Clinically, there is 1 reported case of successful simultaneous unipolar RF ablation (a patient with incessant septal VT secondary to nonischemic cardiomyopathy). A nonirrigated 8 mm ablation catheter delivered 55 W of RF energy opposed to an irrigated 3.5 mm ablation catheter delivering 50 W determining termination of VT.[20] However, bipolar RF using 2 irrigated 3.5 mm ablation catheters delivering up to 40 W of energy has been successfully used in a few cases of refractory septal VT (ischemic and nonischemic), free-wall VT (ischemic), and outflow tract VT (idiopathic), with good acute but mixed long-term results (**Table 2**).[21–23] Studies directly comparing these various different modalities of RF delivery are needed to determine their true additional value.

SURGICAL ABLATION

Surgical treatment of VT was the first used for drug-resistant VT. Aneurysmectomy, encircling endocardial ventriculostomy, and subendocardial resection have been used for decades, before the advent of electroanatomical mapping made transcatheter ablation of VT feasible.[24–26] Over the years, mapping-guided surgical ablation has emerged as an alternative strategy for the surgical management of VT because it allows delivery of

Table 2
Clinical studies on bipolar radiofrequency ablation

Author, Year	N	Age (y)	ICM	Acute Success	Complications	Follow-up	Recurrence
Koruth et al,[21] 2012	6	~65	67%	67% any VT	17% (CHB)	1 y	50%
Gizurarson et al,[22] 2014	1	56	100%	100% clinical VT 0% any VT	0%	1 y	0%
Iyer et al,[20] 2014	1	56	100%	100% any VT	0%	1 mo	0%
Teh et al,[23] 2014	4	~53	0%	75%	0%	4 mo	25%

Abbreviations: CHB, complete heart block; ICM, ischemic cardiomyopathy; N, number.

RF or cryoenergy after precise localization of the arrhythmogenic focus or substrate. Moreover, epicardial surgical ablation might be the only feasible alternative in case of difficult pericardial access (adhesions from prior cardiac surgery or extensive epicardial ablation), especially when the substrate is not limited to a single coronary branch distribution.

Surgical access can be minimally invasive, achieved either with a subxiphoid window or with a limited anterior or left thoracotomy, allowing preferential exposure of the inferior versus anterior or lateral left ventricular walls. Alternatively, a full median sternotomy may be used to expose the whole heart, with or without cardiopulmonary bypass. Surgically based ablation is mainly a substrate-based ablation, due to the difficulty of inducing the clinical arrhythmia in this setting and the impossibility to compare the QRS morphology on the electrocardiogram. Although visual inspection can be used to detect the scar, it is often not easy to do so given the presence of epicardial fat; therefore, intraprocedural electroanatomic guidance, ideally with image integration, is useful. Once the substrate is localized, both RF (bipolar or unipolar) and cryoablation can be applied epicardially using standard electrophysiological ablation catheters or dedicated surgical ablation tools.[27,28]

Few observational studies have systematically reported the results of surgical ablation (**Table 3**). Although acute success is achieved in a good number of patients, complication rates, and long-term success are poor, influenced by the invasiveness of the procedure and the highly selected high-risk population.[10,27–34]

STEREOTACTIC ABLATIVE RADIOSURGERY

Stereotactic ablative radiosurgery (SABR) is a form of radiotherapy that focuses high-dose ionizing radiation beams to be delivered in a small, localized area of the body and it is widely used for the

Table 3
Clinical studies on surgical ablation

Author, Year	N	Age (y)	ICM	Acute Success	Complications	Follow-up	Recurrence
Soejima et al,[29] 2004	6	57 ± 10	33%	67%	33% (1 prolonged pericarditic pain, 1 hemorrhagic effusion)	106–675 d	33%
Maury et al,[30] 2007	1	74	100%	100%	0%	6 mo	0%
Steven et al,[10] 2009[a]	2	NA	NA	100%	0%	NA	NA
Maury et al,[31] 2009[b]	1	62	0%	100%	100% (pleural effusion)	9 mo	0%
Michowitz et al,[32] 2010	14	63 ± 10	71%	57%	29% (3 hemorrhagic effusion, 1 wound infection)	19 ± 12 mo	50%
Anter et al,[33] 2011	8	58 ± 11	0%	NA	25% (2 deaths, sepsis and progressive HF)	23 ± 6 mo	25%
Mathuria et al,[27] 2011	1	62	100%	100% clinical VT 0% any VT	0%	6 mo	0%
Mulloy et al,[28] 2013	7	48 ± 11	29%	NA	57% (tamponade, prolonged ventilation, pneumonia, GI bleeding, AF)	5 ± 3 mo	0%
Patel et al,[34] 2016	5	60 ± 11	40%	60% any VT	10% (mediastinal bleeding)	12 ± 12 mo	0%

Abbreviations: AF, atrial fibrillation; GI, gastrointestinal; HF, heart failure; ICM, ischemic cardiomyopathy; N, number.
[a] Part of a case series on VT originating from the aortomitral continuity in structural heart disease.
[b] Lateral thoracotomy approach.

treatment of various types of cancers. In contrast to traditional radiotherapy, SABR creates radiation-induced necrosis in the targeted tissue, minimizing the exposure to surrounding tissues.[35] Compared with other forms of ablation, SABR is noninvasive and can be used in patients whose comorbidities render them unsuitable for invasive treatment (RF ablation or cardiac surgery).[36,37] So far, SABR has been used in 2 patients with refractory VT. A 25 Gy dose was delivered to the target volume, corresponding to the ventricular arrhythmogenic substrate as determined with electrophysiological-imaging integration, without acute complications. At follow-up, no late complications (eg, extracardiac toxicity) occurred and both patients showed a clinical benefit with substantial VT burden reduction.

REFERENCES

1. Reek S, Geller JC, Schildhaus HU, et al. Catheter ablation of ventricular tachycardia by intramyocardial injection of ethanol in an animal model of chronic myocardial infarction. J Cardiovasc Electrophysiol 2004;15:332–41.
2. Segal OR, Wong T, Chow AWC, et al. Intra-coronary guidewire mapping - a novel technique to guide ablation of human ventricular tachycardia. J Interv Card Electrophysiol 2007;18:143–54.
3. Baher A, Shah DJ, Valderrabano M. Coronary venous ethanol infusion for the treatment of refractory ventricular tachycardia. Heart Rhythm 2012;9:1637–9.
4. Verna E, Repetto S, Saveri C, et al. Myocardial dissection following successful chemical ablation of ventricular tachycardia. Eur Heart J 1992;13:844–6.
5. Brugada P, de Swart H, Smeets JL, et al. Transcoronary chemical ablation of ventricular tachycardia. Circulation 1989;79:475–82.
6. Dailey SM, Kay GN, Epstein AE, et al. Modification of late potentials by intracoronary ethanol infusion. Pacing Clin Electrophysiol 1992;15:1646–50.
7. Kay GN, Epstein AE, Bubien RS, et al. Intracoronary ethanol ablation for the treatment of recurrent sustained ventricular tachycardia. J Am Coll Cardiol 1992;19:159–68.
8. Nellens P, Gürsoy S, Andries E, et al. Transcoronary chemical ablation of arrhythmias. Pacing Clin Electrophysiol 1992;15:1368–73.
9. Sacher F, Sobieszczyk P, Tedrow U, et al. Transcoronary ethanol ventricular tachycardia ablation in the modern electrophysiology era. Heart Rhythm 2008;5:62–8.
10. Steven D, Roberts-Thomson KC, Seiler J, et al. Ventricular tachycardia arising from the aortomitral continuity in structural heart disease characteristics and therapeutic considerations for an anatomically challenging area of origin. Circ Arrhythm Electrophysiol 2009;2:660–6.
11. Tokuda M, Sobieszczyk P, Eisenhauer AC, et al. Transcoronary ethanol ablation for recurrent ventricular tachycardia after failed catheter ablation: an update. Circ Arrhythmia Electrophysiol 2011;4:889–96.
12. Okishige K, Andrews TC, Friedman PL. Suppression of incessant polymorphic ventricular tachycardia by selective intracoronary ethanol infusion. Pacing Clin Electrophysiol 1991;14:188–95.
13. de Paola AA, Gomes JA, Miyamoto MH, et al. Transcoronary chemical ablation of ventricular tachycardia in chronic chagasic myocarditis. J Am Coll Cardiol 1992;20:480–2.
14. Qi XQ, Gao RL, Wang FZ, et al. Transcoronary chemical ablation of ventricular tachycardia. Chin Med J (Engl) 1992;105:247–50.
15. Gursoy S, Nellens P, Guiraudon G, et al. Epicardial and subselective transcoronary chemical ablation of incessant ventricular tachycardia. Cathet Cardiovasc Diagn 1993;28:323–7.
16. Miller MA, Kini AS, Reddy VY, et al. Transcoronary ethanol ablation of ventricular tachycardia via an anomalous first septal perforating artery. Heart Rhythm 2011;8:1606–7.
17. Inada K, Seiler J, Roberts-Thomson KC, et al. Substrate characterization and catheter ablation for monomorphic ventricular tachycardia in patients with apical hypertrophic cardiomyopathy. J Cardiovasc Electrophysiol 2011;22:41–8.
18. Tholakanahalli VN, Bertog S, Roukoz H, et al. Catheter ablation of ventricular tachycardia using intracoronary wire mapping and coil embolization: description of a new technique. Heart Rhythm 2012;10:292–6.
19. Sivagangabalan G, Barry MA, Huang K, et al. Bipolar ablation of the interventricular septum is more efficient at creating a transmural line than sequential unipolar ablation. Pacing Clin Electrophysiol 2010;33:16–26.
20. Iyer V, Gambhir A, Desai SP, et al. Successful simultaneous unipolar radiofrequency ablation of septal ventricular tachycardia using 2 ablation catheters. Heart Rhythm 2014;11:710–3.
21. Koruth JS, Dukkipati S, Miller MA, et al. Bipolar irrigated radiofrequency ablation: a therapeutic option for refractory intramural atrial and ventricular tachycardia circuits. Heart Rhythm 2012;9:1932–41.
22. Gizurarson S, Spears D, Sivagangabalan G, et al. Bipolar ablation for deep intra-myocardial circuits: human ex vivo development and in vivo experience. Europace 2014;16:1684–8.
23. Teh AW, Reddy VY, Koruth JS, et al. Bipolar radiofrequency catheter ablation for refractory ventricular outflow tract arrhythmias. J Cardiovasc Electrophysiol 2014;25:1093–9.

24. Couch OJ. Cardiac aneurysm with ventricular tachycardia and subsequent excision of aneurysm; case report. Circulation 1959;20:251–3.

25. Guiraudon G, Fontaine G, Frank R, et al. Encircling endocardial ventriculotomy: a new surgical treatment for life-threatening ventricular tachycardias resistant to medical treatment following myocardial infarction. Ann Thorac Surg 1978;26:438–44.

26. Josephson ME, Harken AH, Horowitz LN. Endocardial excision: a new surgical technique for the treatment of recurrent ventricular tachycardia. Circulation 1979;60:1430–9.

27. Mathuria NS, Vaseghi M, Buch E, et al. Successful ablation of an epicardial ventricular tachycardia using a surgical ablation tool. Circ Arrhythmia Electrophysiol 2011;4:e84–6.

28. Mulloy DP, Bhamidipati CM, Stone ML, et al. Cryoablation during left ventricular assist device implantation reduces postoperative ventricular tachyarrhythmias. J Thorac Cardiovasc Surg 2013;145:1207–13.

29. Soejima K, Couper G, Cooper JM, et al. Subxiphoid surgical approach for epicardial catheter-based mapping and ablation in patients with prior cardiac surgery or difficult pericardial access. Circulation 2004;110:1197–201.

30. Maury P, Leobon B, Duparc A, et al. Epicardial catheter ablation of ventricular tachycardia using surgical subxyphoid approach. Europace 2007;9:212–5.

31. Maury P, Marcheix B, Duparc A, et al. Surgical catheter ablation of ventricular tachycardia using left thoracotomy in a patient with hindered access to the left ventricle. Pacing Clin Electrophysiol 2009; 32:556–60.

32. Michowitz Y, Mathuria N, Tung R, et al. Hybrid procedures for epicardial catheter ablation of ventricular tachycardia: value of surgical access. Heart Rhythm 2010;7:1635–43.

33. Anter E, Hutchinson MD, Deo R, et al. Surgical ablation of refractory ventricular tachycardia in patients with nonischemic cardiomyopathy. Circ Arrhythmia Electrophysiol 2011;4:494–500.

34. Patel M, Rojas F, Shabari FR, et al. Safety and feasibility of open chest epicardial mapping and ablation of ventricular tachycardia during the period of left ventricular assist device implantation. J Cardiovasc Electrophysiol 2016;27:95–101.

35. Sharma A, Wong D, Weidlich G, et al. Noninvasive stereotactic radiosurgery (CyberHeart) for creation of ablation lesions in the atrium. Heart Rhythm 2010;7:802–10.

36. Cvek J, Neuwirth R, Knybel L, et al. Cardiac radiosurgery for malignant ventricular tachycardia. Cureus 2014;6:e190.

37. Loo BW, Soltys SG, Wang L, et al. Stereotactic ablative radiotherapy for the treatment of refractory cardiac ventricular arrhythmia. Circ Arrhythmia Electrophysiol 2015;8:748–50.

Ablation of Ventricular Tachycardia in Arrhythmogenic Right Ventricular Dysplasia

Rajeev K. Pathak, MBBS, PhD, Fermin C. Garcia, MD*

KEYWORDS

- Arrhythmogenic right ventricular cardiomyopathy • Catheter ablation • Electroanatomical mapping

KEY POINTS

- Endocardial and epicardial electroanatomical mapping and ablation is a safe and effective therapy in the treatment of right ventricle arrhythmias occurring in the setting of arrhythmogenic right ventricular cardiomyopathy.
- Careful mapping and ablation plans should be tailored for each individual patient based on their comorbidities and ventricular tachycardia (VT) morphologies.
- Activation and entrainment mapping are the preferred techniques to identify critical parts of VT circuits and targeted for ablation.
- In the event of unmappable VTs, substrate mapping and pace mapping will help identifying the potential surrogate markers and landmarks that will serve as references for linear ablation.
- Strict hemodynamic monitoring during the ablation procedure will help minimize the complications associated to endocardial and epicardial VT ablation.

INTRODUCTION

Arrhythmogenic right ventricular cardiomyopathy (ARVD) is an heterogeneous genetically determined heart muscle disease clinically characterized by life-threatening ventricular tachycardias (VTs) and/or heart failure that mostly involves the right ventricle (RV) but may have involved the left ventricle (LV) in the initial stages of the disease.[1]

The RV myocardial abnormalities that favor the occurrence of VT are concentrated to the RV free-wall, usually sparing the RV septum. The affected regions are usually the anterior infundibular portion of the RV, the basal inferior RV (in the proximity of the acute angle of the heart), and the RV apex, completing the so-called triangle of dysplasia.[2] Although histologically affected, the RV apex is not a frequent site of origin of VTs in the setting of ARVD.[3]

In the overall management of ARVD, recognition of ARVD as the underlying pathologic condition in a patient presenting with RV tachycardia is pivotal. The diagnosis is based on reported task force criteria, including RV dilatation and dysfunction, and identification of multiple RV tachycardia morphologies and baseline electrocardiogram (ECG) abnormalities (**Fig. 1**). These baseline ECG signs include incomplete or complete right bundle branch block, T-wave inversion in the anterior precordial leads (V1 to V4), postexcitation Epsilon waves, and selective prolongation (25 ms) of the QRS duration in leads V1 to V3 compared with lead V6. After establishing the diagnosis, the next

Clinical Cardiac Electrophysiology, Cardiovascular Medicine Division, Hospital of the University of Pennsylvania, 9 Founders Pavilion – Cardiology, 3400 Spruce Street, Philadelphia, PA 19104, USA
* Corresponding author.
E-mail address: fermin.garcia@uphs.upenn.edu

Card Electrophysiol Clin 9 (2017) 99–106
http://dx.doi.org/10.1016/j.ccep.2016.10.007
1877-9182/17/Published by Elsevier Inc.

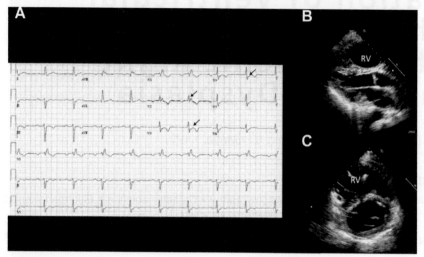

Fig. 1. (*A*) Characteristic baseline 12-lead ECG in a patient with ARVD. Note the abnormalities in depolarization (Epsilon waves, *arrows*) and T-wave inversion across the precordium. (*B, C*) Two-dimensional echocardiograms show enlarged RV and normal LV in the same patient.

step is accurate risk stratification of patients for sudden cardiac death and need for intracardiac defibrillator (ICD). Another component of management is the treatment of ventricular arrhythmias (VAs) with medication or catheter ablation (CA). The final component of management is preventing progression of the disease. Although all these steps are equally important and warrant discussion, this review focuses on the CA for VA in patients with ARVD.[4]

VENTRICULAR TACHYCARDIA ABLATION APPROACH

Although endocardial VT mapping and ablation frequently result in adequate arrhythmia control, notorious discrepancies have arisen regarding the long-term outcome of these patients. As a result, for a long time, CA in the setting of ARVD was considered as a palliative treatment of patients with drug refractory and recurrent or incessant VAs. However, limited efficacy of antiarrhythmic drugs (AAD), as well as the progressive nature of the arrhythmogenic substrate, remained a major challenge. Recently, better understanding of the pathologic state and due to rapid advancement in the ablation strategies, CA has become the treatment of choice in ARVD patients developing VAs.[5–7]

In the past, especially due to the more extensive epicardial pathologic substrate, endocardial-only approaches may have led to limited results, with a noninducibility rate at the end of the procedure ranging from 46% to 75%, and a VT recurrence rate up to 91% during a 3-year follow-up.[3,8,9]

Approaches using a combination of endocardial and epicardial ablation have shown to significantly improve the long-term VT-free survival with limited need for AADs, particularly amiodarone, in most patients.[6,10,11] The current approach of CA in ARVD comprises the abolition of all inducible VTs and an extensive modification on both endocardial and epicardial substrate. Only this approach has been demonstrated to reduce AAD-free VT recurrences.[5,10]

However, due to technical challenges, at this stage CA should only be performed in expert centers and should only be considered in patients symptomatic for frequent premature ventricular complex or nonsustained ventricular tachycardia, or recurrent sustained drug-refractory VT.[8,12]

Preprocedural Planning

When CA is considered in an ARVD patient presenting with RV-VT, preprocedural planning is prudent. An individualized preparation of the mapping and ablation strategy should be planned based on the initial clinical evaluation and cardiac hemodynamic status, including the degree of RV and/or LV function. If possible, optimization of fluid status should be attempted to minimize the incidence of intraprocedural complications related to pump failure. Additionally, it is important to assess for the hemodynamic tolerance of the clinical VT to anticipate the possibility of intraprocedural collapse. Moreover, 12-lead ECG documentation of all VT morphologies, as well as ICD electrograms (EGMs), if available, can be used to compare spontaneous and induced VT during the procedure. The 12-lead ECG characteristics are important predictors of the location of the arrhythmia and aid in preparing for an early epicardial approach, for which specific patient's preparation, including the need for general anesthesia, is of special concern.[13–15]

Ablation Procedure

The procedure is usually started under conscious sedation because general anesthesia can make the VT less inducible. General anesthesia and mechanical ventilation are reserved for cases in which the epicardial approach is necessary. Epicardial procedures under deep sedation with midazolam and remifentanil have been described; however, in ARVD patient general anesthesia is preferred due to a lower complication rate (ie, avoiding patient movement during long procedures) and better patient management in case of severe complications such as RV wall perforation at the time of epicardial access.[16] Whenever possible, AADs are discontinued at least 5 half-lives before the procedure.

Endocardial Voltage Mapping

Careful identification of valvular and intracavitary structures is critical during RV-VT mapping. At the outset, intracardiac echocardiograph (ICE)-guided biventricular 3-dimensional geometry should be constructed. Also, ICE is helpful and permits for real-time monitoring of catheter position to anatomically guide the mapping and ablation procedures.

After ICE reconstruction of the endocardial surface, a detailed voltage mapping of the RV should be performed. A sinus or paced rhythm endocardial high-density point-by-point voltage map of the RV is made with particular attention to the perivalvular regions that are frequently involved in the disease (**Fig. 2**). A cut-off for normal tissues of 1.5 mV and 5.5 mV (8.3 mV for the LV) are widely accepted for the definition of abnormal bipolar and unipolar voltage, respectively (see **Fig. 2** A, B).[17,18] A wider extension of the abnormal unipolar voltage area than the abnormal bipolar 1 is common in ARVD and indicates a larger substrate in the midwall and subepicardium (away from the endocardium).[19] Abnormal signals representing diseased myocardial tissue and border zone are considered between 0.5 to 1.5 mV. Fractionated and late potentials extending beyond the QRS are tagged in the map and are of particular utility when pace mapping is used to correlate the arrhythmia with the diseased myocardium that incorporates a critical portion of the reentrant VT circuit. It is useful to tag these sites to rapidly direct attention to these areas during VT mapping because, frequently, these abnormal EGM sites represent a critical component of the VT or to target for ablation later in the procedure.[20] Late or fractionated potentials are usually distributed in clusters within the

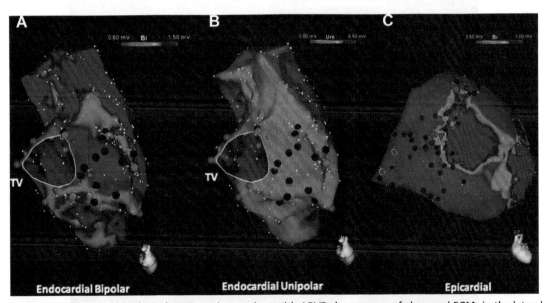

Fig. 2. (*A*) Endocardial bipolar voltage map in a patient with ARVD shows areas of abnormal EGMs in the lateral wall at the level of tricuspid valve. (*B*) The endocardial unipolar voltage map suggests a much larger abnormal substrate in the epicardium. (*C*) The epicardial bipolar voltage map confirms a very extensive abnormal substrate in the epicardium, as opposed to the endocardial counterpart. Black dots represent areas with late potentials. Blue dots represent areas with fractionated signals.

abnormal voltage area but sometimes they can be found even in areas with higher voltage. Thus, careful attention should be paid to the EGMs at every voltage point taken during mapping (**Fig. 3**).[21] Additionally, pace mapping is performed at sites where pathologic potentials were recorded, a good matching between paced QRS with spontaneous VT in presence of a long stimulus to QRS time leads to the identification of critical isthmuses that should be targeted.

Epicardial Mapping

Epicardial access

Access to the pericardial space is commonly obtained using the percutaneous subxiphoid approach originally described by Sosa and colleagues.[22] The skin in the subxiphoid region is sterilized and anesthetized. A 17-gauge Tuohy needle (originally designed for epidural access) is used to perform the puncture. The needle is directed to the left shoulder and oriented to the left border of the subxiphoid process and the left rib. The angle between the needle and the thorax determines the area of the ventricle accessed. The posterior approach to pericardial puncture is preferred because a dilated RV may increase the risks associated with an anterior needle pass.

However, in case of accidental RV perforation, identification is critical because withdrawing the wire before advancing the sheath is usually of no consequence. Additionally, during a posterior approach, careful attention has to be given to the orientation of the needle, given the potential risk of liver damage as the needle is directed deeper in the subxiphoid area.

The needle is slowly advanced under fluoroscopic and/or ICE guidance through the area between the diaphragm and the chest wall until the cardiac pulsation may be appreciated because the pericardium is indented. At this point, a small amount of contrast fluid is injected to appreciate the location of the needle tip and the tension of the pericardium. The perforation of the pericardium is then performed using a floppy guidewire passed through the Tuohy needle and used as a probe. Once in the pericardial space, the wire should be visualized in multiple fluoroscopic projections using ICE to ensure that it surrounds the cardiac silhouette before insertion of the pericardial sheath. At this point, the sheath could be advanced over the guidewire into the pericardial space. This sheath is then attached to a suction system to avoid fluid accumulation during mapping and ablation while using an irrigated catheter.

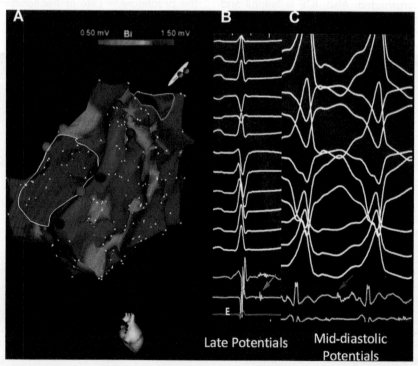

Fig. 3. (A) Bipolar endocardial voltage map shows an area of abnormal voltage and scar (0.5–1.5 mV). The star indicates the area of late potentials. (B) Low-voltage EGMs (*green arrow*) and late potentials are recorded from the area of late potentials. (C) Mid-diastolic potentials (*red arrow*) are seen in the area.

Epicardial mapping

After the epicardial access is obtained, a sinus or paced rhythm epicardial high-density point-by-point voltage map should be made with more rigid voltage criteria to limit the influence of epicardial fat and coronary vasculature. The reference value reported for defining abnormal EGMs in the epicardium is less than 1.0 mV.[10] To further limit the influence of epicardial fat and small-vessel coronary vasculature (ie, vessels that cannot be directly appreciated by coronary angiogram) on the low-voltage region, the contiguous low-voltage EGMs has to demonstrate not only a low amplitude but also signals with discrete late potentials (recorded after the QRS of the surface ECG) and demonstrate broad multicomponent or split signals within the boundary of the defined contiguous low-voltage abnormality (see **Fig. 2**C). Signals larger than 1.0 mV that also demonstrate abnormal, multicomponent, or split or late signal should also be tagged and, if adjacent to confluent areas of low voltage, included in substrate-based ablation targets.

Catheter Ablation

A programmed ventricular stimulation protocol should be performed to induce VT with up to 3 extrastimuli delivered from at least 2 different RV sites (usually RV apex and RV outflow tract) of at least 2 drive cycle lengths. Twelve-lead morphology and ICD EGMs morphology of all induced VTs are compared with those occurring spontaneously. An induced VT is identified as clinical when it matches the cycle length and morphology of stored ICD EGMs (near-field and far-field) and/or the 12-lead ECG, when available.

Stable Ventricular Tachycardias

The primary end point of the ablation is to eliminate all the mappable clinical and nonclinical VTs. All the induced VTs with a cycle length greater than 250 milliseconds should be considered potentially relevant and consequently addressed for ablation. For hemodynamically tolerated VTs, activation and entrainment mapping is performed at sites showing diastolic activity to identify critical sites of the VT reentrant circuit. Critical sites showing entrainment with concealed QRS fusion and return cycle within 30 milliseconds of the VT cycle length with matching stimulus to QRS interval and local EGM to QRS interval are defined as appropriate target sites for ablation.[23] Catheter contact and lesion formation are monitored with the use of ICE and effective lesion creation is indexed by bipolar signal attenuation; increase in local pace-capture threshold; and, very importantly, by the

disappearance of isolated potentials or high-frequency late EGM components after ablation.[3,24]

Unstable Ventricular Tachycardias

Ablation of hemodynamically unstable VTs requires a substrate modification approach. The site of origin of VT can be approximated using pace mapping to reproduce the VT QRS complex morphology and to identify sites with a long stimulus to QRS interval, fractionated potentials, late potentials, and local abnormal ventricular activity, especially within the low-voltage zone, with the aim to eliminate the critical components of the potential circuits.

Tagging of abnormal EGMs could also be used to identify conducting channels within the scar, between 2 confluent scar areas, or between a scar and the tricuspid annulus. These channels represent slow pathways orthodromically activated inside the scar during sinus rhythm and are defined by the presence of at least 2 recordings of isolated late potentials with the delayed component showing sequential orthodromic activation.[6,25,26] Entrance and exit sites could also be identified at the conducting channel level, with the entrance site having the shortest delay between the far-field component and the delayed local component.[6] The presence and site of conducting channels could also be approximated by a color-coded voltage map adjustment of the lower and upper thresholds (voltage channels). Once the voltage map is completed, the amplitude scale can be adjusted by setting the lower value at 0.2 mV and the upper value at 0.5 mV, allowing the identification of voltage channels differentiated from the surrounding scar tissue by a higher amplitude, bounded by 2 scar areas or 1 scar area and the tricuspid annulus, and connected to normal myocardium by at least 2 sites.[25,26]

Characteristically, linear and/or cluster lesions can be placed targeting previously identified critical sites by pace mapping, abnormal EGMs, or through channels transecting the abnormal myocardium and extending from the valve annulus to normal myocardium.[5,24] All recorded markedly abnormal fractionated split and late potentials should be targeted by ablation, with a specific emphasis on abnormal potentials recorded within a 2- to 3-cm radius of the site of origin, defined by entrainment mapping or the best pace map with the endpoint of signal modification or elimination in addition to any linear lesion. An extensive substrate modification is pursued on the epicardium, where linear lesions anchored to the valve annulus are limited by proximity to the right coronary artery.

Evidence suggests that, in patients with ARVD, RV activation is modified by the presence of confluent scar with a delayed epicardial activation suggestive of possible independent rather than direct transmural activation. This may predispose to VT circuits contained entirely within the epicardium. Successful endocardial ablation of such VT may be less likely given the poor transmural penetration of current ablation energy sources.[8] This is particularly likely to be a limitation when burning in the thickened, densely scarred RVs is seen in this condition. Though no randomized comparisons are available, the incorporation of epicardial mapping seems to be associated with better outcomes for ARVD-related VT ablation than does endocardial ablation alone. This is likely related to the increased ability to directly ablate the substrate for confined epicardial VT circuits when approaching these with a transpericardial, rather than transmural, strategy.[27]

Radiofrequency Ablation

Radiofrequency energy is usually applied with an open irrigated tip catheter using powers up to 40 W with a goal of 12 to 15 Ohm impedance drop or 10% decrease from the baseline impedance. Lesion duration is typically set for 60 to 90 seconds but further increases to greater than or equal to 3 minutes in duration can be applied at sites associated with transient suppression of VT, with monitoring to confirm stable impedance drop. Regarding epicardial ablation, coronary artery angiography should be performed before radiofrequency delivery to assess a safest distance of ablation sites from main epicardial coronary vessels (at least 1 cm). Moreover, sites of phrenic nerve capture during pacing should be marked to avoid the risk of permanent nerve injury during RF delivery. After the procedure, triamcinolone acetate is usually injected into the pericardial space to prevent postprocedure pericarditis and consequent adhesion formation.[28] The pericardial drain usually is left in place for 24 hours and should be removed only after echocardiographic confirmation of the absence of significant pericardial effusion.

Assessment of Acute Procedural Outcomes

Acute procedural success is usually assessed by programmed ventricular stimulation at the end of the procedure performed from at least 2 RV sites with at least 2 drive cycle lengths and defined as lack of inducibility of any VT with cycle length greater than 250 milliseconds. The predictive value of noninducibility at the end of the procedure is still a matter of debate with discordant reports.[29,30] Several factors may affect VT inducibility at the end of the procedure, including changes in AADs after ablation, particularly concerning amiodarone; changes in autonomic tone and/or the use of general anesthesia; and dynamical changes in ablation lesions that may either expand as a result of disruption of microcirculation, with consequent myocyte loss, or regress secondary to healing and resolution of acute edema.[31,32] Moreover, the patient may not be able to tolerate the stimulation protocol after a long ablation procedure. Recently, noninvasive programmed stimulation performed through the ICD in the days following the ablation procedure in patients without spontaneous VT recurrence, has been reported of great value in identifying patients at high risk of recurrence that may need more extensive ablation.[5,33]

Procedural Complications

Complications of VT ablation can be prevented by careful preprocedural preparation and patient individualization. Fluid status, ventricular function, and hemodynamic condition are evaluated noninvasively and invasively before the mapping and ablation procedure. During mapping and ablation, careful attention to the hemodynamics and constant monitoring under ICE to assess catheter position, and early recognition of a pericardial effusion are essential. By these means, early drainage of pericardial fluid and anticoagulation reversal will prevent cardiac tamponade. Risk of pulmonary embolism, RV perforation (anterior route epicardial access), liver laceration (posterior route epicardial access), and damage to the coronary artery and phrenic nerve are other potential complications that operators must bear in mind during mapping and ablation. Coronary angiography and high output pacing should be performed before any RF lesion is deployed on the epicardial RV surface. Assessment for phrenic nerve capture, although less frequently observed compared with epicardial LV mapping and ablation, is also recommended but usually not a limitation for energy delivery.

Postprocedure Care

Acute pericarditis, with its common signs and symptoms, is frequent after pericardial mapping and ablation. Treatments of pericarditis after ablation focus on pain relief and inflammation control. The cornerstone for the treatment is nonsteroidal anti-inflammatory drugs (NSAIDs), with ibuprofen being the preferred medication. Pain control is also managed with intravenous infusion of opioids. Intrapericardial administration of corticosteroids, usually triamcinolone (2 mg/kg or up to 300 mg/m^2) immediately on completion of the case while pericardial access is still available has been reported to effectively decrease inflammation and is routinely used in the authors' laboratory for pericardial mapping procedure.[28,34]

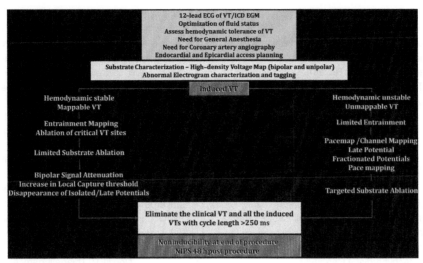

Fig. 4. Flow chart of the VT ablation approach in ARVD.

SUMMARY

Endocardial and epicardial electroanatomical mapping and ablation is a safe and effective therapy in the treatment of RV arrhythmias occurring in the setting of ARVD. Careful mapping and ablation plan should be tailored for each individual patient based on their comorbidities and VT morphologies (**Fig. 4**). Activation and entrainment mapping are the preferred techniques to identify critical parts of VT circuits and targeted for ablation. In the event of unmappable VTs, substrate mapping and pace mapping will help identify the potential surrogate markers and landmarks that will serve as references for linear ablation. Strict hemodynamic monitoring during the ablation procedure will help minimize the complications associated with endocardial and epicardial VT ablation.

REFERENCES

1. Basso C, Corrado D, Bauce B, et al. Arrhythmogenic right ventricular cardiomyopathy. Circ Arrhythm Electrophysiol 2012;5:1233–46.
2. Fontaine G, Fontaliran F, Hebert JL, et al. Arrhythmogenic right ventricular dysplasia. Annu Rev Med 1999;50:17–35.
3. Marchlinski FE, Zado E, Dixit S, et al. Electroanatomic substrate and outcome of catheter ablative therapy for ventricular tachycardia in setting of right ventricular cardiomyopathy. Circulation 2004;110: 2293–8.
4. Marcus FI, McKenna WJ, Sherrill D, et al. Diagnosis of arrhythmogenic right ventricular cardiomyopathy/dysplasia: proposed modification of the Task Force Criteria. Eur Heart J 2010;31:806–14.
5. Santangeli P, Zado ES, Supple GE, et al. Long-term outcome with catheter ablation of ventricular tachycardia in patients with arrhythmogenic right ventricular cardiomyopathy. Circ Arrhythm Electrophysiol 2015;8:1413–21.
6. Berruezo A, Fernandez-Armenta J, Mont L, et al. Combined endocardial and epicardial catheter ablation in arrhythmogenic right ventricular dysplasia incorporating scar dechanneling technique. Circ Arrhythm Electrophysiol 2012;5:111–21.
7. Marcus GM, Glidden DV, Polonsky B, et al. Efficacy of antiarrhythmic drugs in arrhythmogenic right ventricular cardiomyopathy: a report from the North American ARVC Registry. J Am Coll Cardiol 2009; 54:609–15.
8. Dalal D, Jain R, Tandri H, et al. Long-term efficacy of catheter ablation of ventricular tachycardia in patients with arrhythmogenic right ventricular dysplasia/cardiomyopathy. J Am Coll Cardiol 2007;50:432–40.
9. Verma A, Kilicaslan F, Schweikert RA, et al. Short- and long-term success of substrate-based mapping and ablation of ventricular tachycardia in arrhythmogenic right ventricular dysplasia. Circulation 2005; 111:3209–16.
10. Garcia FC, Bazan V, Zado ES, et al. Epicardial substrate and outcome with epicardial ablation of ventricular tachycardia in arrhythmogenic right ventricular cardiomyopathy/dysplasia. Circulation 2009; 120:366–75.
11. Bai R, Di Biase L, Shivkumar K, et al. Ablation of ventricular arrhythmias in arrhythmogenic right ventricular dysplasia/cardiomyopathy: arrhythmia-free survival after endo-epicardial substrate based mapping and ablation. Circ Arrhythm Electrophysiol 2011;4:478–85.
12. Philips B, Madhavan S, James C, et al. Outcomes of catheter ablation of ventricular tachycardia in

arrhythmogenic right ventricular dysplasia/cardiomy-opathy. Circ Arrhythm Electrophysiol 2012;5:499–505.

13. Josephson ME, Callans DJ. Using the twelve-lead electrocardiogram to localize the site of origin of ventricular tachycardia. Heart Rhythm 2005;2:443–6.

14. Tada H, Tadokoro K, Ito S, et al. Idiopathic ventricular arrhythmias originating from the tricuspid annulus: prevalence, electrocardiographic characteristics, and results of radiofrequency catheter ablation. Heart Rhythm 2007;4:7–16.

15. Bazan V, Bala R, Garcia FC, et al. Twelve-lead ECG features to identify ventricular tachycardia arising from the epicardial right ventricle. Heart Rhythm 2006;3:1132–9.

16. Mandel JE, Hutchinson MD, Marchlinski FE. Remi-fentanil-midazolam sedation provides hemodynamic stability and comfort during epicardial ablation of ventricular tachycardia. J Cardiovasc Electrophysiol 2011;22:464–6.

17. Campos B, Jauregui ME, Park KM, et al. New unipolar electrogram criteria to identify irreversibility of nonischemic left ventricular cardiomyopathy. J Am Coll Cardiol 2012;60:2194–204.

18. Hutchinson MD, Gerstenfeld EP, Desjardins B, et al. Endocardial unipolar voltage mapping to detect epicardial ventricular tachycardia substrate in patients with nonischemic left ventricular cardiomyopathy. Circ Arrhythm Electrophysiol 2011;4:49–55.

19. Polin GM, Haqqani H, Tzou W, et al. Endocardial unipolar voltage mapping to identify epicardial substrate in arrhythmogenic right ventricular cardiomyopathy/dysplasia. Heart Rhythm 2011;8:76–83.

20. de Bakker JM, van Capelle FJ, Janse MJ, et al. Fractionated electrograms in dilated cardiomyopathy: origin and relation to abnormal conduction. J Am Coll Cardiol 1996;27:1071–8.

21. Berte B, Sacher F, Cochet H, et al. Postmyocarditis ventricular tachycardia in patients with epicardial-only scar: a specific entity requiring a specific approach. J Cardiovasc Electrophysiol 2015;26:42–50.

22. Sosa E, Scanavacca M, d'Avila A, et al. A new technique to perform epicardial mapping in the electrophysiology laboratory. J Cardiovasc Electrophysiol 1996;7:531–6.

23. Hsia HH, Lin D, Sauer WH, et al. Relationship of late potentials to the ventricular tachycardia circuit defined by entrainment. J Interv Card Electrophysiol 2009;26:21–9.

24. Marchlinski FE, Callans DJ, Gottlieb CD, et al. Linear ablation lesions for control of unmappable ventricular

tachycardia in patients with ischemic and nonischemic cardiomyopathy. Circulation 2000;101:1288–96.

25. Arenal A, del Castillo S, Gonzalez-Torrecilla E, et al. Tachycardia-related channel in the scar tissue in patients with sustained monomorphic ventricular tachycardias: influence of the voltage scar definition. Circulation 2004;110:2568–74.

26. Hsia HH, Lin D, Sauer WH, et al. Anatomic characterization of endocardial substrate for hemodynamically stable reentrant ventricular tachycardia: identification of endocardial conducting channels. Heart Rhythm 2006;3:503–12.

27. Haqqani HM, Tschabrunn CM, Betensky BP, et al. Layered activation of epicardial scar in arrhythmogenic right ventricular dysplasia: possible substrate for confined epicardial circuits. Circ Arrhythm Electrophysiol 2012;5:796–803.

28. d'Avila A, Neuzil P, Thiagalingam A, et al. Experimental efficacy of pericardial instillation of anti-inflammatory agents during percutaneous epicardial catheter ablation to prevent postprocedure pericarditis. J Cardiovasc Electrophysiol 2007;18:1178–83.

29. Tokuda M, Tedrow UB, Kojodjojo P, et al. Catheter ablation of ventricular tachycardia in nonischemic heart disease. Circ Arrhythm Electrophysiol 2012;5:992–1000.

30. Piers SR, Leong DP, van Huls van Taxis CF, et al. Outcome of ventricular tachycardia ablation in patients with nonischemic cardiomyopathy: the impact of noninducibility. Circ Arrhythm Electrophysiol 2013;6:513–21.

31. Fenelon G, Brugada P. Delayed effects of radiofrequency energy: mechanisms and clinical implications. Pacing Clin Electrophysiol 1996;19:484–9.

32. Nath S, Whayne JG, Kaul S, et al. Effects of radiofrequency catheter ablation on regional myocardial blood flow. Possible mechanism for late electrophysiological outcome. Circulation 1994;89:2667–72.

33. Frankel DS, Mountantonakis SE, Zado ES, et al. Noninvasive programmed ventricular stimulation early after ventricular tachycardia ablation to predict risk of late recurrence. J Am Coll Cardiol 2012;59:1529–35.

34. Maisch B, Seferovic PM, Ristic AD, et al. Guidelines on the diagnosis and management of pericardial diseases executive summary; the Task force on the diagnosis and management of pericardial diseases of the European society of cardiology. Eur Heart J 2004;25:587–610.

Ablation of Ventricular Tachycardia in Congenital and Infiltrative Heart Disease

CrossMark

Adrianus P. Wijnmaalen, MD, PhD,
Katja Zeppenfeld, MD, PhD*

KEYWORDS

- Ventricular tachycardia • Catheter ablation • Congenital heart disease • Cardiac sarcoidosis

KEY POINTS

- Slow conducting anatomic isthmuses bordered by surgical scars, prosthetic material, and valve annuli are the dominant substrate for VT in repaired congenital heart disease.
- Identification and transsection of these anatomic isthmuses by catheter or surgical ablation leads to long-term VT-free survival in patients with repaired CHD and preserved biventricular function.
- Among infiltrative cardiac disease, cardiac sarcoidosis is the most important cause of ventricular arrhythmias.
- Catheter ablation in the advanced stage of cardiac sarcoidosis is challenging because of complex ventricular scars and an active inflammation.
- In most patients with cardiac sarcoidosis a significant decrease of the VT burden is achieved often requiring multiple procedures.

INTRODUCTION

Ventricular arrhythmias (VA) are frequently encountered in patients with structural heart disease and are an important cause of morbidity and sudden cardiac death (SCD). Most VAs in patients with ventricular scars are caused by reentry, which is facilitated by barriers of functional or fixed conduction block and zones of slow conduction. Radiofrequency catheter ablation (RFCA) targets the substrate and has the potential to prevent ventricular tachycardia (VT) recurrence. The nature and cause of ventricular scars and the prevalence and characteristics of VTs vary widely according to the underlying heart disease and surgical interventions. This article focuses on the substrate of VA and RFCA for VT in patients with surgically corrected congenital heart disease (CHD) and infiltrative heart disease.

VENTRICULAR ARRHYTHMIAS IN CONGENITAL HEART DISEASE

The incidence of moderate to severe CHD is 6 in 1000 live births.[1] Because of earlier surgical interventions and advances in medical care over the last decades more patients with repaired CHD (rCHD) survive to adulthood.[2] Accordingly, an increasing number of patients may be at risk for arrhythmias and SCD later in life.[3–5] SCD accounts for 19% of all deaths in adults with rCHD, often occurring in the fourth and fifth decades of life.[6] Sustained monomorphic VT and polymorphic VT/ventricular fibrillation (VF) are thought to be the dominant cause of SCD in this population.[6] Repaired cardiac defects associated with a high risk for VA and presumed arrhythmic deaths are tetralogy of Fallot (TOF) and transposition of the great arteries (TGA).[3,4,6,7] In patients with CHD

Department of Cardiology, Leiden University Medical Center, Leiden, The Netherlands
* Corresponding author. Department of Cardiology, Leiden University Medical Center, Albinusdreef 2, 2333ZA Leiden, The Netherlands
E-mail address: K.Zeppenfeld@lumc.nl

Card Electrophysiol Clin 9 (2017) 107–117
http://dx.doi.org/10.1016/j.ccep.2016.10.008
1877-9182/17/© 2016 Elsevier Inc. All rights reserved.

ventricular dysfunction has been associated with the occurrence of VA and SCD as in other cardiac disease with increased wall stress and interstitial and replacement fibrosis.[5,6] However, two-thirds of patients with rCHD who died suddenly had a preserved ventricular function before the event.[6] This suggests that non-heart-failure-related VT mechanisms and substrates may play an important role.[8,9] Because VTs often recur despite anti-arrhythmic drugs, and implantable cardioverter defibrillators (ICD) terminate but do not prevent arrhythmia recurrence, RFCA is an important treatment option.[10] A thorough understanding of the underlying mechanism and substrate of VT is crucial for risk stratification and treatment.

Tetralogy of Fallot

TOF is the most common form of cyanotic CHD.[1] It encompasses a subpulmonary stenosis, a sub-aortic ventricular septal defect (VSD), dextraposition of the aortic orifice, and as a consequence right ventricular (RV) hypertrophy. Since the 1960s a two-stage surgical procedure has been performed with initial palliative shunt operations and total repair later in childhood. Total repair includes patch closure of the VSD and relief of the infundibular or valvular RV outflow tract (RVOT) obstruction and was initially accomplished through a vertical or transverse right ventriculotomy often combined with the use of a large (transannular) patches. This often led to RV dysfunction and pulmonary regurgitation with chronic volume overload and subsequent RV dilatation and further functional impairment. Consequently, a transatrial-transpulmonary approach performed earlier in life, avoiding RV incision and the use of smaller transannular patches, has become the treatment of choice.[11] The type and timing of repair are decisive factors for the substrate of the late VTs.

Ventricular Arrhythmias and Anatomic Isthmus

The reported prevalence of monomorphic VT in the adult TOF population was 14.2% in a recent multicenter study accounting for 97.5% of all documented VAs.[12] Similarly, more than 80% of appropriate ICD therapy in patients with TOF with ICDs implanted for primary and secondary prevention is triggered by monomorphic VT.[13] These VTs are generally fast with heart rates greater than 200 bpm and may therefore cause hemodynamic compromise and SCD.[9,10,13,14]

Areas of dense fibrosis after surgical incisions, patch material, and valve annuli are the unexcitable borders of anatomic isthmuses (AI) that have been shown to contain critical isthmuses of VT reentry circuits. Four AI have been identified. Isthmus 1 is bordered by the tricuspid annulus and scar or patch material in the anterior RVOT/RV, isthmus 2 by the pulmonary annulus and the RVOT/RV incision or patch sparing the pulmonary annulus, isthmus 3 by the pulmonary annulus and the VSD patch, and isthmus 4 by the VSD patch and the tricuspid annulus in patient with a muscular VSD (**Fig. 1**).[14]

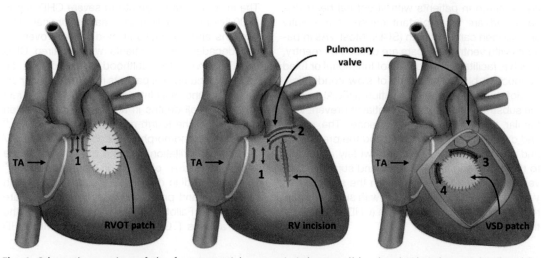

Fig. 1. Schematic overview of the four potential anatomic isthmuses (*blue brackets*): isthmus 1 bordered by tricuspid annulus and right ventricular outflow tract patch/right ventricular incision, isthmus 2 by right ventricular incision and pulmonary valve, isthmus 3 by pulmonary valve and ventricular septal defect patch, and isthmus 4 by ventricular septal defect patch and tricuspid annulus. TA, tricuspid annulus. (*Adapted from* Kapel GF, Sacher F, Dekkers OM, et al. Arrhythmogenic anatomic isthmuses identified by electroanatomical mapping are the substrate for ventricular tachycardia in repaired tetralogy of Fallot. Euro Heart J 2016. [Epub ahead of print]; with permission.)

Not all AIs are related to VT. Specific isthmus characteristics depending on the malformation but also pathologic remodeling over time may be important to form the substrate for VT decades after surgery. A recent detailed voltage and activation mapping study in patients with repaired TOF (rTOF) with and without spontaneous and/or inducible VT has further elucidated the specific isthmus characteristics required to sustain monomorphic VT (**Fig. 2**).[9] Of the 41 spontaneous and induced VTs in 28 patients, 37 were proven related to an AI with specific characteristics, referred to as arrhythmogenic isthmus. Most VTs were related to isthmus 3.

The best discriminator between arrhythmogenic and nonarrhythmogenic isthmuses was slow conduction (<0.5/ms) through the isthmus during sinus rhythm.[9] Of importance, none of the 44 patients with rTOF without documented and/or inducible VT had such a slow conducting AI (SCAI). This strong association between SCAI and VT has important implications. First, in symptomatic patients SCAI can be targeted by RFCA even if VT is not inducible or not tolerated. Second, electroanatomic mapping to identify SCAI may be an important tool for risk stratification, in particular in patients with preserved biventricular function.

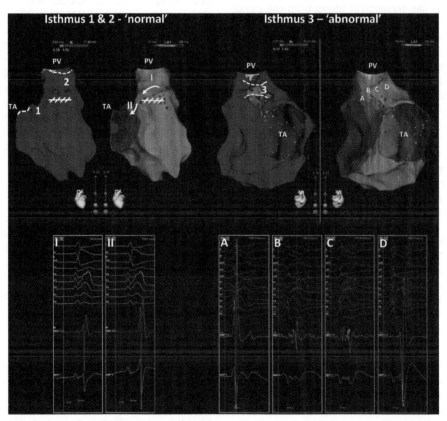

Fig. 2. Electroanatomic assessment of anatomic isthmus 1, 2, 3, and 4. (*Left Side*) Example of electroanatomic normal isthmuses 1 and 2 in a patient without inducible VT. (*Top Left*) 3D electroanatomic reconstruction of the right ventricle (anterior view) displayed as color-coded voltage map (*left, purple* indicates normal voltages) and activation map (*right, red* indicates early activation, *purple* late activation). The gray tags (electrically unexcitable scar) correspond to a previous right ventricular incision (marked with the *white line*). (*Lower Left*) Normal bipolar electrograms with a peak-to-peak amplitude of greater than or equal to 1.5 mV recorded from isthmus 1 (site II) and isthmus 2 (site I). (*Right Side*) Isthmus 3 of a patient with inducible VT is shown. (*Top Right*) 3D electroanatomic reconstruction of the right ventricle (posterior view) displayed as voltage map and activation map. The gray tags correspond with the ventricular septal defect patch. (*Lower Right*) Electrograms recorded through isthmus 3 (sites A–B–C–D) are shown as indicated. The first and last electrogram (*A* and *D*) are normal, the second and third electrogram (*B* and *C*) are abnormal. EGM, electrogram; PV, pulmonary valve; TA, tricuspid annulus. (*Adapted from* Kapel GF, Sacher F, Dekkers OM, et al. Arrhythmogenic anatomic isthmuses identified by electroanatomical mapping are the substrate for ventricular tachycardia in repaired tetralogy of Fallot. Eur Heart J 2016. [Epub ahead of print]; with permission.)

Transposition of the Great Arteries

Dextro-TGA (d-TGA) is the second most common form of cyanotic heart disease.[1] In d-TGA there is a concordant atrioventricular (AV) connection with ventriculararterial discordance with the aorta connecting to the morphologic RV and the pulmonary trunk to the morphologic left ventricle. D-TGA can occur as an isolated defect (simple d-TGA) or in combination with other congenital malformations (complex d-TGA). In complex TGA the most common associated malformations are VSD and right or left ventricular (LV) outflow obstruction.

From 1959 until the 1980s most newborns with TGA underwent an atrial switch procedure in the first year of life, redirecting blood from the caval veins to the LV using the atrial septum, pericardial, or synthetic material. Nowadays, the arterial switch procedure, in which the aorta and pulmonary trunk are disconnected and switched to the correct ventricle, is the treatment of choice. In complex d-TGA ventricular scar and/or patch material may be the consequence of the repair of associated lesions and can form the substrate for VTs similar to rTOF.[15–17]

Following the atrial switch operation reported SCD rates are 4% to 9% 20 years after surgery.[7] VT or VF have been recorded in patients presenting with (aborted) SCD, which may be the primary arrhythmia, but may also be the consequence of rapid conducted atrial arrythmias.[7,15] In simple rTGA without ventricular scars or patches monomorphic VT amendable to RFCA is uncommon.[7,16] In complex d-TGA, however, cases of AIs between a VSD patch and the pulmonary valve and between a basoseptal dense scar and the aortic valve serving as substrate for VT successfully targeted by RFCA have been reported.[10,17]

Catheter Ablation

RFCA has been shown to be an effective treatment of monomorphic VT in patients with rCHD. **Table 1** summarizes data on RFCA in rCHD published over the last decades.

Detailed knowledge of the malformation and prior surgical records that usually provide information on the location of surgical incisions and patch material that may define reentry circuit borders is important. In addition, preprocedural evaluation of ventricular function and residual lesions that may require surgery is mandatory. Contrast-enhanced (CE) MRI has been shown to enhance substrate identification before RFCA in morphologic normal hearts.[17–19] In a patient with repaired complex d-TGA, CE-MRI-derived reconstruction of an AI related to

VT has been reported.[17] Whether current MRI technology is able to identify SCAI requires further studies.

A cornerstone of substrate mapping and ablation of VT in rCHD is the identification and reconstruction of SCAI during sinus rhythm or paced rhythm facilitated by three-dimensional (3D) mapping systems.[9,14,20] High-output pacing is performed at sites with bipolar voltage amplitudes less than 0.5 mV to identify unexcitable tissue. Sites with noncapture have been shown to coincide with patch material or surgical scars, which can serve as boundaries of AI.[10,14,21] 3D maps can be displayed as voltage and activation maps and information on specific isthmus characteristics (length, widths, conduction velocity) is retrieved to identify SCAI that are potentially related to VT (see **Fig. 2**).

Ventricular programmed electrical stimulation is still used to induce VT and obtain the 12-lead electrocardiogram morphology. If VT is well tolerated the critical VT circuit isthmus site is identified by activation and entrainment mapping. For hemodynamically poorly tolerated VT pace-mapping is used to determine whether an AI is related to a reentry circuit. Arrhythmogenic AI is transected by a linear RF lesion connecting the adjoining anatomic boundaries.[10,14,20]

End Points and Outcome

Complete ablation success after RFCA of VT in structural heart disease is often defined as noninducibility of any monomorphic VT; however, VTs may recur even if this end point has been reached.[22] Considering the importance of AI as substrate for VT in rCHD a combined end point of noninducibility and successful transection of the VT-related AI has been proposed.[10] Transection of an isthmus is confirmed by noncapture at high-output pacing along the ablation line. Conduction block of the isthmus is further supported by the presence of double potentials; a change in the activation sequence; and, most reliably, differential pacing.[10] The first study reporting on the combined end point included 34 patients with rCHD. VT related AIs were identified for all but 2 of 61 induced VTs. In 25 (74%) patients all VT-related isthmus could be successfully transected resulting in noninducibility of any VT. None of these patients experienced any monomorphic VT during follow-up of 46 months.[10] In another study 14 of the 21 patients with various CHD (48% rTOF) had an AI-dependent VT, which could be successfully transected in 8 of 14 patients. None of the patients with confirmed transection of the VT-related isthmus and

Table 1
RFCA in CHD, cohort studies

Author Year	Type and Number CHD	Patients (n)	Method	Mean VTCL (ms)	Successful RFCA, n (%)	Spontaneous VT After RFCA, n (%)	Follow-up (mo)
Gonska et al,[42] 1996	7 TOF, 1 TGA + VSD, 1 VSD, 2 PS	11	AM	377	9 (82)	1 (9)	20 ± 9
Morwood et al,[43] 2004	8 TOF, 3 VSD, 3 miscellaneous	14	NR	NR	10 (50)	Only successful RFCA reported: 4 (40)	NR
Furushima et al,[44] 2006	4 TOF, 3 DORV	7	AM, LL	346	4 (57)	0 (0)	61 ± 29
Kriebel et al,[20] 2007	TOF	10	AM, SM	270	8 (80)	2 (20)	35 (range 3–52)
Zeppenfeld et al,[14] 2007	9 TOF, 1 AVSD, 1 TGA + VSD	11	AM, SM, LL	276	11 (100)	0 (0)	30 ± 29
Kapel et al,[10] 2015	TOF 28, TGA + sPS 1, TGA + VSD 1 VSD + sPS 1, PS 1 VSD + bAV 1, AVSD 1	34	AM, SM, LL	295	25 (74)	0 (0) (success) 4 (44) (no success)	46 ± 29
Van Zyl et al,[21] 2016	TOF 10, TGA 4, VSD 2, Ebstein 2, PS 1, TA 1, AS 1	21	AM, SM, LL	300	17 (81)	3 (14)	33 ± 7

Abbreviations: AM, activation mapping; AS, aortic stenosis; AVSD, atrioventricular septal defect; bAV, bicuspid aortic valve; DORV, double outlet right ventricle; LL, linear lesions; NR, not reported; PS, pulmonary stenosis; SM, substrate mapping; sPS, (sub)pulmonary stenosis; TA, truncus arteriosus; VTCL, ventricular tachycardia cycle length.
Adapted from Kapel GF, Reichlin T, Wijnmaalen AP, et al. Re-entry using anatomically determined isthmuses: a curable ventricular tachycardia in repaired congenital heart disease. Circ Arrhythm Electrophysiol 2015;8:102–9; with permission.

noninducibility experienced VT recurrence; in contrast, in two of six patients without confirmed isthmus block but noninducibility after ablation VT recurred.[21]

Inability to achieve isthmus block may be caused by the hypertrophoid myocardium or the prosthetic material both preventing transmural lesions. Pulmonary homografts or patch material covering the infundibular septum are important reasons for a failed ablation procedure of isthmus 3 and 4.[10,23] The proximity of the His bundle is another anatomic reason for withholding RFCA to avoid total AV block.[10] If ablation from the RV side fails a left-sided approach should be considered for AI with a septal location. Ablation from the LV outflow tract and the right- and noncoronary aortic cusps has improved ablation outcome in one series.[23]

Preventive Isthmus Ablation

The strong association between SCAI and macrorentrant VT and the reported failure to transect isthmus 3 by RFCA after pulmonary valve replacement may justify preventive isthmus ablation in those that undergo reoperation. Preoperative mapping can identify SCAI that can be transected intraoperatively. The feasibility of surgical cryoablation has been demonstrated in a series of 22 patients scheduled for pulmonary valve replacement. During surgery the VSD patch and pulmonary valve were connected (isthmus 3) and in selected patients additional cryolesions were applied connecting the verticulotomy with the tricuspid annulus (isthmus 1) and pulmonary annulus (isthmus 2). VT recurred in only one patient during 7 years of follow-up after surgery. In this study conduction block along the line has not been confirmed. Whether this approach is sufficient to transect arrhythmogenic isthmuses without being proarrhythmic if previously nonarrhythmogenic isthmuses are targeted requires further evaluation.[24]

INFILTRATIVE DISEASE

Infiltrative cardiomyopathies include rare inherited or acquired diseases, characterized by the deposition of abnormal substances in the heart altering normal structure and function. Diffuse deposition in the interstitium or myocytes can result in increased wall thickness, typical for amyloidosis and Fabry disease. In contrast, localized cell death, granulomatous inflammation, and myocardial fibrosis may lead to regional wall motion abnormalities as found in cardiac sarcoidosis (CS).[25,26] Monomorphic VA can be caused by reentry facilitated by localized myocardial scar but may also be the consequence of abnormal automaticity of triggered activity.

Amyloidosis

Amyloidosis results from deposition of fibrils composed of a variety of low-molecular-weight proteins in extracellular tissue. Cardiac involvement is associated with a poor prognosis caused by heart failure and, less frequently, SCD.[27] In a cohort of 133 patients with biopsy-proven AL amyloidosis total mortality was 53% at 1 year, and 22 of 71 were sudden death.[27] Small series of ICD carriers, however, revealed a low prevalence of VA with 11% to 28% appropriate ICD therapies for any sustained VA during follow-up of greater than 2 years.[28,29] Data on RFCA for VA in cardiac amyloidosis is limited to two reports of a total of three patients.[30,31] In two patients recurrent PVCs (premature ventricular contraction) inducing VF and in one patient a monomophic VT were successfully targeted by ablation. All three arrhythmias had a focal source mapped to an LV area with normal electrograms, potentially related to the Purkinje system in one.[30,31]

Fabry Disease

Fabry disease is a rare lysosome storage disorder with X-chromosomal inheritance resulting in accumulation of glycolipids in multiple cell types with the development of a cardiomyopathy at middle age.[25] Myocardial hypertrophy is the predominant phenotype. However, localized fibrosis involving the inferolateral and mid-basal segments with a mesocardial distribution is a frequent finding.[32] The observed fibrosis pattern may serve as a substrate for reentry VA. A single case has been published describing endocardial and epicardial RFCA for two scar-related reentry VTs in a patient with Fabry disease. One circuit was mapped to the subepicardial LV lateral wall successfully targeted by ablation and a second likely intramural circuit could not be abolished. This case may suggest a similar substrate for VT in Fabry disease as described for other forms of LV nonischemic cardiomyopathies with a dominant intramural or subepicardial basolateral scar location.[18]

Sarcoidosis

Sarcoidosis is an inflammatory granulomatous disease of unknown cause. A total of 3% to 5% of patients diagnosed with sarcoidosis have clinically evident cardiac involvement.[26] CS can affect any part of the heart. Clinical manifestations depend on the location, extent, and activity of CS and may be suspected in patients with AV conduction abnormalities, VA, and progressive heart failure.[26]

Table 2
RFCA in infiltrative cardiomyopathy

Author, Year	Diagnosis	Method	Patients (n)	Sus-VT (n)	VTCL Mean (ms)	Acute Success, n (%)	Recurrence, n (%)	Follow-Up (mo)
Mlcochova, et al,[31] 2006	Amyloidosis	AM, SM	2	PVC-induced VF	NR	2 (100)	0 (100)	0.75
Seethala et al,[30] 2010	Amyloidosis	AM, SM	1	1	400	1 (100)	0 (100)	18
Higashi et al,[45] 2011	Fabry disease	AM, SM, EPI	1	2	430	0 (0)	0 (100)	24
Koplan et al,[38] 2006	Sarcoidosis	AM, SM	8	34	NR	2 (25)	6 (75)	6–84
Jefic et al,[37] 2009	Sarcoidosis	AM, SM, EPI	9	44	348	4 (44)	4 (9)	20 ± 20
Dechering et al,[39] 2013	Sarcoidosis	AM, SM, EPI	8	30	326	5 (44)	NR	NR
Naruse et al,[35] 2014	Sarcoidosis	AM, SM	14	37	400	NR	6 (43)	33 (IQR 26–460)
Kumar et al,[36] 2015	Sarcoidosis	AM, SM, EPI	21	99	355	16 (76)	18 (86)	58 ± 61
Muser et al,[40] 2016	Sarcoidosis	AM, SM, EPI	31	93	369	23 (74)	20 (64)	30 (IQR 16–62)

Abbreviations: AM, activation mapping; EPI, epicardial; IQR, interquartile range; NR, not reported; PVC, premature ventricular contraction; SM, substrate mapping; VTCL, ventricular tachycardia cycle length.

Ventricular Tachycardia and Sudden Cardiac Death in Cardiac Sarcoidosis

Acute myocardial inflammation may result in VT or ventricular ectopy caused by abnormal automaticity or triggered activity similar to the findings in active myocarditis.[33] These arrhythmias can occur in the early stage of CS and corticosteroids suppressing the inflammatory process have been associated with a reduced VA burden.[34] VTs in the more advanced stage of the disease are often caused by scar-related reentry.[35,36]

A stepwise approach for the treatment of VT associated with CS has been suggested. Corticosteroid therapy combined with antiarrhythmic drug treatment was effective to prevent VT recurrence in 57% to 62% of patients. In the remaining patients RFCA was subsequently performed to control recurrent VTs, which was successful in 13 of 23 patients.[35,37] RFCA is recommended in patients with monomorphic VT or VT storm refractory to immunosuppressive and antiarrhythmic therapy and in patients with incessant VT.[26]

Radiofrequency Catheter Ablation for Ventricular Tachycardia in Cardiac Sarcoidosis

The number of patients with CS referred for VT ablation is small. In one VT ablation series of patients with an NICM (non ischemic cardiomyopathy) only 5% fulfilled the diagnostic criteria of CS.[36] To date, six studies have reported on RFCA for VT in a total of 83 patients with CS **(Table 2)**.[35–40] Ten percent to one-third of patients present with incessant VT or VT storm.[36,37,40] Most VTs were attributed to scar-related reentry, but Purkinje-related VTs have been reported in patients with

affected infrahissian conduction system. The underlying mechanisms for the latter were bundle branch reentry, microreentry, or a nonreentrant source, which could be mapped to one of the three fascicles and successfully ablated.[35]

Frequently, multiple scar-related VT morphologies are inducible in CS. Most VTs have a left bundle branch block–like morphology indicating an RV or septal origin. In most patients areas with low-voltage electrograms are identified by electroanatomic mapping. RV scars are often large and confluent in advanced disease.[36] However, predilection for the peritricuspid region, RVOT, or the RV apex has been reported and may be observed in earlier stages of the disease.[37,39,40] In the LV pattern of low voltage and abnormal electrograms tend to be more patchy with involvement of the septum and the basal anterior and lateral wall **(Fig. 3)**.[36,40,41] Epicardial scar is predominantly found at the basal lateral LV and RV and anterior basal LV wall[40] and may overlay and exceed RV low-voltage areas but may also be unrelated to low-voltage endocardial LV areas.[36] VT reentry circuit sites are typically related to areas of electroanatomic scar.[35–40]

A first procedure resulted in noninducibility of the clinical VT in 63% to 77% of patients.[36,39,40] Importantly, RFCA can eliminate incessant VT or VT storm in most patients. However, clinical or nonclinical VT remained inducible in up to 76% of patients.[36] VT recurrences rates are high occurring in up to 65% to 86% of patients after a first procedure.[36,40] Patients with an active and ongoing inflammation are at high risk for VT recurrence.[39] Second and third ablation procedures are common in this challenging population.[35–37,40] Failure to abolish all VTs may be caused by intramural septal

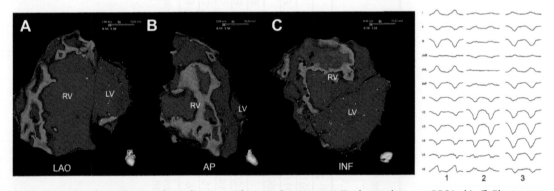

Fig. 3. Example of a patient with cardiac sarcoidosis and recurrent VT who underwent RFCA. (A–C) Electroanatomic voltage maps of the LV and RV in (A) left anterior oblique (LAO), (B) anterior (AP), and (C) inferior (INF) views. Bipolar voltages are color coded according to bar. Normal voltage electrograms (>1.5 mV) are color-coded purple. There is a confluent, dense scar of the inferior RV wall (C) that extends to the RV free wall and anterior RVOT (A). The LV shows only a small patchy apical scar (A, B). The patient was inducible for three VTs (1–3, cycle length 340 ms, 300 ms, and 345 ms) with matching pacemaps of VT1 and three in the RV inferior low voltage area. Because of hemodynamically instability substrate guided ablation was performed after which only fast (cycle length 250 ms, not shown) nonclinical VT remained inducible.

circuits, extensive RV scar with multiple reentry circuits, but also proximity of the coronary arteries or the conduction system.[36] In many patients a significant decrease in number of VT episodes during long-term follow-up can be achieved after one to three procedures.[36,40] Even though CE-MRI often shows a midwall and subepicardial scar distribution, epicardial mapping and ablation has only been performed in 36% of the patients.[36,40] Further prospective evaluation is needed to assess whether a systematic epicardial approach impacts outcome in CS. A significant proportion of patients referred for ablation died or required heart transplant during follow-up reflecting the poor outcome of the advanced stage of CS.[36,37,40]

SUMMARY

RFCA is an important treatment modality to prevent VT recurrence in patients with rCHD. Over the last decade progress has been made to understand and delineate the dominant substrate for monomorphic VTs. Macroreentry is facilitated by regions of slow conduction that are typically protected by surgical scars and prosthetic material. Ablation of these SCAI with bidirectional conduction block and defined end point results in long-term freedom of VT recurrence in patients with preserved cardiac function.

RFCA for VT in patients with infiltrative disease is rarely reported and CS seems to be the most important cause for an arrhythmogenic substrate. Catheter ablation in patients in the advanced stage of CS in whom complex ventricular scars remain after myocardial inflammation is challenging. Active and ongoing inflammation may further impact efficacy. RFCA reduces the VT burden but multiple procedures are often required and the long-term outcome is less favorable in those with advanced CS.

Better understanding and visualization of the complex substrate by advanced imaging modalities in conjunction with improved ablation techniques and earlier and more effective treatment of the ongoing inflammation is needed to improve the long-term outcome.

REFERENCES

1. Hoffman JI, Kaplan S. The incidence of congenital heart disease. J Am Coll Cardiol 2002;39:1890–900.
2. Khairy P, Ionescu-Ittu R, Mackie AS, et al. Changing mortality in congenital heart disease. J Am Coll Cardiol 2010;56:1149–57.
3. Verheugt CL, Uiterwaal CS, van der Velde ET, et al. Mortality in adult congenital heart disease. Eur Heart J 2010;31:1220–9.
4. Diller GP, Kempny A, Alonso-Gonzalez R, et al. Survival prospects and circumstances of death in contemporary adult congenital heart disease patients under follow-up at a large tertiary centre. Circulation 2015;132:2118–25.
5. Gallego P, Gonzalez AE, Sanchez-Recalde A, et al. Incidence and predictors of sudden cardiac arrest in adults with congenital heart defects repaired before adult life. Am J Cardiol 2012;110:109–17.
6. Koyak Z, Harris L, de Groot JR, et al. Sudden cardiac death in adult congenital heart disease. Circulation 2012;126:1944–54.
7. Silka MJ, Hardy BG, Menashe VD, et al. A population-based prospective evaluation of risk of sudden cardiac death after operation for common congenital heart defects. J Am Coll Cardiol 1998;32:245–51.
8. Zeppenfeld K, Schalij MJ, Bartelings MM, et al. Catheter ablation of ventricular tachycardia after repair of congenital heart disease: electroanatomic identification of the critical right ventricular isthmus. Circulation 2007;116:2241–52.
9. Kapel GF, Sacher F, Dekkers OM, et al. Arrhythmogenic anatomical isthmuses identified by electroanatomical mapping are the substrate for ventricular tachycardia in repaired tetralogy of Fallot. Eur Heart J 2016. [Epub ahead of print].
10. Kapel GF, Reichlin T, Wijnmaalen AP, et al. Re-entry using anatomically determined isthmuses: a curable ventricular tachycardia in repaired congenital heart disease. Circ Arrhythm Electrophysiol 2015;8:102–9.
11. Chowdhury UK, Sathia S, Ray R, et al. Histopathology of the right ventricular outflow tract and its relationship to clinical outcomes and arrhythmias in patients with tetralogy of Fallot. J Thorac Cardiovasc Surg 2006;132:270–7.
12. Khairy P, Aboulhosn J, Gurvitz MZ, et al. Arrhythmia burden in adults with surgically repaired tetralogy of Fallot: a multi-institutional study. Circulation 2010;122:868–75.
13. Khairy P, Harris L, Landzberg MJ, et al. Implantable cardioverter-defibrillators in tetralogy of Fallot. Circulation 2008;117:363–70.
14. Zeppenfeld K, Schalij MJ, Bartelings MM, et al. Catheter ablation of ventricular tachycardia after repair of congenital heart disease: electroanatomic identification of the critical right ventricular isthmus. Circulation 2007;116:2241–52.
15. Kammeraad JA, van Deurzen CH, Sreeram N, et al. Predictors of sudden cardiac death after Mustard or Senning repair for transposition of the great arteries. J Am Coll Cardiol 2004;44:1095–102.
16. Schwerzmann M, Salehian O, Harris L, et al. Ventricular arrhythmias and sudden death in adults after a Mustard operation for transposition of the great arteries. Eur Heart J 2009;30:1873–9.

17. Piers SR, Dyrda K, Tao Q, et al. Bipolar ablation of ventricular tachycardia in a patient after atrial switch operation for dextro-transposition of the great arteries. Circ Arrhythm Electrophysiol 2012;5:e38–40.

18. Piers SR, Tao Q, van Huls van Taxis CF, et al. Contrast-enhanced MRI-derived scar patterns and associated ventricular tachycardias in nonischemic cardiomyopathy: implications for the ablation strategy. Circ Arrhythm Electrophysiol 2013;6:875–83.

19. Wijnmaalen AP, van der Geest RJ, van Huls van Taxis CF, et al. Head-to-head comparison of contrast-enhanced magnetic resonance imaging and electroanatomical voltage mapping to assess post-infarct scar characteristics in patients with ventricular tachycardias: real-time image integration and reversed registration. Eur Heart J 2011;32:104–14.

20. Kriebel T, Saul JP, Schneider H, et al. Noncontact mapping and radiofrequency catheter ablation of fast and hemodynamically unstable ventricular tachycardia after surgical repair of tetralogy of Fallot. J Am Coll Cardiol 2007;50:2162–8.

21. van Zyl M, Kapa S, Padmanabhan D, et al. Mechanism and outcomes of catheter ablation for ventricular tachycardia in adults with repaired congenital heart disease. Heart Rhythm 2016;13:1449–54.

22. Stevenson WG, Wilber DJ, Natale A, et al. Irrigated radiofrequency catheter ablation guided by electroanatomic mapping for recurrent ventricular tachycardia after myocardial infarction: the multicenter thermocool ventricular tachycardia ablation trial. Circulation 2008;118:2773–82.

23. Kapel GF, Reichlin T, Wijnmaalen AP, et al. Left-sided ablation of ventricular tachycardia in adults with repaired tetralogy of Fallot: a case series. Circ Arrhythm Electrophysiol 2014;7:889–97.

24. Sabate Rotes A, Connolly HM, Warnes CA, et al. Ventricular arrhythmia risk stratification in patients with tetralogy of Fallot at the time of pulmonary valve replacement. Circ Arrhythm Electrophysiol 2015;8:110–6.

25. Seward JB, Casaclang-Verzosa G. Infiltrative cardiovascular diseases: cardiomyopathies that look alike. J Am Coll Cardiol 2010;55:1769–79.

26. Birnie DH, Sauer WH, Bogun F, et al. HRS expert consensus statement on the diagnosis and management of arrhythmias associated with cardiac sarcoidosis. Heart Rhythm 2014;11:1305–23.

27. Dubrey SW, Bilazarian S, LaValley M, et al. Signal-averaged electrocardiography in patients with AL (primary) amyloidosis. Am Heart J 1997;134:994–1001.

28. Lin G, Dispenzieri A, Kyle R, et al. Implantable cardioverter defibrillators in patients with cardiac amyloidosis. J Cardiovasc Electrophysiol 2013;24:793–8.

29. Kristen AV, Dengler TJ, Hegenbart U, et al. Prophylactic implantation of cardioverter-defibrillator in patients with severe cardiac amyloidosis and high risk for sudden cardiac death. Heart Rhythm 2008;5:235–40.

30. Seethala S, Jain S, Ohori NP, et al. Focal monomorphic ventricular tachycardia as the first manifestation of amyloid cardiomyopathy. Indian Pacing Electrophysiol J 2010;10:143–7.

31. Mlcochova H, Saliba WI, Burkhardt DJ, et al. Catheter ablation of ventricular fibrillation storm in patients with infiltrative amyloidosis of the heart. J Cardiovasc Electrophysiol 2006;17:426–30.

32. Kramer J, Niemann M, Stork S, et al. Relation of burden of myocardial fibrosis to malignant ventricular arrhythmias and outcomes in Fabry disease. Am J Cardiol 2014;114:895–900.

33. Tai YT, Lau CP, Fong PC, et al. Incessant automatic ventricular tachycardia complicating acute coxsackie B myocarditis. Cardiology 1992;80:339–44.

34. Yodogawa K, Seino Y, Ohara T, et al. Effect of corticosteroid therapy on ventricular arrhythmias in patients with cardiac sarcoidosis. Ann Noninvasive Electrocardiol 2011;16:140–7.

35. Naruse Y, Sekiguchi Y, Nogami A, et al. Systematic treatment approach to ventricular tachycardia in cardiac sarcoidosis. Circ Arrhythm Electrophysiol 2014;7:407–13.

36. Kumar S, Barbhaiya C, Nagashima K, et al. Ventricular tachycardia in cardiac sarcoidosis: characterization of ventricular substrate and outcomes of catheter ablation. Circ Arrhythm Electrophysiol 2015;8:87–93.

37. Jefic D, Joel B, Good E, et al. Role of radiofrequency catheter ablation of ventricular tachycardia in cardiac sarcoidosis: report from a multicenter registry. Heart Rhythm 2009;6:189–95.

38. Koplan BA, Soejima K, Baughman K, et al. Refractory ventricular tachycardia secondary to cardiac sarcoid: electrophysiologic characteristics, mapping, and ablation. Heart Rhythm 2006;3:924–9.

39. Dechering DG, Kochhauser S, Wasmer K, et al. Electrophysiological characteristics of ventricular tachyarrhythmias in cardiac sarcoidosis versus arrhythmogenic right ventricular cardiomyopathy. Heart Rhythm 2013;10:158–64.

40. Muser D, Santangeli P, Pathak RK, et al. Long-Term outcomes of catheter ablation of ventricular tachycardia in patients with cardiac sarcoidosis. Circ Arrhythm Electrophysiol 2016;9.

41. Pedrotti P, Ammirati E, Bonacina E, et al. Ventricular aneurysms in cardiac sarcoidosis: from physiopathology to surgical treatment through a clinical case presenting with ventricular arrhythmias. Int J Cardiol 2015;186:294–6.

42. Gonska BD, Cao K, Raab J, et al. Radiofrequency catheter ablation of right ventricular tachycardia late after repair of congenital heart defects. Circulation 1996;94:1902–8.

43. Morwood JG, Triedman JK, Berul CI, et al. Radiofrequency catheter ablation of ventricular tachycardia in children and young adults with congenital heart disease. Heart Rhythm 2004;1:301–8.

44. Furushima H, Chinushi M, Sugiura H, et al. Ventricular tachycardia late after repair of congenital heart disease: efficacy of combination therapy with radiofrequency catheter ablation and class III antiarrhythmic agents and long-term outcome. J Electrocardiol 2006;39:219–24.

45. Higashi H, Yamagata K, Noda T, et al. Endocardial and epicardial substrates of ventricular tachycardia in a patient with Fabry disease. Heart Rhythm 2011; 8:133–6.

Epicardial Catheter Ablation of Ventricular Tachycardia

Arash Aryana, MS, MD[a], André d'Avila, MD, PhD[b],*

KEYWORDS

- Catheter ablation • Epicardial • Pericardium • Radiofrequency

KEY POINTS

- Epicardial ventricular tachycardia (VT) ablation should be performed using cooled-tip radiofrequency (RF) using a reduced irrigation flow rate within a relatively "dry" pericardial milieu.
- Epicardial fat thickness of greater than 5 mm may attenuate peak-to-peak myocardial electrogram amplitude, augment tissue impedance and pacing capture, and impede RF energy delivery.
- Unlike epicardial fat, electrograms associated with epicardial scar are more likely to exhibit fractionated and longer duration as well as late potentials.
- Although contact force is critical to endocardial VT ablation, catheter orientation remains more pertinent to the efficacy and safety of epicardial VT ablation.
- Hemopericardium remains the most frequent adverse event related to epicardial VT ablation; its presenting timeline can be used to identify the nature of this complication.

INTRODUCTION

The concept of the epicardial ventricular tachycardia (VT) substrate was originally postulated owing to the disproportionately poor success rates associated with endocardial ablation of VT in patients with Chagasic heart disease. Encouraged by the observation that in approximately 15% of patients with ischemic VT the critical anatomic substrate supporting reentry could occur either intramurally or epicardially,[1] Sosa and colleagues[2] introduced the percutaneous epicardial ablation strategy nearly 2 decades ago. Aside from elucidating the usefulness of this then new ablation strategy, Sosa and colleagues[3] further exposed the necessity of this approach illustrating that although interruption of an epicardial VT may be feasible through endocardial delivery of radiofrequency (RF) energy, epicardial ablation is almost always required to successfully abolish a VT arising from an epicardial circuit irrespective of the left ventricular (LV) wall thickness[4] (**Fig. 1**). Since then, this approach has been extended to the treatment of VTs in a variety of disorders including ischemic, nonischemic, idiopathic, inheritable, and infiltrative cardiomyopathy substrates.[5] This article provides a comprehensive overview of the epicardial approach to catheter ablation of VT.

EPICARDIAL ACCESS
Subxiphoid Percutaneous Access

Although epicardial ablation of myocardial targets via the coronary sinus is feasible, this approach is entirely limited by the inherent distribution of the

Disclosure Statement: The authors have nothing to disclose relevant to this submission.
[a] Department of Cardiology and Cardiovascular Surgery, Mercy General Hospital, Dignity Health Heart and Vascular Institute, 3941 J Street, Suite #350, Sacramento, CA 95819, USA; [b] Cardiac Arrhythmia Service, Instituto de Pesquisa em Arritmia Cardiaca, Hospital Cardiologico – Florianopolis, Florianopolis, Rodovia SC 401, 121 – Itacorubi, Florianópolis – Santa Catarina 88030, Brazil
* Corresponding author.
E-mail address: andredavila@mac.com

Card Electrophysiol Clin 9 (2017) 119–131
http://dx.doi.org/10.1016/j.ccep.2016.10.009
1877-9182/17/© 2016 Elsevier Inc. All rights reserved.

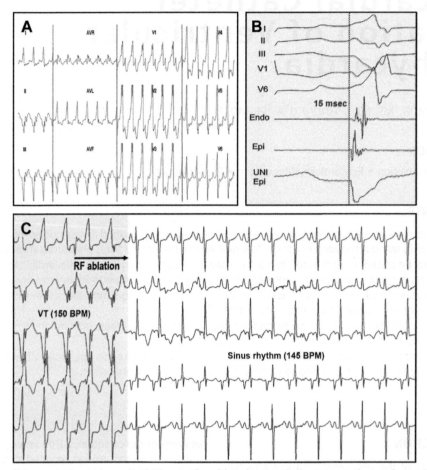

Fig. 1. Epicardial ventricular tachycardia (VT) must be ablated epicardially. A case of an infant with incessant epicardial VT with a left ventricular (LV) wall thickness of 5 mm. (*A*) A 12-lead electrocardiogram (ECG) of VT in an 11-month-old infant with an LV wall thickness of only 5 mm, incessant VT at a rate of 150 bpm and associated heart failure, status post previously failed endocardial ablation. (*B*) ECG and intracardiac recordings demonstrating an epicardial activation site (Epi) 15 ms earlier than the earliest endocardial activation site (Endo), with a completely negative unipolar epicardial (UNI Epi) electrogram. (*C*) Immediate termination of VT upon delivery of radiofrequency energy epicardially to the site of the earliest activation. This successfully abolished the clinical tachycardia rendering it permanently noninducible. This case clearly illustrates that for successful outcomes an epicardial VT must be ablated epicardially. Furthermore, this is independent of the LV wall thickness. (*Adapted from* Sosa E, Scanavacca M, d'Avila A, et al. Nonsurgical transthoracic mapping and ablation in a child with incessant ventricular tachycardia. J Cardiovasc Electrophysiol 2000;11:210; with permission.)

coronary sinus anatomy. Thus, the subxiphoid percutaneous approach to the pericardium is the only method that allows unrestricted epicardial catheter mapping and ablation of the arrhythmia targets. Presently, there are 2 similar strategies used for gaining epicardial access in this setting: (i) the Sosa approach[2] and (ii) the "needle-in-needle" technique.[6] The Sosa approach involves the use of a "blunt" 17- or 18-G, 12- to 15-cm Tuohy needle which bears a specific design to reduce vascular injury (**Fig. 2**A). This needle was devised originally for accessing the epidural space with the intent to specifically reduce the risk of epidural vascular puncture. In contrast, the needle-in-

needle technique uses a smaller 21-G needle (**Fig. 2**B). Briefly, a 21-G, 15- to 20-cm long micropuncture needle (Cook Medical, Bloomington, IN) is used for gaining epicardial access which is in turn inserted through a 7-cm, standard 18-G needle (Cook Medical) for the purpose of stability. Once epicardial access has been established using the micropuncture needle, an 0.018″ long guide wire is advanced into the pericardium which is subsequently replaced/upsized to accommodate the insertion of the larger bore epicardial introducer sheath. In a recent study comparing the outcomes from 316 procedures performed using the Sosa technique against 23 cases using the

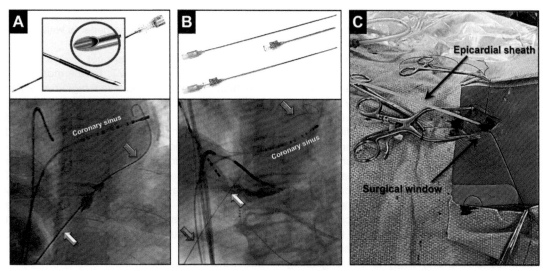

Fig. 2. Tools and strategies for percutaneous and surgical epicardial access. (*A, top*) An 18-G Tuohy needle used for epicardial access using the Sosa technique. As seen in the inset, this needle bears a blunt tip designed specifically for accessing the epidural space thereby reducing the risk of epidural vascular puncture. (*Bottom*) Left anterior oblique Cine of epicardial puncture and access attained using a Tuohy needle (*white arrow*), through which a 0.032″ guide wire is advanced into the pericardial space (*yellow arrow*). (*B, top*) A 21-G, 15-cm micropuncture needle (*green*) and a 7-cm, standard 18-G needle (*pink*) used for epicardial access using the 'needle-in-needle' technique. (*Bottom*) A left anterior oblique Cine showing epicardial access using this approach. Briefly, the micropuncture needle (*white arrow*) is inserted through the 18-gauge needle (*blue arrow*) for stability while epicardial access is obtained using the former. Next, an 0.018″ guide wire is advanced through the micropuncture needle into the pericardial space (*yellow arrow*). (*C*) A surgical pericardial window created in the electrophysiology laboratory using a limited thoracotomy approach in a patient with diffuse, extensive pericardial adhesions, thereby limiting percutaneous epicardial access. As seen, a deflectable epicardial introducer sheath can be subsequently inserted through the surgical window to allow percutaneous epicardial mapping and ablation. This approach may be used effectively in patients with difficult-to-access pericardia such as those with a prior history of cardiac surgery.

needle-in-needle technique, no differences were observed with regard to efficacy or safety between the 2 strategies.[6]

Surgical Access

It should be emphasized that, in patients who have evidence of pericardial adhesions, as most commonly encountered after prior cardiac surgery or percutaneous instrumentation, a limited thoracotomy approach (surgical window) can often be effectively used to allow percutaneous epicardial mapping and ablation (**Fig. 2C**).[7] This is indeed an important consideration, because a great proportion of the catastrophic complications that may be encountered during epicardial procedures occur in those with a history of prior cardiac surgery, which virtually obliterates the anterior pericardial space and greatly distorts the normal anatomy.[8]

DIAGNOSING EPICARDIAL VENTRICULAR TACHYCARDIA

Prior knowledge about whether an epicardial VT is present is always invaluable when performing

VT ablation. Although it is always ideal to secure epicardial access before systemic anticoagulation, this may not always be the case. The presence of an epicardial VT circuit/exit site may be ascertained through different methodologies, including preprocedural imaging modalities (ie, computed tomography or MRI), electrocardiography (ECG) or intraprocedural activation mapping. Several investigators have attempted to propose precise ECG criteria to distinguish an epicardial VT. One study[9] largely investigating patients with ischemic cardiomyopathy identified the presence of a pseudo delta wave interval greater than 34 ms (sensitivity: 83%, specificity: 95%), an intrinsicoid deflection time of greater than 85 ms in the precordial lead V_2 (sensitivity, 87%; specificity, 90%) and an RS complex duration greater than 121 ms (sensitivity, 76%; specificity, 85%) as significant predictors of an epicardial VT. Although no specific criterion based on the QRS duration itself was defined, all those with a QRS duration of greater than 211 ms were virtually found to have an epicardial VT. However, the most recent inspection of these predictors in patients with an ischemic substrate suggests that none of these or other criteria could reliably predict the existence of an epicardial VT.[10] Similarly, Bazan and colleagues[11] proposed and examined several ECG criteria for epicardial VT in the absence of myocardial infarction. The authors found that the criteria were largely region specific, with sensitivity ranging between 14% and 99% and specificity in the range of 20% to 94%.[12] More recently, Valles and colleagues[13] assessed these criteria in a cohort of patients with nonischemic cardiomyopathy using both endocardial and epicardial pacing and clinical VT. As a result, a stepwise algorithm (**Fig. 3**) was developed which was subsequently prospectively validated (sensitivity, 96%; specificity, 93%). It should be emphasized that these criteria only apply to VTs originating

from the superior and lateral perivalvular aortic/mitral valve regions in those patients with a non-ischemic substrate.

Therefore, ECG criteria are not always reliable in diagnosing epicardial VT. Furthermore, they are highly substrate and even region specific. Nonetheless, detailed endocardial mapping in some cases, itself, may prove of potential benefit. Hutchinson and colleagues[14] found that, among those with nonischemic cardiomyopathy, endocardial unipolar low-voltage areas were directly opposite to an area of epicardial bipolar low-voltage in approximately 60% of cases. The latter may in fact prove especially valuable when contemplating an epicardial puncture in patients with nonischemic cardiomyopathy and no clear endocardial substrate.

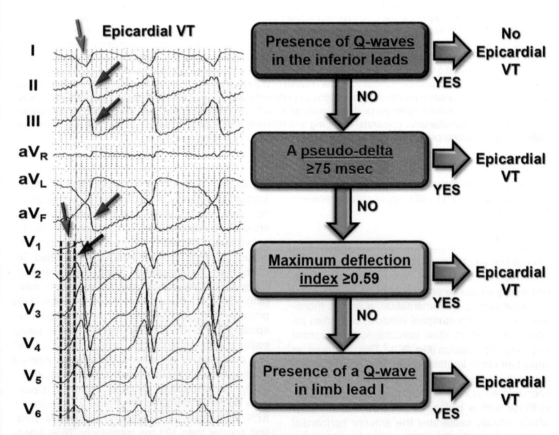

Fig. 3. Stepwise algorithm for identifying an epicardial origin from the basal superior and lateral LV in patients with non-ischemic cardiomyopathy. A 12-lead ECG of an epicardial VT in a patient with non-ischemic cardiomyopathy is shown on the right. On the left, a 4-step algorithm is shown for identifying an epicardial origin from the basal superior and lateral LV in the setting of non-ischemic cardiomyopathy. The algorithm examines for presence/absence of inferior Q-waves (*red arrows*), a pseudo-delta wave ≥75 msec (*yellow arrow*), a maximum deflection index ≥0.59 (*blue arrow*) and a Q-wave in limb lead I (*green arrow*). The overall sensitivity and specificity of the algorithm for pace-map localization was 96% and 93%, respectively.

COMMON ANATOMIC LOCATIONS AND DISEASE STATES EXHIBITING AN EPICARDIAL VENTRICULAR TACHYCARDIA SUBSTRATE

Epicardial VTs in normal hearts are ablated frequently in locations clustered around the atrioventricular and interventricular grooves, along the middle cardiac vein, the anterior interventricular vein, and the course of the major epicardial vessels.[5] Meanwhile, VTs in patients with ischemic substrates typically occur as a consequence of a right coronary or a left circumflex artery-related inferior wall infarction.[1] In contrast, patients with nonischemic cardiomyopathy commonly present with VTs arising from the ventricular base within the perivalvular region.[15] Furthermore, those with nonischemic substrates are more likely to exhibit larger surface area scars epicardially versus endocardially.[16,17] The latter cohort also typically exhibits a lower prevalence of late potentials.[18] Two additional disease states that yield a relatively high predilection for epicardial VT substrates include hypertrophic cardiomyopathy[19] and arrhythmogenic right ventricular (RV) cardiomyopathy.[20] More recently, Berruezo and colleagues[21] reported on the outcomes of combined endocardial and epicardial VT ablation as first-line therapy in a cohort of patients with arrhythmogenic RV cardiomyopathy. The authors found that a combined endocardial/epicardial ablation approach incorporating "scar dechanneling" significantly improved the success rate of VT ablation. Furthermore, epicardial ablation may also be required to successfully abolish VT in 25% to 30% of patients with myocarditis[22] and also sarcoidosis.[23] Last, Nademanee and colleagues[24] reported recently on a new application for epicardial ablation in those with type I Brugada syndrome and recurrent ventricular fibrillation. In their study, detailed endocardial/epicardial mapping uncovered areas of low voltage with prolonged duration/fractionation epicardially along the anterior aspect of the RV outflow tract. RF ablation at these sites rendered the ventricular arrhythmias noninducible in approximately 80% with normalization of the ECG pattern in approximately 90% of patients.

EPICARDIAL ABLATION OF VENTRICULAR TACHYCARDIA

Although the biophysical variables that predict an effective epicardial ablation (ie, power and impedance) are similar to those that govern endocardial ablation, there are indeed certain fundamental differences between these 2 ablation strategies. Next, we review the underlying rationales and

conditions that differentiate an epicardial from an endocardial RF ablation procedure.

Radiofrequency Ablation

Epicardial ablation can be performed using standard (nonirrigated) RF, cooled (ie, irrigated) RF,[25] or even cryoablation.[26] Focused ultrasound and electroporation have also been evaluated experimentally but not yet adopted clinically. Cooled-tip or irrigated RF ablation can generate more effective lesions epicardially as compared with standard RF ablation.[25] In a direct head-to-head comparison performed in vivo, cooled-tip RF ablation created lesions larger than those formed using standard RF. Although the presence of epicardial fat interposed between the catheter tip and myocardium further attenuated the lesions created by cooled-tip RF, this completely abrogated lesion formation using standard RF (**Fig. 4**). More recently, in the era of force-sensing technologies, a recent study investigated the role and impact of contact force (CF) during epicardial ablation.[27] Although the optimal CF for ventricular mapping and ablation has yet to be determined, Jesel and colleagues[27] provided important insights into regional variations in CF and catheter orientation relating to endocardial and epicardial mapping. First, these authors showed that bipolar signal amplitude in healthy endocardial and epicardial tissue may increase with CF of up to 10 g, but not beyond. As such, based on a general linear mixed model analysis, the best CF cutoff value for obtaining a signal amplitude of greater than 1.5 mV was determined to be 7 g in the LV endocardium (sensitivity, 80%; specificity, 75%), 9 g in the RV endocardium (sensitivity, 65%; specificity, 83%), and 4 g in the epicardium (sensitivity, 83%; specificity, 64%). These findings are consistent with other published reports. For instance, Mizuno and colleagues[28] similarly found that the optimal CF cutoff in predicting adequate tissue contact during LV endocardial and epicardial mappings was 9 g. Second, Jesel and colleagues[27] also found that the degree of CF exerted during endocardial mapping (13 g inside the RV and 15 g within the LV) was significantly greater than that applied during epicardial mapping (8 g). Furthermore, the catheter orientation was directed toward the myocardium more than 90% of the time during endocardial mapping, but less than 50% while mapping epicardially. This was particularly apparent during epicardial mapping of the LV apical and basal regions where optimal catheter orientation was only achieved less than one-third of the time. As such, suboptimal catheter orientation during epicardial mapping was associated

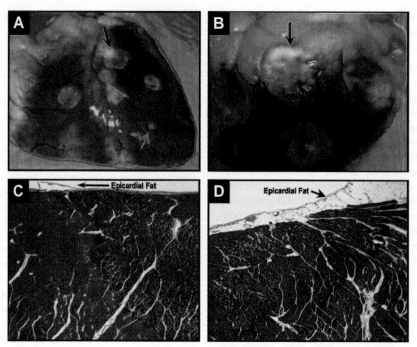

Fig. 4. Gross and histologic examination of epicardial lesions created in vivo using standard versus cooled-tip radiofrequency (RF) in the presence and absence of epicardial fat. (*A*) In vivo epicardial lesions created using cooled-tip (*black arrows*) and standard (*yellow arrow*) RF ablation. As noted, lesions created using cooled-tip RF are visibly much larger than with standard RF. (*B*) An ablation lesion created using cooled-tip RF on the epicardial surface covered with (*black arrow*) and without epicardial fat. As seen, cooled-tip RF is capable of still creating RF lesions over epicardial fat. (*C*) Histologic examination of an epicardial RF lesion created using standard RF. As seen, epicardial fat interposed between the ablation catheter tip and myocardium prevented creation of deep lesions. This is particularly evident by the distinct lesion corresponding with the location of the epicardial fat layer. (*D*) In contrast, when using cooled-tip RF, the presence of epicardial fat significantly attenuated but did not completely abrogate lesion formation. (*Adapted from* d'Avila A, Houghtaling C, Gutierrez P, et al. Catheter ablation of ventricular epicardial tissue: a comparison of standard and cooled-tip radiofrequency energy. Circulation 2004;109:2365; with permission.)

frequently with higher CF measurements (ie, 16 g when pointing away from the epicardial surface vs 8 g when directed toward the myocardium; $P < .0001$). Consequently, this finding suggests that increased CF during epicardial mapping does not necessarily imply adequate myocardial contact. On the contrary, application of higher CF epicardially can in fact redirect the ablation catheter away from the myocardium toward extracardiac structures (ie, parietal pericardium, lungs), which could in fact result in undesired complications.[29] These observations are also entirely consistent with results from the same authors' prior in vivo study,[30] which demonstrated that total CF was greater endocardially as a result of increased axial force. Conversely, assessment of lateral CF seems more relevant when ablation is performed epicardially. It is also plausible that such differences could account for certain lesion characteristics considered more typical of epicardial ablation (ie, shallower and wider RF lesions).

Hence, these findings are of key importance, indicating that although CF is more relevant to endocardial ablation, catheter orientation is in fact more pertinent to the efficacy and safety of epicardial ablation.[31]

Another factor distinguishing epicardial from endocardial ablation has to do with the extravascular nature of the pericardial space. That is, absence of blood flow within the pericardium can lead to premature heating of the ablation catheter tip, thereby limiting the delivery of sufficient power during RF ablation. Although historically during epicardial ablation most operators have typically used conventional irrigation flow rates similar to those recommended endocardially (13–30 mL/min), in a recent study[32] the authors illustrated that reduced irrigation flow during epicardial RF ablation in the range of 5 to 7 mL/min can in fact yield lesion sizes similar to those created with conventionally higher flow rates without a substantial increase in steam pop or tissue disruption. Furthermore, in the same study the authors also showed that RF ablation in presence of intrapericardial fluid at a fixed CF can in fact lead to a significant reduction in the lesion size (**Fig. 5**). In other words, not only can epicardial ablation at higher irrigation flow rates ($\geq$10 mL/min) result in significant intrapericardial fluid accumulation, but this can impact RF lesion formation adversely. Thus, it seems that epicardial RF ablation should be performed ideally using a reduced irrigation flow rate (ie, 5 mL/min) within a relatively "dry" pericardial milieu.

Cryoablation

There are limited data on the role and value of epicardial cryoablation of ventricular arrhythmia substrates. In a prior in vivo study,[26] the authors found that in a chronic postinfarction porcine model focal cryoablation was in fact capable of creating deep ventricular epicardial lesions, comparable in size and depth with those formed endocardially. As such, it was concluded that the ability to rapidly create deep linear epicardial cryolesions may offer an alternative strategy to substrate-based RF ablation of ventricular arrhythmias. However, this approach failed to emerge as a safer modality for ablation in close proximity to the epicardial vessels.[33] Thus, this approach has yet to evolve into a practical and advantageous ablation methodology in clinical practice.

Epicardial Fat

Another characteristic that exclusively differentiates epicardial from endocardial ablation is the presence of epicardial fat. In essence, epicardial fat can undesirably affect pacing, recording, and impedance measurements as well as the ability to deliver RF energy. As illustrated by Abbara and colleagues,[34] the mean epicardial fat in the adult human measures approximately 5.3 mm in thickness. However, the mean thickness of the epicardial fat may be greater in women, those older than 65 years of age, and along the RV anterior free wall and the LV lateral wall. Furthermore, several studies have demonstrated that the presence of epicardial fat measuring less than 5 mm in thickness does not significantly impact recording of peak-to-peak myocardial electrogram amplitude or duration, nor the pacing threshold.[35,36] Conversely, epicardial fat measuring greater than 5 mm can deceptively diminish the peak-to-peak electrogram amplitude and further impede pacing capture.[35,36]

Moreover, epicardial fat, unlike scar, typically exhibits an higher impedance as the resistivity of fat greatly exceeds that of scar tissue and even muscle.[37] Conversely, the extracellular matrix contains fibrous proteins (ie, collagen, elastin, and fibronectin) immersed in an amorphous substance composed of water and electrically charged glycoproteins (proteoglycans). As a result of its biochemical composition, the extracellular matrix within the fibrous tissue affords a greater ionic diffusibility and, thereby, a lower tissue electrical resistivity than fat. Meanwhile, computer modeling has illustrated a direct linear relationship between epicardial fat thickness and impedance measurements, such that the thicker the epicardial fat, the greater impedance.[38] In actuality, epicardial fat can be distinguished more easily from epicardial scar based on electrogram duration. That is, although the presence of critically thick fat can reduce the electrogram amplitude

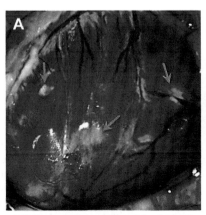 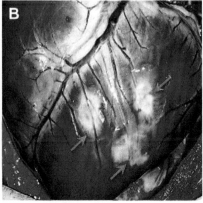

Fig. 5. Gross analysis of in vivo epicardial radiofrequency (RF) lesions. Shown are epicardial RF lesions (*arrows*) created in presence (*A*) and absence (*B*) of intrapericardial fluid using fixed irrigation flow (5 mL/min), contact force (10 gm), at fixed power (40 Watts) and duration (60 s). As seen, the lesions generated in the absence of pericardial fluid (*B*) are significantly larger than those in presence of intrapericardial fluid (*A*).

markedly, the epicardial fat does not in any way affect the electrogram duration. Conversely, electrograms associated with epicardial scar are more likely to exhibit fractionated and longer duration as well as late potentials as compared with epicardial fat.[39] Last, as previously described, the presence of epicardial fat can also seriously impede the passage of RF current into the underlying tissue/myocardium, such that the thicker the epicardial fat, the smaller (shallower) the lesions created using RF.[40] Along these lines, Desjardins and colleagues[41] studied the 3-dimensional distribution of epicardial fat on computed tomography imaging with electroanatomic voltage maps created during epicardial mapping to determine the estimated cutoff for epicardial fat thickness capable of attenuating voltage measurement and ablation lesion. The authors found that a fat thickness of 3 mm or greater could indeed result in voltage attenuation, and that ablations over sites bearing greater than 10 mm of epicardial fat was virtually ineffective. Hypothetically, ablation at these sites containing "thick" epicardial fat may be attempted through prolonged delivery of RF energy in an effort to "liquefy" the inherent adipose tissue, to reduce its burden on effectual ablation of the underlying myocardial substrate.

ADVERSE EVENTS AND MITIGATING COMPLICATIONS

The rate of major complications associated with epicardial VT ablation typically ranges between 5% and 10%, with hemopericardium representing the most common serious adverse event, followed by intraabdominal bleeding and epicardial vascular and phrenic nerve injuries.[42–44] One of the most common markers of a complication in the setting of an epicardial procedure is a history of prior cardiac surgery/instrumentation, which can lead to the development of dense pericardial adhesions. As a result, detailed knowledge about the patient's prior history including cardiac surgery, pericarditis, or pericardial instrumentation is absolutely critical to this procedure. Furthermore, ensuring normal coagulation parameters at the time of the procedure and prompt access to echocardiography (ie, intracardiac, surface, or transesophageal), blood products and a cardiac surgery/surgical team can all help in turn enhance the safety of the procedure. Additionally, the operator should always have a low threshold for pursuing a surgical window in place of a subxiphoid percutaneous approach to mitigate potential complications in those with pericardial adhesions. Having said that, despite the best efforts, complications cannot be avoided entirely. Therefore,

knowledge regarding the presenting timeline of hemopericardium is in fact relevant because it may be used to effectively diagnose or classify the specific etiology for the underlying complication.[45] As such, the timeline of hemopericardium may be classified as (i) early after the epicardial puncture, (ii) during the procedure, (iii) at the end of the procedure, or (iv) late after the procedure. Overall, 3 possible etiologies may account for the hemopericardium that is encountered early after an epicardial puncture: (i) an inadvertent RV puncture, (ii) disruption of pericardial adhesions, or (iii) puncture/perforation of an epicardial vessel. Although bleeding related to an inadvertent RV puncture and disruption of pericardial adhesions is generally self-limiting and can be managed invariably within the electrophysiology laboratory without major clinical sequelae, puncture or perforation of an epicardial vessel often requires a surgical repair or at the very least percutaneous intervention.[46] Furthermore, percutaneous intervention is characterized commonly by continuous, rapid, bright red bleeding from a perforated epicardial arterial source. Meanwhile, bleeding that is encountered some time during the procedure is commonly related to either an inadvertent RV puncture "blossoming" after systemic anticoagulation or an epicardial steam pop. Once again, these complications are in general self-limiting and can be managed adequately in the electrophysiology laboratory. However, delayed pericardial bleeding at the end of the procedure is generally uncommon and typically more ominous. Although this bleeding could be related to the accumulation of blood within the pericardium from injury to the subcutaneous vessels within the tract created using the catheters and introducer sheaths, the other troublesome possibility may be that of a "double RV perforation." A double RV perforation could occur if the needle or guide wire enters and exits the RV free wall at 2 different sites at the time of epicardial puncture. If unrecognized and the introducer sheath is advanced over the guide wire, the introducer tip could in theory still be positioned inside the pericardium without recognizing this complication. As a result, the entire procedure may be completed uneventfully. But, upon removal of the introducer sheath, torrential intrapericardial bleeding would appear suddenly from the 2 perforation sites within the RV (**Fig. 6**). Such a complication is luckily rare. If encountered, however, it requires urgent cardiac surgical repair. Two other clinical scenarios that similarly constitute surgical emergencies are (i) the presence of a hemodynamically significant loculated pericardial effusion not accessible to percutaneous needle aspiration and (ii) pericardial

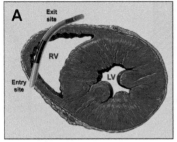
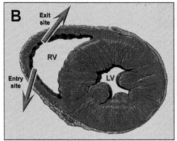
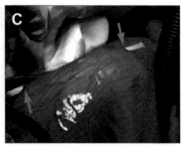

Fig. 6. Double right ventricular (RV) puncture. (*A*) A cross-sectional schematic of the heart showing advancement of the epicardial introducer sheath into the pericardial space using an "inferior puncture approach" after entering and then exiting the RV. (*B*) A cross-sectional schematic of the heart showing the RV perforation entry and exit sites after removal of the introducer sheath. Upon removal of the introducer, torrential intrapericardial bleeding will be observed from both the introducer entry and exit sites within the RV (*arrows*). (*C*) A case of double RV puncture as confirmed at cardiac surgery in a patient who underwent epicardial ventricular tachycardia ablation. The arrows point to the entry and exit sites in the RV, with the introducer sheath clearly visible as it enters and exits this structure at these 2 different sites.

clot formation associated with hemodynamic compromise, which is also not subject to aspiration or drainage (**Fig. 7**). Last, bleeding may also occur late after an epicardial procedure. The etiology for this bleeding is commonly owing to postprocedure pericarditis while on systemic anticoagulation or Dressler's syndrome. In fact, it should be highlighted that by far the most common adverse event related to epicardial ablation is that of pericarditis. Generally, postprocedure pericarditis after epicardial ablation can be managed conservatively. Having said that, an isolated case of constrictive pericarditis has been described in a patient subjected to multiple epicardial ablations.[47] An in vivo animal study strongly supports the use of intrapericardial corticosteroids (ie, 2 mg/kg triamcinolone) to minimize postprocedure pericarditis in those who undergo an epicardial ablation (**Fig. 8**).[48] Despite the lack of a randomized clinical trial, it remains common practice to administer intrapericardial steroids directly into the pericardium upon completion of the procedure. The authors' clinical experience suggests that this measure, coupled with postprocedure use of nonsteroidal antiinflammatory drugs, can help to effectively reduce postablation pericarditis.

Other, less common adverse events related to epicardial ablation include intraabdominal bleeding and coronary vascular or phrenic nerve injury. Nevertheless, when present, intraabdominal bleeding may pose a significant clinical dilemma. This complication is often a direct consequence of diaphragmatic or subdiaphragmatic structures (ie, the liver). In fact, the triad of hypotension in the setting of an epicardial procedure in the absence of pericardial effusion heralds

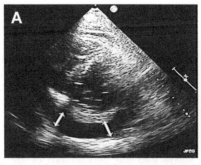
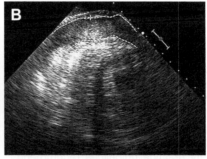

Fig. 7. Complications that may arise from epicardial ventricular tachycardia ablation that require urgent cardiac surgical intervention. (*A*) An echocardiographic image of loculated hemopericardium (*arrows*) in a patient with a history of prior cardiac surgery and pericardial adhesions. (*B*) An echocardiographic image of pericardial clot in a patient with hemopericardium and resultant cardiac tamponade. The echogenic material (outlined) inside the pericardium represents clot within this space. If hemodynamically significant, both of these types of complications require urgent cardiac surgical attention. (*Adapted from* Koruth JS, d'Avila A. Management of hemopericardium related to percutaneous epicardial access, mapping, and ablation. Heart Rhythm 2011;8:1653; with permission.)

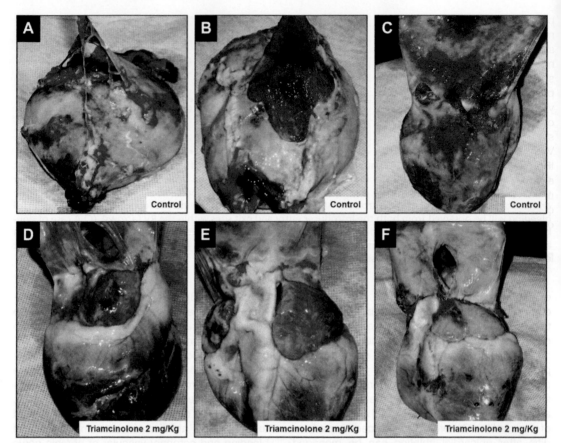

Fig. 8. Pericarditis after epicardial ablation and the effect of intrapericardial corticosteroids. Swine hearts harvested after epicardial ablation in control animals without corticosteroid treatment (*A–C*) and in animals treated with intrapericardial triamcinolone 2 mg/kg (*D–F*). As seen, in the control animals there are marked adhesions between the parietal and visceral pericardium, obscuring the tissue planes and the pericardial anatomy. Additionally, in these animals extrapericardial adhesions were also discovered between the pleura and the parietal pericardium. In contrast, in animals treated with triamcinolone either no adhesions or only loose, filmy adhesions were observed disrupted easily using gentle blunt dissection. As a result, triamcinolone (2 mg/kg) is commonly used to attenuate the postprocedural pericarditis that commonly occurs in those who undergo epicardial ventricular tachycardia ablation.

intraabdominal bleeding until proven otherwise. Of course, the management of this type of complication is entirely guided by its clinical scenario and the magnitude of bleeding. Coronary vascular injury may be avoided to a great extent by adopting the routine practice of coronary angiography whenever delivering energy current in the vicinity of the coronary vascular system. Accordingly, the European Heart Rhythm Association and the Heart Rhythm Society practice guidelines recommend maintaining a distance of 5 mm or more from an epicardial vessel during delivery of energy to the myocardium.[49] Last, phrenic nerve palsy represents another rare complication that may ensue from epicardial ablation. Phrenic nerve palsy may occur because the left phrenic nerve descends on the fibrous pericardium along one of the

following 3 courses: (i) over the anterior surface of the LV (18% of cases), (ii) over the lateral margin of the LV (59% of cases), or (iii) in a posterior–inferior direction (23% of cases).[50] In any case, injury may be avoided with simple precautionary measures such as high-output pacing whenever ablating in the phrenic nerve territory. Additionally, the phrenic nerve may be insulated or even displaced from the ablation site by injecting air and/or saline into the pericardium or by positioning a balloon catheter between the ablation site and the phrenic nerve.[51–53]

SUMMARY

Since its adoption nearly 2 decades ago, epicardial catheter ablation has steadily evolved into a practical and widely used approach for the treatment of VT in a broad range of disease substrates. During the first decade, strides were made in characterizing the epicardial substrate itself and the disease processes that bear a higher predilection for epicardial VT; the last decade has yielded incremental improvements in the methodology for energy delivery to the epicardial VT substrate. Nevertheless, the outcomes of epicardial VT ablation remain far from perfect. As such, there is tremendous need and potential for exploring alternate energy sources and delivery methods to further improve the results and success associated with epicardial catheter ablation of VT.

REFERENCES

1. Svenson RH, Littmann L, Gallagher JJ, et al. Termination of ventricular tachycardia with epicardial laser photocoagulation: a clinical comparison with patients undergoing successful endocardial photocoagulation alone. J Am Coll Cardiol 1990;15: 163–70.
2. Sosa E, Scanavacca M, d'Avila A, et al. A new technique to perform epicardial mapping in the electrophysiology laboratory. J Cardiovasc Electrophysiol 1996;7:531–6.
3. Sosa E, Scanavacca M, d'Avila A, et al. Endocardial and epicardial ablation guided by nonsurgical transthoracic epicardial mapping to treat recurrent ventricular tachycardia. J Cardiovasc Electrophysiol 1998;9:229–39.
4. Sosa E, Scanavacca M, d'Avila A, et al. Nonsurgical transthoracic mapping and ablation in a child with incessant ventricular tachycardia. J Cardiovasc Electrophysiol 2000;11:208–10.
5. Boyle NG, Shivkumar K. Epicardial interventions in electrophysiology. Circulation 2012;126:1752–69.
6. Kumar S, Bazaz R, Barbhaiya CR, et al. "Needle-in-needle" epicardial access: preliminary observations with a modified technique for facilitating epicardial interventional procedures. Heart Rhythm 2015;12: 1691–7.
7. Soejima K, Couper G, Cooper JM, et al. Subxiphoid surgical approach for epicardial catheter-based mapping and ablation in patients with prior cardiac surgery or difficult pericardial access. Circulation 2004;110:1197–201.
8. Koruth JS, Aryana A, Dukkipati SR, et al. Unusual complications of percutaneous epicardial access and epicardial mapping and ablation of cardiac arrhythmias. Circ Arrhythm Electrophysiol 2011;4: 882–8.
9. Berruezo A, Mont L, Nava S, et al. Electrocardiographic recognition of the epicardial origin of ventricular tachycardias. Circulation 2004;109:1842–7.
10. Martinek M, Stevenson WG, Inada K, et al. QRS characteristics fail to reliably identify ventricular tachycardias that require epicardial ablation in ischemic heart disease. J Cardiovasc Electrophysiol 2012;23:188–93.
11. Bazan V, Bala R, Garcia FC, et al. Twelve-lead ECG features to identify ventricular tachycardia arising from the epicardial right ventricle. Heart Rhythm 2006;3:1132–9.
12. Bazan V, Gerstenfeld EP, Garcia FC, et al. Site-specific twelve-lead ECG features to identify an epicardial origin for left ventricular tachycardia in the absence of myocardial infarction. Heart Rhythm 2007;4:1403–10.
13. Valles E, Bazan V, Marchlinski FE. ECG criteria to identify epicardial ventricular tachycardia in nonischemic cardiomyopathy. Circ Arrhythm Electrophysiol 2010;3:63–71.
14. Hutchinson MD, Gerstenfeld EP, Desjardins B, et al. Endocardial unipolar voltage mapping to detect epicardial ventricular tachycardia substrate in patients with nonischemic left ventricular cardiomyopathy. Circ Arrhythm Electrophysiol 2011;4:49–55.
15. Hsia HH, Callans DJ, Marchlinski FE. Characterization of endocardial electrophysiological substrate in patients with nonischemic cardiomyopathy and monomorphic ventricular tachycardia. Circulation 2003;108:704–10.
16. Soejima K, Stevenson WG, Sapp JL, et al. Endocardial and epicardial radiofrequency ablation of ventricular tachycardia associated with dilated cardiomyopathy: the importance of low-voltage scars. J Am Coll Cardiol 2004;43:1834–42.
17. Cano O, Hutchinson M, Lin D, et al. Electroanatomic substrate and ablation outcome for suspected epicardial ventricular tachycardia in left ventricular nonischemic cardiomyopathy. J Am Coll Cardiol 2009;54:799–808.
18. Nakahara S, Tung R, Ramirez RJ, et al. Characterization of the arrhythmogenic substrate in ischemic and nonischemic cardiomyopathy implications for catheter ablation of hemodynamically unstable ventricular tachycardia. J Am Coll Cardiol 2010;55: 2355–65.
19. Dukkipati SR, d'Avila A, Soejima K, et al. Long-term outcomes of combined epicardial and endocardial ablation of monomorphic ventricular tachycardia related to hypertrophic cardiomyopathy. Circ Arrhythm Electrophysiol 2011;4:185–94.
20. Garcia FC, Bazan V, Zado ES, et al. Epicardial substrate and outcome with epicardial ablation of ventricular tachycardia in arrhythmogenic right ventricular cardiomyopathy/dysplasia. Circulation 2009;120:366–75.
21. Berruezo A, Fernández-Armenta J, Mont L, et al. Combined endocardial and epicardial catheter ablation in arrhythmogenic right ventricular dysplasia

incorporating scar dechanneling technique. Circ Arrhythm Electrophysiol 2012;5:111–21.

22. Dello Russo A, Casella M, Pieroni M, et al. Drug-refractory ventricular tachycardias following myocarditis: endocardial and epicardial radiofrequency catheter ablation. Circ Arrhythm Electrophysiol 2012;5:492–8.

23. Koplan BA, Soejima K, Baughman K, et al. Refractory ventricular tachycardia secondary to cardiac sarcoid: electrophysiologic characteristics, mapping, and ablation. Heart Rhythm 2006;3:924–9.

24. Nademanee K, Veerakul G, Chandanamattha P, et al. Prevention of ventricular fibrillation episodes in Brugada syndrome by catheter ablation over the anterior right ventricular outflow tract epicardium. Circulation 2011;123:1270–9.

25. d'Avila A, Houghtaling C, Gutierrez P, et al. Catheter ablation of ventricular epicardial tissue: a comparison of standard and cooled-tip radiofrequency energy. Circulation 2004;109:2363–9.

26. d'Avila A, Aryana A, Thiagalingam A, et al. Focal and linear endocardial and epicardial catheter-based cryoablation of normal and infarcted ventricular tissue. Pacing Clin Electrophysiol 2008;31:1322–31.

27. Jesel L, Sacher F, Komatsu Y, et al. Characterization of contact force during endocardial and epicardial ventricular mapping. Circ Arrhythm Electrophysiol 2014;7:1168–73.

28. Mizuno H, Vergara P, Maccabelli G, et al. Contact force monitoring for cardiac mapping in patients with ventricular tachycardia. J Cardiovasc Electrophysiol 2013;24:519–24.

29. Mathuria N, Buch E, Shivkumar K. Pleuropericardial fistula formation after prior epicardial catheter ablation for ventricular tachycardia. Circ Arrhythm Electrophysiol 2012;5:e18–9.

30. Sacher F, Wright M, Derval N, et al. Endocardial versus epicardial ventricular radiofrequency ablation: utility of in vivo contact force assessment. Circ Arrhythm Electrophysiol 2013;6:144–50.

31. Aryana A, d'Avila A. Contact force during VT ablation: vector orientation is key. Circ Arrhythm Electrophysiol 2014;7:1009–10.

32. Aryana A, O'Neill PG, Pujara DK, et al. Impact of irrigation flow rate and intrapericardial fluid on cooled-tip epicardial radiofrequency ablation. Heart Rhythm 2016;13(8):1602–11.

33. Lustgarten DL, Bell S, Hardin N, et al. Safety and efficacy of epicardial cryoablation in a canine model. Heart Rhythm 2005;2:82–90.

34. Abbara S, Desai JC, Cury RC, et al. Mapping epicardial fat with multi-detector computed tomography to facilitate percutaneous transepicardial arrhythmia ablation. Eur J Radiol 2006;57:417–22.

35. d'Avila A, Dias R, Scanavacca M, et al. Epicardial fat tissue does not modify amplitude and duration of the epicardial electrograms and/or ventricular stimulation threshold [abstract]. Eur J Cardiol 2002;23:109.

36. Saba MM, Akella J, Gammie J, et al. The influence of fat thickness on the human epicardial bipolar electrogram characteristics: measurements on patients undergoing open-heart surgery. Europace 2009;11:949–53.

37. Jacobson JT, Hutchinson MD, Cooper JM, et al. Tissue-specific variability in human epicardial impedance. J Cardiovasc Electrophysiol 2011;22:436–9.

38. González-Suárez A, Hornero F, Berjano EJ. Impedance measurement to assess epicardial fat prior to RF intraoperative cardiac ablation: a feasibility study using a computer model. Physiol Meas 2010;31:N95–104.

39. Tung R, Nakahara S, Ramirez R, et al. Distinguishing epicardial fat from scar: analysis of electrograms using high-density electroanatomic mapping in a novel porcine infarct model. Heart Rhythm 2010;7:389–95.

40. Suárez AG, Hornero F, Berjano EJ. Mathematical modeling of epicardial RF ablation of atrial tissue with overlying epicardial fat. Open Biomed Eng J 2010;4:47–55.

41. Desjardins B, Morady F, Bogun F. Effect of epicardial fat on electroanatomical mapping and epicardial catheter ablation. J Am Coll Cardiol 2010;56:1320–7.

42. Sacher F, Roberts-Thomson K, Maury P, et al. Epicardial ventricular tachycardia ablation a multicenter safety study. J Am Coll Cardiol 2010;55:2366–72.

43. Della Bella P, Brugada J, Zeppenfeld K, et al. Epicardial ablation for ventricular tachycardia: a European multicenter study. Circ Arrhythm Electrophysiol 2011;4:653–9.

44. Tung R, Michowitz Y, Yu R, et al. Epicardial ablation of ventricular tachycardia: an institutional experience of safety and efficacy. Heart Rhythm 2013;10:490–8.

45. Koruth JS, d'Avila A. Management of hemopericardium related to percutaneous epicardial access, mapping, and ablation. Heart Rhythm 2011;8:1652–7.

46. Hsieh CH, Ross DL. Case of coronary perforation with epicardial access for ablation of ventricular tachycardia. Heart Rhythm 2011;8:318–21.

47. Javaheri A, Glassberg HL, Acker MA, et al. Constrictive pericarditis presenting as a late complication of epicardial ventricular tachycardia ablation. Circ Heart Fail 2012;5:e22–3.

48. d'Avila A, Neuzil P, Thiagalingam A, et al. Experimental efficacy of pericardial instillation of anti-inflammatory agents during percutaneous epicardial catheter ablation to prevent postprocedure pericarditis. J Cardiovasc Electrophysiol 2007;18:1178–83.

49. Aliot EM, Stevenson WG, Almendral-Garrote JM, et al, European Heart Rhythm Association (EHRA),

Registered Branch of the European Society of Cardiology (ESC), Heart Rhythm Society (HRS), American College of Cardiology (ACC), American Heart Association (AHA). EHRA/HRS expert consensus on catheter ablation of ventricular arrhythmias: developed in a partnership with the European Heart Rhythm Association (EHRA), a registered branch of the European Society of Cardiology (ESC), and the Heart Rhythm Society (HRS); in collaboration with the American College of Cardiology (ACC) and the American Heart Association (AHA). Heart Rhythm 2009;6:886–933.

50. Sánchez-Quintana D, Ho SY, Climent V, et al. Anatomic evaluation of the left phrenic nerve relevant to epicardial and endocardial catheter ablation: implications for phrenic nerve injury. Heart Rhythm 2009;6:764–8.

51. Di Biase L, Burkhardt JD, Pelargonio G, et al. Prevention of phrenic nerve injury during epicardial ablation: comparison of methods for separating the phrenic nerve from the epicardial surface. Heart Rhythm 2009;6:957–61.

52. Fan R, Cano O, Ho SY, et al. Characterization of the phrenic nerve course within the epicardial substrate of patients with nonischemic cardiomyopathy and ventricular tachycardia. Heart Rhythm 2009;6: 59–64.

53. Buch E, Vaseghi M, Cesario DA, et al. A novel method for preventing phrenic nerve injury during catheter ablation. Heart Rhythm 2007;4:95–8.

Premature Ventricular Complex Ablation in Structural Heart Disease

Rakesh Latchamsetty, MD*, Frank Bogun, MD

KEYWORDS

- Premature ventricular complexes • Ablation • Structural heart disease • Cardiomyopathy

KEY POINTS

- Frequent premature ventricular complexes (PVCs) portend a worse outcome in patients with structural heart disease, particularly in patients after myocardial infarction.
- The use of antiarrhythmic drugs in patients after myocardial infarction with frequent PVCs does not improve, and in some instances, can worsen mortality.
- Frequent PVCs can cause or worsen an existing cardiomyopathy in patients with underlying cardiac disease.
- PVCs, often originating from the Purkinje system, have been implicated in triggering ventricular fibrillation in postinfarction patients and can be successfully mapped and ablated.
- Further studies are needed to define risk for sustained ventricular arrhythmias after PVC ablation in patients with structural heart disease.

INTRODUCTION

The significance of premature ventricular complexes (PVCs) in the setting of structural heart disease, particularly in patients with a history of myocardial infarction, has long been studied. Early analyses suggested a worse prognosis in patients with a recent myocardial infarction with frequent PVCs, multiform PVCs, or nonsustained ventricular tachycardia (VT). Initial attempts to eliminate or reduce this ventricular ectopy, however, was met with disappointing results and the use of antiarrhythmic drugs (AADs) resulted in an increase in mortality. The conclusion was that the presence of PVCs in this setting represented a worse prognosis but was not an underlying, and moreover, a modifiable cause.

More recently, frequent PVCs have been verified to cause a decrease in left ventricular ejection fraction as well as chamber dilatation. Furthermore,

elimination of these PVCs with successful catheter ablation can abate and usually reverse this process. Although the majority of data focus on patients with idiopathic PVCs, there are also data verifying the ability of PVCs to worsen preexisting cardiomyopathy and the ability of successful ablation to provide an improvement in cardiac function in patients with underlying structural heart disease.

Occasionally, PVCs can also be implicated in triggering malignant and potentially lethal ventricular arrhythmias, including ventricular fibrillation (VF). In patients with underlying structural heart disease, particularly ischemic disease, these PVCs often originate in or near the Purkinje conduction system and can be mapped and ablated to prevent recurrent ventricular tachyarrhythmias.

In this review of PVC ablation in patients with structural heart disease, we start with a historical perspective describing our evolving knowledge

The authors have nothing to disclose.
Division of Electrophysiology, Department of Internal Medicine, University of Michigan Health System, CVC, SPC 5853, 1500 East Medical Center Drive, Ann Arbor, MI 48109-5853, USA
* Corresponding author.
E-mail address: rakeshl@med.umich.edu

Card Electrophysiol Clin 9 (2017) 133–140
http://dx.doi.org/10.1016/j.ccep.2016.10.010
1877-9182/17/© 2016 Elsevier Inc. All rights reserved.

cardiacEP.theclinics.com

of the role of frequent PVCs in the setting of structural heart disease. We then focus on the impact of frequent PVCs on the development of cardiomyopathy and the mechanism of PVCs and sudden cardiac death in postinfarction patients and discuss the benefit and outcomes of PVC ablation in these patients. We also discuss risk assessment in patients with structural heart disease undergoing PVC ablation.

PREMATURE VENTRICULAR COMPLEX MECHANISMS

PVCs can initiate from various mechanisms including automaticity, reentry, or triggered activity. The predominant mechanism depends on the underlying cardiac substrate. Patients with a previous myocardial infarction may have the potential to develop PVCs or VT through a reentrant mechanism with signal propagation around or through existing scar. Although described in animal postinfarction models,[1] this is yet to be verified in humans.

Triggered activity occurs when ectopic impulses are generated through early or late afterdepolarizations. Early afterdepolarizations occur before the end of phase 3 of the action potential and delayed afterdepolarizations occur during phase 4. Early afterdepolarizations have been described to trigger PVCs causing polymorphic VT in patients with long QT syndrome. Purkinje fibers have also been noted to generate early afterdepolarizations, which can lead to PVCs triggering VF in patients after myocardial infarction.[2]

PROGNOSIS OF PATIENTS WITH PREMATURE VENTRICULAR COMPLEXES AND STRUCTURAL HEART DISEASE

Patients with myocardial infarction and frequent PVCs have long been recognized to have a poor prognosis. In 1967, Lown and colleagues[3] reported that patients after an acute myocardial infarction with PVCs were at risk of malignant ventricular arrhythmias if they displayed PVCs with short coupling intervals, multiform PVCs, or more than 5 PVCs per minute. In 1993, Maggioni and colleagues[4] reported that patients after an acute myocardial infarction with more than 10 PVCs per hour had an increased 6-month mortality.

This recognition naturally led to attempts at suppression of PVCs and the use of class Ic AADs for this purpose was tested in the CAST study (Cardiac Arrhythmia Suppression Trial).[5] Surprisingly, this resulted in a mortality increase likely owing to the proarrhythmic effects of the AADs. PVCs in the setting of coronary artery disease and previous myocardial infarction were viewed more as a marker, rather than a cause, of poor outcome and attempts to suppress or eliminate PVCs in this setting were reserved for symptomatic improvement. This finding, along with a long-held belief that frequent PVCs in the absence of other underlying cardiac disease was benign,[6] precluded aggressive attempts at PVC suppression or elimination except in the setting of significant symptoms associated with PVCs.

It was not until the recognition of frequent PVCs as a cause of cardiomyopathy that more aggressive efforts at PVC reduction or elimination were renewed. Coincident with this recognition were the technological advances of catheter ablation, which provided greater success in elimination of PVCs without the need for long-term pharmacotherapy. Because most of the studies on PVC-induced cardiomyopathy were performed in patients with idiopathic PVCs, our discussion includes studies evaluating the pathophysiology and risk factors for PVC-induced cardiomyopathy in patients without structural heart disease before we focus on PVC mechanisms, characteristics, and ablation in patients with structural heart disease.

The risk of sudden cardiac death associated with frequent PVCs remains low, but case reports have been published in patients with and without underlying structural heart disease. Quantifying this risk remains a challenge given its low occurrence, but we discuss elsewhere in this article the suspected mechanisms in patients with underlying structural disease as well as management of these patients.

PREMATURE VENTRICULAR COMPLEX–INDUCED CARDIOMYOPATHY
Mechanisms

Frequent PVCs often cause a reversible cardiomyopathy in patients without structural heart disease and can worsen an existing cardiomyopathy in patients with structural heart disease. Multiple factors can determine which patients are at higher risk for the development of cardiomyopathy.

Initial descriptions of PVC-induced cardiomyopathy equated the mechanism to tachycardia-induced cardiomyopathy,[7] as is seen frequently in patients with atrial fibrillation or other tachyarrhythmias. This description has been abandoned, largely after the observation that patients with frequent PVCs develop cardiomyopathy in the absence of tachycardia (or even in the presence of bradycardia). There are multiple current theories explaining the potential mechanisms by which frequent PVCs cause cardiomyopathy and the true mechanism may be multifactorial, incorporating several of these theories.[8] Among the proposed mechanisms are:

- Promotion of ventricular dyssynchrony;
- Increased oxygen consumption[9–11];
- Autonomic dysregulation[12]; and
- Impaired contractility with altered intracellular calcium currents.[13]

Most of these proposed mechanisms are based on animal models and remain to be verified in human studies. Ultimately, the reversibility of the cardiomyopathy seems to favor an initial functional over a structural abnormality. However, over time, structural abnormalities may also develop, possibly owing to continued remodeling.

Risk Factors for Premature Ventricular Complex–Induced Cardiomyopathy

It remains unknown why some patients with frequent PVCs develop cardiomyopathy whereas others retain normal function. Risk factors for developing PVC-induced cardiomyopathy in patients with idiopathic PVCs include high PVC frequency, epicardial PVC location, duration of PVC exposure, increased QRS width, interpolated PVCs, male gender, absence of circadian fluctuation of the PVC burden, and asymptomatic status. While discussing the role of some of these risk factors, one should remember that the existing data are largely from patients with idiopathic PVCs and that whether the risk factors would remain the same in patients with underlying structural heart disease needs to be verified.

In a retrospective study of patients referred for ablation of idiopathic PVCs, Baman and colleagues[14] identified a PVC burden cutoff of 24% as showing the best sensitivity and specificity to identify patients at risk of developing cardiomyopathy (**Fig. 1**). It should be noted, however, that some patients with significantly greater PVC burdens had normal cardiac function and occasional patients with much lesser PVC burdens were seen to develop cardiomyopathy. Whether this correlation of PVC burden and cardiomyopathy holds for patients with other underlying structural disease, or whether a lower PVC percentage may be sufficient to worsen cardiac function in such patients, remains to be determined. The same is the case for other factors that are correlated with the development of PVC-induced cardiomyopathy.

The development of PVC-induced cardiomyopathy is generally a slow process and the longer the duration of exposure to frequent PVCs, the greater the likelihood of cardiomyopathy. Patients

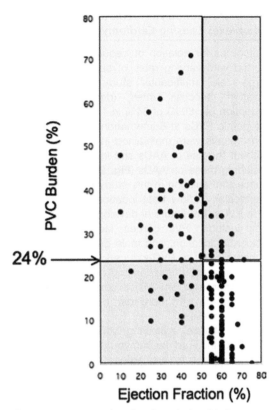

Fig. 1. Scattergram showing the relationship between the premature ventricular complex (PVC) burden and ejection fraction in a cohort of patients referred for catheter ablation. A cutoff of 24% showed the best sensitivity and specificity separating those who did or did not have evidence of cardiomyopathy. (*From* Baman TS, Lange DC, Ilg KJ, et al. Relationship between burden of premature ventricular complexes and left ventricular function. Heart Rhythm 2010;7:867; with permission.)

asymptomatic from PVCs may reflect a longer exposure time before their diagnosis of PVCs.[15] A recent study also suggests that low PVC variability throughout a 24-hour period may also be an independent risk factor for the development of cardiomyopathy.[16]

An epicardial location and greater QRS duration have also been predictive of developing cardiomyopathy and this finding supports the theory of ventricular dyssynchrony as a potential mechanism contributing to the development of cardiomyopathy.[17,18] Interpolated PVCs have also been shown to correlate with a greater chance of developing cardiomyopathy, although the mechanism involved is unclear.[19] A recent study on outcomes of PVC ablation suggested male gender as an independent risk factor for development of PVC-induced cardiomyopathy.[20]

Catheter Ablation for Premature Ventricular Complexes Causing Cardiomyopathy

Outcomes for ablation of frequent PVCs are reported with varying rates of success. A recent, large-scale, multicenter study reported acute ablation success rates (defined as PVC reduction of >80%) of 84% in 1185 patients with idiopathic PVCs at 8 international centers. Long-term results were maintained in 73% of patients without the use of AADs and in 83% of patients including those on AADs (**Fig. 2**).[20] Predictors of successful ablation in this study included a right ventricular outflow tract location and monomorphic PVCs. Predictors of developing cardiomyopathy included PVC burden, lack of symptoms, epicardial location, and male gender. In the 245 patients with a PVC-induced cardiomyopathy, the mean ejection fraction improved from 38% to 50% after ablation. Major complications were seen in 2.4% with more than one-half related to femoral access.

Most studies evaluating ablation in patients with PVC-induced cardiomyopathy have included primarily patients with idiopathic PVCs where the causal relationship between PVCs and cardiomyopathy and the reversibility can be established clearly after successful ablation. Patients with underlying structural heart disease, in addition to frequent PVCs, may have a mixed or multifactorial etiology causing their cardiomyopathy. In such patients, although cardiomyopathy may not resolve completely after successful ablation, the majority do show some improvement in ejection fraction.

Sarrazin and colleagues[21] reported on 15 patients with previous myocardial infarction, frequent PVCs, and decreased ejection fraction who were referred for implantable cardioverter-defibrillator (ICD) placement and found to have frequent PVCs. In these patients, the mean ejection fraction increased from 38% to 51% ($P = .001$; **Fig. 3**) after successful catheter ablation and only 5 patients still required ICD implantation. Of note, compared with a control patient population with ischemic cardiomyopathy without frequent PVCs, these patients were found to have a significantly smaller scar burden as detected by MRI. The amount of scarring in patients with prior myocardial infarction is helpful in estimating whether an ablation will likely improve the ejection fraction or not. In the presence of significant scarring, the likelihood of an improved ejection fraction after the ablation is small. The amount of scarring is also an indicator of risk for life-threatening arrhythmias[22] and this factor needs to be considered in patients without ICD implantation who do have a compromised ejection fraction and no history of VT. Therefore, preprocedural MRIs are beneficial for risk stratification in these patients.

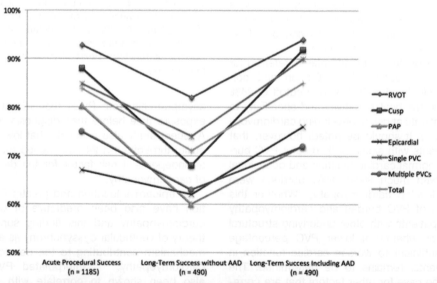

Fig. 2. Acute and long-term success rates after ablation of idiopathic premature ventricular complexes (PVCs) with and without the use of antiarrhythmic drugs (AAD). Acute procedural success data are for the entire cohort of 1185 patients whereas the long-term success data are for 490 patients at centers where Holter monitors were performed routinely after ablation. Results are shown by PVC location and single versus multiple PVCs. PAP, papillary muscle; RVOT, right ventricular outflow tract. (*From* Latchamsetty R, Yokokawa M, Morady F, et al. Multicenter outcomes for catheter ablation of idiopathic premature ventricular complexes. JACC Clinical Electrophysiol 2015;1:119; with permission.)

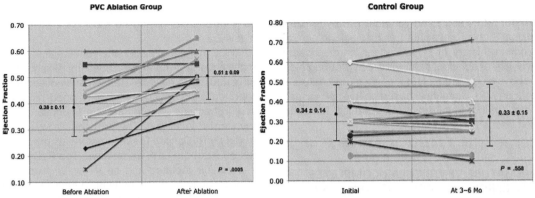

PVC Ablation Group

Control Group

Fig. 3. (*Left*) Left ventricular ejection fractions before and after premature ventricular contraction (PVC) ablation in patients with previous myocardial infarction. (*Right*) Left ventricular ejection fractions at baseline and 3 to 6 months later in the control group. (*From* Sarrazin JF, Labounty T, Kuhne M, et al. Impact of radiofrequency ablation of frequent post-infarction premature ventricular complexes on left ventricular ejection fraction. Heart Rhythm 2009;6:1547; with permission.)

A recent study of patients with nonischemic cardiomyopathy based on scarring detected by MRI or patients with cardiomyopathy preceding the development of frequent PVCs, showed that the elimination of PVCs by catheter ablation can also provide a significant improvement in the ejection fraction.[23] Ablation in these patients, however, can be more challenging, may have lower success rates than in patients with idiopathic PVCs, and even when successful can often fail to normalize the ejection fraction. The lower success rates in this cohort may be related to the location of the PVCs and, in most patients with nonischemic cardiomyopathy, scar identified by MRI is often located intramurally.[24] With nonischemic cardiomyopathy, it has also been shown that increased transmurality of scar encompassing 26% to 75% of the wall thickness can identify higher risk patients more likely to have inducible VT.[25] The intramural location of scar on preprocedural MRI correlates well with mapping during ablation where PVCs were also intramurally located in the majority of patients in whom the site of origin could be identified (**Fig. 4**).[23] Despite the lower success rates associated with these locations, ablation can still be of benefit and successful ablation in 18 out of 30 patients in this study resulted in a mean increase in the ejection fraction from 33.9% to 45.7% (*P*<.0001).

Frequent PVCs in patients with underlying cardiac disease can worsen or be the primary cause for cardiomyopathy. Moreover, elimination of these PVCs with successful ablation can improve and at times normalize cardiac function. Clues to the contribution of PVCs to the cardiomyopathy can include low scar burden by MRI, particularly in patients with underlying ischemic disease, or other high-risk PVC features such as a high PVC burden.

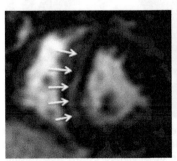
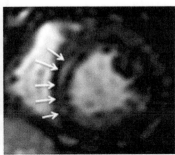
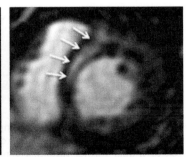

Fig. 4. Delayed enhanced MRI with a short axis view of the basal left ventricle of a patient with nonischemic cardiomyopathy. There is intramural delayed enhancement in the basal septum (*arrows*). This patient had pleomorphic premature ventricular complexes, and ablation was ineffective. (*From* El Kadri M, Yokokawa M, Labounty T, et al. Effect of ablation of frequent premature ventricular complexes on left ventricular function in patients with nonischemic cardiomyopathy. Heart Rhythm 2015;12:708; with permission.)

In patients without an ICD, assessing a patient's risk for future sustained ventricular arrhythmias is critical. Tools to evaluate this risk include cardiac function, history of VT or sudden cardiac death, success of ablation, inducibility of VT during electrophysiologic study, and the extent and nature of scar on MRI. Ultimately, based on this risk assessment, an individualized decision on ICD implantation needs to be made.

PREMATURE VENTRICULAR COMPLEXES TRIGGERING SUSTAINED VENTRICULAR ARRHYTHMIAS

The risk of sudden cardiac death in most patients with PVCs is quite low, particular in those with idiopathic PVCs. There does exist, however, a subset of patients where PVCs have been identified to trigger sustained VT or VF (**Fig. 5**). This was described more than 20 years ago in a group of patients without structural heart disease by Leenhardt and colleagues,[26,27] where PVCs with very short coupling intervals were seen to induce torsade de pointes.

Haissaguerre and colleagues[28] subsequently described a series of 27 patients who were resuscitated from idiopathic VF and noted to have an initiating complex identical to isolated PVCs after resuscitation. These PVCs were mapped to the Purkinje fiber system in 23 of these patients and to the right ventricular outflow tract in 4 patients.

Successful ablation targeting the PVCs resulted in 89% of patients having no recurrence at 2 years follow-up.

PVCs triggering malignant ventricular arrhythmias have also been described in patients with structural heart disease. Bänsch and colleagues[29] reported on 4 patients who developed recurrent drug-refractory ventricular arrhythmia after myocardial infarction. The arrhythmias were triggered by PVCs with Purkinje potentials preceding the onset of the QRS complexes. The PVCs were successfully ablated and no VT or VF was seen subsequently in these patients during follow-up. It was noted that, in these patients, the Purkinje potentials were found near the border areas of infarction and conduction time between the Purkinje fibers and the ventricular myocardium was prolonged as compared with patients without structural heart disease. It is hypothesized that surviving Purkinje fibers that can give rise to PVCs and subsequently trigger sustained ventricular arrhythmias in this infarct or border areas in patients with ischemic disease may be owing to the fact that Purkinje fibers may be less vulnerable to ischemia than myocardial cells, possibly owing to nourishment by intracavitary blood.[29–31] Targeting and elimination of a PVC-triggering polymorphic VT or VF can result in reduction or abolishment of VF, provided there is a predominant PVC present that triggers these arrhythmias.

Another study by Bogun and colleagues[32] evaluated 13 patients with prior myocardial infarction,

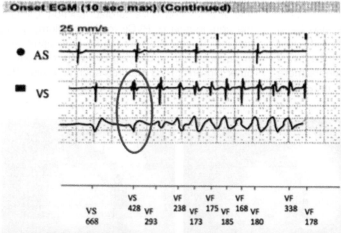
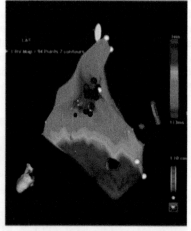

Fig. 5. (*Left*) Encircled in this stored implantable cardioverter defibrillator electrogram is a premature ventricular complex (PVC) triggering an episode of ventricular fibrillation (VF). A similar morphology during ablation was seen to trigger further sustained ventricular arrhythmias. AS indicates the atrial sensed events (*top tracing*) and VS indicates the ventricular sensed events (*middle tracing* from near-field electrograms; lower tracings from far-field electrograms). The PVC originated from the right ventricular outflow tract (activation map; *right*) and was ablated successfully, preventing further episodes of VF. (*From* Latchamsetty R, Bogun F. Premature ventricular complexes. In: Zipes D, Jalife J, editors. Cardiac electrophysiology: from cell to bedside. 6th edition. Philadelphia: Saunders; 2014. p. 809–13; with permission.)

sustained monomorphic VT, and more than 10 PVCs per hour (mean PVC burden of 12%). In these patients, postinfarction PVCs usually arose from within or at the border of the infarct scar and elimination of these PVCs was associated frequently with the elimination of inducible VT as well.[32] PVC morphologies were often similar to the VT morphology (the differences may be explained by faster rates during VT) and suggest a possible similar mechanism of reentry for both the VT and PVCs. Targeting and eliminating PVCs with an identical or very similar morphology to an inducible monomorphic VT can, therefore, potentially eliminate sustained VT owing to a shared critical site.

OTHER INDICATIONS FOR ABLATION OF PREMATURE VENTRICULAR COMPLEXES IN PATIENTS WITH STRUCTURAL HEART DISEASE

Catheter ablation of frequent PVCs has been shown to be beneficial in patients with suspected PVC-induced cardiomyopathy as well as PVCs triggering sustained ventricular arrhythmias. At least 2 other scenarios exist where elimination of PVCs can be beneficial in patients with underlying structural heart disease.

The first scenario is for symptomatic relief in patients with significant symptoms correlated with PVCs. Medical management or catheter ablation may be reasonable in such patients. Factors improving amenability to catheter ablation in these patients include monomorphic PVCs, high frequency PVCs, and more accessible locations (ie, right ventricular outflow tract).

Another scenario where ablation of frequent PVCs may be helpful is in patients with criteria for cardiac resynchronization therapy where frequent PVCs limit the benefit of biventricular pacing. Lakkireddy and colleagues[33] demonstrated that, in 65 patients with cardiac resynchronization therapy and suboptimal biventricular pacing owing to frequent PVCs, ablation of the PVCs improved heart failure symptoms (New York Heart Association functional class 3.0 vs 2.0; $P<.001$), decreased left ventricular volume (178 vs 145 mL; $P<.001$), and improved left ventricular ejection fraction (ejection fraction of 26% vs 33%; $P<.001$).

SUMMARY

In this article, we have highlighted 4 indications for catheter ablation of PVCs in the setting of underlying structural heart disease:

- PVCs are frequent and suspected to be causing or contributing to cardiomyopathy;
- PVCs have triggered sustained arrhythmias;
- PVCs are causing bothersome symptoms; and
- Frequent PVCs are limiting the benefits of biventricular pacing.

Interestingly, these indications are similar to our recommendations for ablation of frequent PVCs in patients without other structural heart disease and highlight the ability of PVCs to affect similarly both groups of patients, despite potential differences in PVC mechanisms. More patients with structural heart disease will have contraindications or limitations for the use of antiarrhythmic medications and may be more amenable to catheter ablation. Improvements in mapping and ablation technology, as well as our understanding of the specific mechanisms behind PVC initiation and how they cause cardiomyopathy and other ventricular arrhythmias, will hopefully improve our ability to manage and treat such patients.

REFERENCES

1. El-Sherif N. Reentrant ventricular arrhythmias in the late myocardial infarction period. 6. Effect of the autonomic system. Circulation 1978;58: 103–10.
2. Haissaguerre M, Shah DC, Jais P, et al. Role of Purkinje conducting system in triggering of idiopathic ventricular fibrillation. Lancet 2002;359:677–8.
3. Lown B, Fakhro AM, Hood WB, et al. The coronary care unit. New perspectives and directions. JAMA 1967;199:188–98.
4. Maggioni AP, Zuanetti G, Franzosi MG, et al. Prevalence and prognostic significance of ventricular arrhythmias after acute myocardial infarction in the fibrinolytic era. GISSI-2 results. Circulation 1993; 87:312–22.
5. Echt DS, Liebson PR, Mitchell LB, et al. Mortality and morbidity in patients receiving encainide, flecainide, or placebo. The Cardiac Arrhythmia Suppression Trial. N Engl J Med 1991;324:781–8.
6. Kennedy HL, Whitlock JA, Sprague MK, et al. Longterm follow-up of asymptomatic healthy subjects with frequent and complex ventricular ectopy. N Engl J Med 1985;312:193–7.
7. Yarlagadda RK, Iwai S, Stein KM, et al. Reversal of cardiomyopathy in patients with repetitive monomorphic ventricular ectopy originating from the right ventricular outflow tract. Circulation 2005;112: 1092–7.
8. Lee GK, Klarich KW, Grogan M, et al. Premature ventricular contraction-induced cardiomyopathy: a treatable condition. Circ Arrhythm Electrophysiol 2012;5:229–36.
9. Hoffman BF, Bartelstone HJ, Scherlag BJ, et al. Effects of postextrasystolic potentiation on normal

and failing hearts. Bull N Y Acad Med 1965;41: 498–534.

10. Chardack WM, Gage AA, Dean DC. Paired and coupled electrical stimulation of the heart. Bull N Y Acad Med 1965;41:462–80.

11. Bogun F, Crawford T, Reich S, et al. Radiofrequency ablation of frequent, idiopathic premature ventricular complexes: comparison with a control group without intervention. Heart Rhythm 2007;4:863–7.

12. Smith ML, Hamdan MH, Wasmund SL, et al. High-frequency ventricular ectopy can increase sympathetic neural activity in humans. Heart Rhythm 2010;7:497–503.

13. Wang Y, Eltit JM, Kaszala K, et al. Cellular mechanism of premature ventricular contraction-induced cardiomyopathy. Heart Rhythm 2014;11:2064–72.

14. Baman TS, Lange DC, Ilg KJ, et al. Relationship between burden of premature ventricular complexes and left ventricular function. Heart Rhythm 2010;7: 865–9.

15. Yokokawa M, Kim HM, Good E, et al. Relation of symptoms and symptom duration to premature ventricular complex-induced cardiomyopathy. Heart Rhythm 2012;9(1):92–5.

16. Bas HD, Baser K, Hoyt J, et al. Effect of circadian variability in frequency of premature ventricular complexes on left ventricular function. Heart Rhythm 2016;13:98–102.

17. Yokokawa M, Kim HM, Good E, et al. Impact of QRS duration of frequent premature ventricular complexes on the development of cardiomyopathy. Heart Rhythm 2012;9(9):1460–4.

18. Yokokawa M, Good E, Crawford T, et al. Recovery from left ventricular dysfunction after ablation of frequent premature ventricular complexes. Heart Rhythm 2013;10:172–5.

19. Olgun H, Yokokawa M, Baman T, et al. The role of interpolation in PVC-induced cardiomyopathy. Heart Rhythm 2011;8:1046–9.

20. Latchamsetty R, Yokokawa M, Morady F, et al. Multicenter outcomes for catheter ablation of idiopathic premature ventricular complexes. JACC Clin Electrophysiol 2015;1:116–23.

21. Sarrazin JF, Labounty T, Kuhne M, et al. Impact of radiofrequency ablation of frequent post-infarction premature ventricular complexes on left ventricular ejection fraction. Heart Rhythm 2009;6:1543–9.

22. Bello D, Kaushal R, Fieno D, et al. Cardiac MRI: infarct size as an independent predictor of mortality in patients with coronary artery disease. J Am Coll Cardiol 2005;45(288A):821–6.

23. El Kadri M, Yokokawa M, Labounty T, et al. Effect of ablation of frequent premature ventricular complexes on left ventricular function in patients with nonischemic cardiomyopathy. Heart Rhythm 2015; 12:706–13.

24. Neilan TG, Coelho-Filho OR, Danik SB, et al. CMR quantification of myocardial scar provides additive prognostic information in nonischemic cardiomyopathy. JACC Cardiovasc Imaging 2013;6: 944–54.

25. Nazarian S, Bluemke DA, Lardo AC, et al. Magnetic resonance assessment of the substrate for inducible ventricular tachycardia in nonischemic cardiomyopathy. Circulation 2005;112:2821–5.

26. Leenhardt A, Glaser E, Burguera M, et al. Short-coupled variant of torsade de pointes. A new electrocardiographic entity in the spectrum of idiopathic ventricular tachyarrhythmias. Circulation 1994;89: 206–15.

27. Willems S, Hoffmann BA, Schaeffer B, et al. Mapping and ablation of ventricular fibrillation-how and for whom? J Interv Card Electrophysiol 2014;40: 229–35.

28. Haissaguerre M, Shoda M, Jais P, et al. Mapping and ablation of idiopathic ventricular fibrillation. Circulation 2002;106:962–7.

29. Bänsch D, Oyang F, Antz M, et al. Successful catheter ablation of electrical storm after myocardial infarction. Circulation 2003;108:3011–6.

30. Friedman PL, Stewart JR, Wit AL. Spontaneous and induced cardiac arrhythmias in subendocardial Purkinje fibers surviving extensive myocardial infarction in dogs. Circ Res 1973;33:612–26.

31. Arnar DO, Bullinga JR, Martins JB. Role of the Purkinje system in spontaneous ventricular tachycardia during acute ischemia in a canine model. Circulation 1997;96:2421–9.

32. Bogun F, Crawford T, Chalfoun N, et al. Relationship of frequent postinfarction premature ventricular complexes to the reentry circuit of scar-related ventricular tachycardia. Heart Rhythm 2008;5:367–74.

33. Lakkireddy D, Di Biase L, Ryschon K, et al. Radiofrequency ablation of premature ventricular ectopy improves the efficacy of cardiac resynchronization therapy in nonresponders. J Am Coll Cardiol 2012; 60:1531–9.

Hemodynamic Support for Ventricular Tachycardia Ablation

Chandrasekar Palaniswamy, MD[a], Marc A. Miller, MD[b],
Vivek Y. Reddy, MD[b], Srinivas R. Dukkipati, MD[b],*

KEYWORDS

- Ventricular tachycardia • Catheter ablation • Hemodynamic support
- Percutaneous left ventricular assist device • Cerebral oximetry

KEY POINTS

- A significant proportion of patients presenting for ablation of scar-related ventricular tachycardia have hemodynamically unstable ventricular tachycardia.
- Percutaneous hemodynamic support during ventricular tachycardia ablation is feasible and safe.
- Hemodynamic support devices used for ventricular tachycardia ablation include intra-aortic balloon pump, Impella, TandemHeart, and venoarterial extracorporeal membrane oxygenation.
- Hemodynamic support aims to maintain adequate end-organ perfusion during prolonged episodes of ventricular tachycardia, thereby allowing detailed mapping of the reentrant circuit.
- Randomized, controlled trials are needed to determine the effect of hemodynamic support on procedural success and clinical outcomes.

INTRODUCTION

Catheter ablation is effective for the treatment of scar-related ventricular tachycardia (VT).[1] The 2 dominant ablation strategies include (1) mapping and ablation of the relevant substrate during stable sinus rhythm (substrate-based) and/or (2) delineation of the VT circuit with activation and entrainment mapping during VT.[2] Substrate-based ablation targets the putative channels during sinus rhythm and can include elimination of fractionated electrograms, late potentials, and local abnormal ventricular activities.[3–5] Although substrate-guided ablation is an effective approach in patients with ischemic cardiomyopathy, it is significantly less effective in patients with nonischemic cardiomyopathy, which comprise more than one-third of patients presenting with scar-related VT.[6] Patients with nonischemic cardiomyopathy have fewer putative channels that can be identified/targeted during sinus rhythm.[7] Furthermore, extensive substrate-based ablation is not an optimal strategy when the potential VT circuits are adjacent to critical anatomic structures, such as the coronary artery or phrenic nerve. Although entrainment and activation mapping may help identify the critical isthmus and avoid potentially unnecessary ablation near critical structures, hemodynamic instability during VT often precludes detailed entrainment or activation mapping.[8] In fact, even repetitive brief episodes of unstable VT may have a detrimental cumulative effect on end-organ perfusion with potential long-term sequelae. Inadequate systemic perfusion also results in lactic acidosis and release of catecholamines and neurohormones,

[a] Division of Cardiology, Department of Medicine, University of California San Francisco Fresno Medical Education Program, 155 N Fresno Street, Fresno, CA 93701, USA; [b] Helmsley Electrophysiology Center, Division of Cardiology, Department of Medicine, Icahn School of Medicine at Mount Sinai, One Gustave L. Levy Place, New York, NY 10029, USA
* Corresponding author.
E-mail address: srinivas.dukkipati@mountsinai.org

Card Electrophysiol Clin 9 (2017) 141–152
http://dx.doi.org/10.1016/j.ccep.2016.10.011
1877-9182/17/© 2016 Elsevier Inc. All rights reserved.

with activation of systemic inflammatory cytokines. These can contribute to further depression of myocardial contractility and worsening end-organ function.[9] Furthermore, prolonged episodes of hemodynamically stable VT may result in venous congestion and acute heart failure post-procedure. Indeed, postprocedural hemodynamic decompensation, which occurs in approximately 10% of patients undergoing scar VT ablation, is associated with higher mortality in long-term follow-up.[10]

Adequate intraprocedural hemodynamic support during the procedure is essential to avoid the adverse hemodynamic effects associated with prolonged episodes of VT. Although intravenous vasopressor and inotropic agents may help support cardiac output and maintain systemic blood pressure during prolonged episodes of VT or repeated attempts (programmed stimulation) to induce an arrhythmia, the extent of hemodynamic support is usually insufficient.[11] Prolonged use of these agents may also be cardiotoxic and may be associated with increased risk for multiorgan dysfunction, morbidity, and mortality.[12] Increasing focus has been placed on use of temporary mechanical circulatory support devices in the electrophysiology laboratory during catheter ablation of scar-related VT.

PERCUTANEOUS DEVICES USED FOR HEMODYNAMIC SUPPORT

The goal of mechanical circulatory support during VT ablation is to maintain adequate cardiac output and end-organ perfusion while promoting diuresis, preventing significant increases in pulmonary pressures, reducing the incidence of acute heart failure and multisystem organ failure, and perhaps improving safety and permitting more rapid recovery after the procedure. The mechanical circulatory support devices that have been used during VT ablation include intra-aortic balloon pump counterpulsation (IABP), the TandemHeart left atrial-to-femoral artery bypass (CardiacAssist Inc, Pittsburgh, PA), and the Impella (Abiomed, Danvers, MA). Although extracorporeal membrane oxygenation/peripheral cardiopulmonary bypass provides the greatest level of hemodynamic support in experimental models of fast-simulated VT or ventricular fibrillation,[13] the largest published experience thus far in hemodynamic support for VT ablation has been with the Impella and TandemHeart systems. **Table 1** provides a comparison of commonly used percutaneous hemodynamic support devices for VT ablation.

Intra-aortic Balloon Pump Counterpulsation

IABPs are the most widely used temporary mechanical circulatory support devices, most commonly for cardiogenic shock or complex percutaneous intervention. The balloon is positioned in the descending aorta with the distal end of the balloon lying a few centimeters distal to the origin of the left subclavian artery and the proximal end above the renal arteries. Inflation of the balloon in diastole augments the diastolic pressure and improves coronary and peripheral blood flow. Decrease in afterload by balloon inflation in systole augments left ventricular (LV) performance. However, IABPs are only able to augment cardiac output by 0.5 L/min, and the increases in mean arterial pressure and stroke volume afforded by the IABP may not be sufficient to meet the hemodynamic demands of patients in ongoing VT. Furthermore, optimal functioning of the IABP depends on timing of balloon inflation and deflation to pressure- or electrocardiogram (ECG)-based triggers. This timing requires a stable, regular, and nontachycardic (>120 bpm) rhythm, and thus is not ideally suited for patients undergoing VT ablation.[14] Synchronization triggers used for balloon inflation during VT should be either a peak of QRS trigger on surface ECG or arterial pressure waveform trigger. The benefits of the IABP are its relatively small arterial sheath size (7.5F–8F), ease of insertion, and familiarity to laboratory personnel.

TandemHeart

The TandemHeart device (CardiacAssist Inc) is a percutaneous left atrial to femoral artery bypass system, which uses an external centrifugal pump that provides up to 3.5 to 5 L/min of output.[14] To access the left atrium, venous access is obtained followed by transseptal puncture and dilation to accommodate the 21F inflow cannula in the left atrium (**Fig. 1**). The position transseptal cannula is then confirmed fluoroscopically by injecting dye into the cannula to make sure that all its side ports are across the interatrial septum. Alternatively, an intracardiac echocardiogram can also be used to confirm the position of the cannula. A femoral artery angiogram is obtained to ensure that the puncture is above the level of common femoral artery bifurcation and to rule out significant peripheral arterial disease. The arteriotomy tract is then dilated with a 6F to 8.5F sheath and 15F to 17F sheath for the arterial perfusion cannula. Before upsizing to the larger sheath, preclosure of the arteriotomy can be performed using 2 orthogonally placed 6F Perclose vascular closure devices (Abbott Laboratories, Abbott Park, IL).[15]

Table 1
Percutaneous hemodynamic support devices for ventricular tachycardia ablation

Device	Insertion Technique	Mechanism of Support	Augmentation of CO	Advantages	Limitations	Contraindications	Major Complications
IABP	Percutaneous or surgical 7.5–8F	Counterpulsation (systolic unloading and diastolic augmentation)	0.5 L/min	Familiarity. Ease of insertion Smaller vascular access	Only modest augmentation of cardiac output Based on ECG or pressure triggers—not optimal for patients in VT	Moderate to severe AI Aortic disease Severe PAD	Limb ischemia Vascular injury Stroke
TandemHeart	Percutaneous or surgical 21F inflow (venous)-transseptal 15 or 17F outflow (arterial)	Centrifugal, continuous flow pump	3.5–5.0 L/min	Partial LV support	Larger vascular cannulae Requires transseptal puncture	Severe PAD Ventricular sepal defect RV failure	Limb ischemia Vascular injury Cardiac tamponade Stroke Residual ASD Bleeding
Impella 2.5	Percutaneous or surgical 13F single arterial access	Axial flow pump delivering blood from LV to aorta	2.5 L/min	Partial LV support	Large arterial cannula	Mechanical aortic valve Aortic stenosis (orifice area of 0.6 cm2 or less) Moderate to severe aortic insufficiency LV thrombus Severe PAD Ventricular sepal defect RV failure	Limb ischemia Vascular injury Perforation Stroke
Impella CP	Percutaneous or surgical 14F single arterial access		3.5 L/min	Partial LV support	Large arterial cannula		Limb ischemia Vascular injury Perforation Stroke
Impella 5.0	Surgical (femoral or axillary artery cutdown) 21F single arterial access		5 L/min	Complete LV support	Larger arterial cannula		Limb ischemia Vascular injury (highest risk) Perforation Stroke
Extracorporeal membrane oxygenation (VA-ECMO) (peripheral CPB)	Percutaneous or surgical 17–22F venous, 15F arterial cannula	Centrifugal continuous flow pump with quadrox oxygenator	>4.5 L/min	Highest level of cardiopulmonary support May be used in severe RV failure	Larger vascular cannulae More complex setup	Severe PAD Uncontrolled coagulopathy	Limb ischemia Vascular injury Bleeding Sepsis Systemic embolism

Abbreviations: AI, aortic insufficiency; ASD, atrial septal defect; CO, cardiac output; CPB, cardiopulmonary bypass; PAD, peripheral arterial disease; RV, right ventricular.

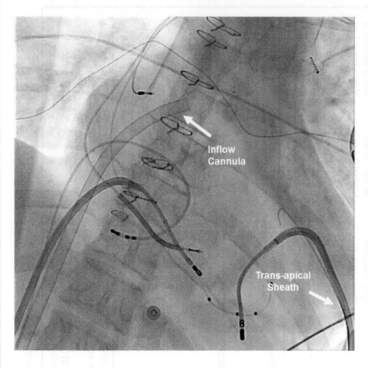

Inflow
Cannula

Trans-apical
Sheath

Fig. 1. Patient with valvular cardiomyopathy, mechanical mitral and aortic valves, and electrical storm caused by hemodynamically unstable VT. Because of electrical storm and severe LV dysfunction, hemodynamic support was used during VT ablation. Because of the presence of 2 metallic valves, a transapical approach was used for LV endocardial mapping. A TandemHeart pLVAD was used for hemodynamic support to facilitate mapping during VT and decrease risk of subsequent heart failure. The 21F inflow cannula is positioned in the left atrium via a transseptal approach. The outlet of the pLVAD is in the femoral artery using a 15F to 17F sheath. The device provides up to 5 L/min of support during VT.

The transseptal and the arterial cannulae are then connected to the respective ports in the external pump. Heparin is given as a bolus before transseptal puncture, followed by infusion to maintain activated clotting time (ACT) of at least 300 seconds. The device is typically programmed to 3000 to 7500 rpm and titrated to achieve desired hemodynamic support. A major limitation of this percutaneous left ventricular assist device (pLVAD) is the need for large venous and arterial accesses thereby increasing the risk of vascular complications. The large transseptal venous cannula can interfere with the transseptal mapping of the left ventricle. Hence, a retrograde aortic approach is usually required for mapping and ablation, which may negatively impact mapping and contact force during ablation. Potential complications of this system include cardiac tamponade, bleeding, critical limb ischemia, sepsis, arrhythmias, and residual atrial septal defects.[14]

Impella

The Impella (Abiomed) is a pLVAD with a miniaturized impeller-driven axial flow pump placed temporarily through the aortic valve to pump blood directly from the left ventricle to the ascending aorta (**Fig. 2**). Most clinical experience with the Impella thus far has been in patients undergoing high-risk percutaneous coronary intervention and those in cardiogenic shock, in whom the Impella

2.5 has provided greater augmentation of cardiac index and mean arterial pressure compared with IABP.[16,17] Three Impella devices with different pump flow capabilities are relevant for hemodynamic support during VT ablation: (1) the Impella 2.5, placed through a 13F introducer sheath in the femoral artery and delivering a maximal flow rate of 2.5 L/min; (2) the Impella CP, placed through a 14F access sheath, allowing flow rate of approximately 3.5 L/min; (3) and the Impella 5.0, that requires a surgical cutdown for arterial access (21F sheath), which is capable of providing a maximal support of about 5.0 L/min. Of these, most clinical experience thus far with VT ablation has been with the Impella 2.5 device.

The implant technique for patients undergoing VT ablation has been described before.[18] Briefly, percutaneous vascular access is obtained in the (usually left) common femoral artery with care to ensure that the puncture is above the level of common femoral artery bifurcation. Contrast is administered to ensure the level of access and to rule out significant peripheral arterial disease. The arteriotomy tract is then dilated with a 6F to 8.5F sheath. Before upsizing to the 13F sheath, preclosure of the arteriotomy is performed using 2 orthogonally placed 6F Perclose vascular closure devices.[15] To accommodate this system, blunt dissection of the subcutaneous tissue with a mosquito clamp can be performed along the arteriotomy tract with the wire in place before insertion of the

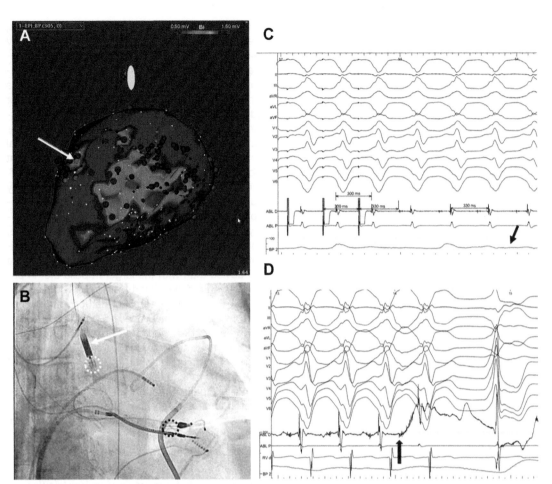

Fig. 2. Patient with nonischemic cardiomyopathy and VT. (*A*) The epicardial bipolar voltage map shows areas of patchy scar with areas of fractionated electrograms (*white circles*) and late potentials (*black points*). An extensive substrate-based ablation approach is limited by the presence of the phrenic nerve (*blue points*). Sites of ablation are shown (*red points*) as is the site of VT termination during ablation (*yellow point, arrow*). (*B*) Fluoroscopy in this patient shows the Impella CP pLVAD, which was used to facilitate entrainment mapping during otherwise hemodynamically unstable VT. The pLVAD inlet (*black circle*), outlet (*white circle*), and motor (*arrow*) are shown. (*C*) During VT, a site with a middiastolic potential (*yellow point* and *arrow* in panel A) was identified. Entrainment of VT at this site showed concealed fusion with a postpacing interval (330 milliseconds) that was equivalent to the VT cycle length. Furthermore, the stim-QRS interval is equivalent to the egm-QRS, which is consistent with the ablation catheter (ABL) being located at the isthmus site for the VT. Note that the mean femoral arterial blood pressure during VT with pLVAD support is approximately 55 to 60 mm Hg (*arrow*). (*D*) Ablation at the VT isthmus site resulted termination of VT (<1 sec; *arrow* denotes start of ablation). In this case, the extended duration of mapping during VT facilitated by the hemodynamic support from Impella was necessary to target an otherwise hemodynamically unstable VT. The Impella CP provides up to 3.5 L/min of support during VT.

Perclose. Preclosure helps with rapid hemostasis after removal of the arterial sheath at the end of the procedure. After upsizing the sheath to the final large-bore introducer needed to accommodate the pLVAD system, anticoagulation with intravenous heparin is initiated to achieve target ACT of greater than 250 seconds. Achieving an ACT ≥250 seconds before removing the dilator will help prevent a thrombus from entering the catheter and causing a sudden stop on startup. The

pLVAD is advanced retrograde through the aorta over a 0.018-inch guidewire (inserted through JR4, AL-1, multipurpose, or pigtail catheters), and across the aortic valve such that the inlet of the device is positioned in the left ventricle approximately 4 cm below the aortic valve annulus, with the outlet in the aortic root. After confirming the appropriate positioning of the device with fluoroscopy and intracardiac echocardiography, the device is turned on and titrated up to its full support capability. Proper device positioning should then be reconfirmed using the positioning waveform on the console. As the device position may change during episodes of VT or after abrupt termination of tachycardia, the positioning of the device should be monitored throughout the procedure and can typically be corrected with minor manipulation of the shaft at the level of the femoral access sheath.

The timing of anticoagulation initiation depends on whether pericardial access and epicardial mapping or ablation is planned. If epicardial mapping and ablation is planned as the primary strategy, pericardial access may be obtained at the start of the procedure, and the Impella placement is withheld until the lack of pericardial bleeding is confirmed. If there is evidence of pericardial bleeding that can be easily drained and controlled, epicardial mapping may be performed to allow tissue healing before initiating anticoagulation and placement of Impella. Alternatively, if pericardial access is considered after Impella is in place, the device can be withdrawn from the left ventricle and anticoagulation reversed before pericardial access. Once the absence of pericardial bleeding is confirmed, anticoagulation can be reinitiated, and the device is repositioned in to the left ventricle. In this latter scenario, the device should either be completely removed or temporarily withdrawn into the descending aorta with the purge solution and a low performance level maintained to avoid clot formation.

Electromagnetic interference (EMI) from Impella may occur with the use of a magnetic-based electroanatomic mapping system such as CARTO (Biosense Webster, Diamond Bar, CA).[11] EMI is usually manifested by a temporary inability to acquire mapping points or distortion of the catheter position on the mapping system. This usually occurs only to a mild extent in most cases. The severity of EMI is related to both the performance level of Impella and the distance between the motor and the magnetic sensor of the mapping catheter. EMI is typically evident during mapping in the ventricular outflow tract regions on the endocardial aspect or the anterior base on the epicardial aspect because of the proximity of the motor to the ablation catheter. Most cases of EMI do not require any additional intervention, aside from reducing the performance level (reducing the revolutions per minute) of the motor. Because EMI is more pronounced during mapping the left ventricle with a retrograde approach, a transseptal approach is preferred for left-sided ablation when the Impella is in place. Anecdotally, Impella CP appears to be associated with a lesser degree of EMI, likely related to improved insulation of the motor.

Because of direct unloading of the left ventricle, the Impella device is more efficient in reducing LV end-diastolic pressure and myocardial oxygen demand compared with the TandemHeart at comparable flow rates.[14] Furthermore, Impella requires smaller arterial sheaths and obviates the need for additional venous access and transseptal puncture, which may reduce the risk of vascular complications and shorten implantation times. Potential complications associated with Impella placement include vascular injury, hematoma, pseudoaneurysm, retroperitoneal bleeding, aortic valve injury during device placement, stroke or systemic embolism, iatrogenic induction of nonspecific arrhythmias, difficulty with catheter manipulation, and thrombus formation. Vascular access complications are less common with the smaller Impella 2.5 device than with the larger Impella 5.0. In patients with severe heart failure or cardiogenic shock, the greater degree of hemodynamic support provided by the Impella 5.0 or the TandemHeart may be required despite their higher complication rates and longer times to implantation.[14] Contraindications to Impella placement include any mechanical aortic valve, severe aortic stenosis, significant aortic insufficiency (≥2+), LV thrombus, and severe significant aortic or peripheral vascular disease (calcifications, aneurysm, extreme tortuosity).

Clinical Experience with Percutaneous Hemodynamic Support During Ventricular Tachycardia Ablation

Table 2 includes selected case series and studies of percutaneous hemodynamic support during VT ablation.[11,19–24] In a retrospective single-center analysis of 22 VT ablations performed in patients with structural heart disease and hemodynamically unstable VT, Impella 2.5 was used in 10 patients and IABP in was used in 6 patients; hemodynamic support was not used in 7 patients.[11] Compared with the group with IABP or no mechanical support, patients in the Impella group were maintained in VT 2.5-fold longer (66.7 min longer vs 27.5 min, $P = .03$), required fewer premature terminations of the arrhythmia for hemodynamic instability (1.0 vs 4.0, $P<.001$), and had more patients for which at least 1 VT was terminated during ablation (90% vs 38%; $P = .03$). Despite the longer duration of mapping during VT in the Impella group, there were no deleterious effects on end-organ perfusion or LV filling. However, there were no differences in the frequency of recurrent VT at 3-month follow-up, regardless of the type of support used.

A prospective study was performed in 20 consecutive patients undergoing catheter ablation for unstable VT using hemodynamic support with Impella 2.5 (PERMIT1 study) to assess the safety and efficacy of this approach.[22] Entrainment mapping with ablation was used as the principal strategy in all patients inducible for sustained monomorphic VT, with additional substrate modification performed at the discretion of the operator. A mean of 3.5 VTs were induced per patient with cycle length of 372 ± 117 milliseconds. Using cerebral oximetry threshold of 55% as the safety limit, sustained VT was tolerated for nearly 1 hour, with detailed entrainment mapping in these patients. Termination of VT during radiofrequency ablation occurred in two-thirds of patients. Complete procedural success (defined as termination of the clinical VT during ablation and noninducible for any VT after ablation) was achieved in 50% of patients, and partial procedural success (defined as either termination of the clinical VT during ablation but persistent inducibility or no termination of the clinical VT but no longer inducible for VT after ablation) was achieved in an additional 37%. At 1-month follow-up, 80% of patients were free of clinical recurrence of VT. Importantly, despite extended periods of mapping during VT, there were no instances of end-organ damage.[22]

In a multicenter observational study of 66 patients who underwent VT ablation with hemodynamic support, IABP, Impella 2.5, and TandemHeart were used in 22, 25, and 19 patients respectively.[23] In the pLVAD group (Impella 2.5 or TandemHeart), more patients underwent entrainment/activation mapping (82% vs 59%; $P = .046$), more unstable VTs were mapped and ablated per patient (1.05 ± 0.78 vs 0.32 ± 0.48; $P<.001$), and more VTs were terminated by ablation (1.59 ± 1.0 vs 0.91 ± 0.81; $P = .007$). However, acute procedural success, recurrence of VT, or 1-year mortality was similar in both groups.

In a retrospective study of 68 consecutive ablation procedures for unstable VT in 63 patients, mean age 66 years, 88% men, and 53% with ischemic cardiomyopathy, pLVAD was used in 34 patients.[24] With pLVAD use, the patients were sustained in VT for a longer duration (27.4 min vs 5.3 min; $P<.001$) and more VTs were terminated during ablation (1.2 vs 0.4; $P<.001$). Similar to other studies, procedural success rates and recurrence at 19 months of follow-up were not different between both groups. However, it was intriguing that the combined endpoint of 30-day rehospitalization, repeat VT ablation, recurrent implantable cardioverter defibrillator (ICD) therapies, and all-cause mortality (at 3 months) was lower in the pLVAD group (12% vs 35%, $P = .043$).

Hemodynamic Assessment During Ablation

Despite the availability of various tools, monitoring the adequacy of systemic perfusion in patients with hemodynamic support can be challenging. Arterial blood pressure and pulse oximetry alone are suboptimal for hemodynamic monitoring during VT ablation, especially in patients on continuous flow mechanical support devices. Pulse oximetry requires both pulsatile flow and adequate peripheral perfusion. As such, it is a relatively late warning sign of hypoperfusion. Moreover, the lower limits of blood pressure necessary to safely maintain end-organ perfusion during VT is unknown. Although cerebral autoregulation is preserved until mean arterial pressures of 50 to 60 mm Hg, the actual blood pressure levels required to maintain adequate cerebral perfusion in any given individual are highly variable. This finding is further compounded by lower systolic blood pressures and higher diastolic blood pressures resulting from continuous flow pumps.[18,25] Therefore, even with invasive blood pressure monitoring, it is difficult to determine which VT is unstable despite hemodynamic support. Other markers of end-organ perfusion, such as lactate levels, are not dynamic enough to guide decisions regarding termination of VT. Although electroencephalogram can detect early signs of cerebral ischemia, real-time interpretation during VT ablation is difficult. Furthermore, significant interference with the recordings can occur from electrical signals in the laboratory. Continuous bispectral monitoring reflects the depth of anesthesia but is not sensitive enough to detect early hypoperfusion.[26] Transcranial Doppler ultrasonography can detect early cerebral hypoperfusion but is cumbersome and operator dependent.[26] We routinely incorporate cerebral oximetry during scar-VT ablation, irrespective of the use of mechanical hemodynamic support, as it seems to be a reliable, noninvasive method to evaluate cerebral perfusion during VT ablation.[26,27] In contrast to pulse oximetry, cerebral oximetry does not require pulsatile flow for accurate measurement, which is an especially attractive feature when nonpulsatile flow devices are used for hemodynamic support. Although safe lower limits of cerebral tissue oxygen saturation ($SctO_2$) during VT ablation have not been clearly established, $SctO_2$ values less than 50% to 55% are predictive of adverse outcomes in patients undergoing carotid endarterectomy and cardiac surgery.[28] Because cerebral oximetry is an indirect measure of cerebral perfusion pressure (the mean arterial pressure minus central venous pressure), this may provide additional clinically relevant information to guide our decisions regarding volume status, inotrope use, and the timing of extubation.

Table 2
Studies of percutaneous hemodynamic support for ventricular tachycardia ablation

Study	Design	No. of Pts	Device	Substrate	Follow-up	Comments
Carbucicchio et al,[19] 2009	Retrospective	19	Extracorporeal membrane oxygenation (venoarterial) (n = 19)	Nonischemic (42%) Ischemic (58%)	42 mo	62 VTs induced in 19 patients, 56/62 (90%) required support due to hemodynamic instability. Noninducible at end of the procedure in 53%. At 6 mo follow-up, 28% remained VT free. No vascular complications. TIA in 1 patient, anemia in 2 patients.
Miller et al,[11] 2011	Retrospective	22	Impella 2.5 (n = 10) IABP (n = 6), or no support (n = 7)	Nonischemic (50%) Ischemic (50%)	3 mo	Patients in pLVAD group were maintained in VT significantly longer (66.7 min vs 27.5 min; P = .03), required fewer premature terminations of VT for hemodynamic instability (1.0 vs 4.0, P<.001), and had more patients for whom at least 1 VT was terminated during ablation (90% vs 38%; P = .03). No difference was observed in duration of cerebral deoxygenation, hypotension, or perioperative changes in LA pressure, renal function, BNP, or lactate levels.
Bunch et al,[20] 2012	Retrospective	31	TandemHeart (n = 13) vs no support (n = 18)	Nonischemic (35%) Ischemic (65%)	9 ± 3 mo	More VTs induced in pLVAD group (3.2 vs 1.6, P = .04). No difference between the groups in inducibility of VT at end of procedure or ICD therapies for sustained VT on follow-up.
Lu et al,[21] 2013	Retrospective	16	Impella 2.5 (n = 5), peripheral CPB (n = 5) and Heartmate II surgical LVAD (n = 6)	Nonischemic (13%) Ischemic (87%)	3 mo	In the Impella and CPB groups, time in VT was 78 ± 36 min. Hemodynamic support described as adequate (mean arterial pressure >60 mm Hg) to permit sufficient activation mapping in all except for 2 patients with Impella. Clinical VT was terminated at least once by ablation in all patients except 1 case with Impella (due to hemodynamic instability). In Impella group, 1 had hemolysis and 2 had vascular access complications requiring surgical intervention.

Miller et al,[22] 2013	Prospective	20	Impella 2.5 (n = 20)	Nonischemic (65%) Ischemic (35%)	1 mo	Mean VTs per patient - 3.5, tolerated for 58 ± 60 min. Of these, 67% of VTs were terminated during ablation. Complete procedural success in 50%, partial success in 37%. During simulated VT at 300 ms, cerebral desaturation (≤55%) occurred in 53% without pLVAD support vs 5% with pLVAD support (P = .003). Using cerebral oximetry of 55% as safety limit, 3 patients (15%) had mild acute kidney injury (resolved), and 1 (5%) patient had mild cognitive dysfunction (postop MMSE ≥2 from baseline).
Reddy et al,[23] 2014	Prospective multicenter registry	66	IABP (22), Impella 2.5 (25), TandemHeart (19)	Nonischemic (32%) Ischemic (68%)	12 ± 5 mo	In pLVAD group, more patients underwent entrainment/activation mapping (82% vs 59%; P = .046); more unstable VTs mapped and ablated per patient (1.05 ± 0.78 vs 0.32 ± 0.48; P<.001); more VTs terminated by ablation (1.59 ± 1.0 vs 0.91 ± 0.81; P = .007); mortality and VT recurrence similar.
Aryana et al,[24] 2014	Retrospective	68	Impella 2.5 or Impella CP (n = 34) vs no pLVAD (n = 34)	Nonischemic (47%) Ischemic (53%)	19 ± 12 mo	With pLVAD, VT was sustained longer (27.4 vs 5.3, P<.001); higher number of VTs were terminated during ablation (1.2 vs 0.4, P<.001). Similar procedural success rates and recurrence. Composite endpoint of 30-d rehospitalization, redo VT ablation, recurrent ICD therapies, and 3-mo mortality was lower in pLVAD group (12% vs 35%, P = .043).

Abbreviations: BNP, brain natriuretic peptide; CPB, cardiopulmonary bypass; MMSE, mini mental status examination; TIA, transient ischemic attack.

PERMIT1 was the first prospective study to systematically evaluate the use of cerebral oximetry to guide hemodynamic monitoring during pLVAD-assisted VT ablation.[22] Regardless of the arterial blood pressure, VT was allowed to continue as long as the $SctO_2$ remained $\geq$55%. This was feasible in 83% (57 of 69) of inducible VTs, with the remaining 17% of VTs terminated prematurely despite mechanical support by pacing or external defibrillation. Compared with the threshold mean arterial blood pressure of 50 mm Hg, using an $SctO_2$ threshold of 55% helped maintain the patients in VT for significantly longer periods. No significant adverse events or laboratory findings related to end-organ hypoperfusion, left atrial hypertension, congestive heart failure, or neurocognitive dysfunction were noted despite extensive maintenance of VT above this $SctO_2$ threshold. In this study, ventricular pacing was performed in all patients with and without the pLVAD turned on to simulate VT while monitoring the effects on $SctO_2$ and mean arterial blood pressure. With cycle lengths $\geq$400 milliseconds, significant cerebral desaturation was not seen with full pLVAD support, but was seen in 15% with pLVAD off. During fast simulated VT at 300 milliseconds, the benefit of pLVAD was more pronounced with cerebral desaturation occurring 53% of patients with pLVAD off versus 5% when the pLVAD was maintained at full support (P = .003). At this cycle length, patients without pLVAD support had a significantly greater decrease in $SctO_2$ levels compared with those with full pLVAD support (14.1 $\pm$ 6.1% vs 6.3 $\pm$ 4.3%, P<.001). This experiment showed that pLVAD offers better hemodynamic support compared with pharmacologic agents alone, during simulated VT. Maintaining a cerebral oximetry saturation of $\geq$55% or a decrease of 12% to 20% from baseline seems to be safe criteria to guide decisions regarding unstable VT that requires premature termination.[28] Cerebral oximetry thresholds other than 55% have not been studied with pLVAD support. Whether a higher value would offer more safety or if a lower value would offer comparable safety with maintenance of VT for longer duration is not known.

Patient Selection

The potential for complications and the associated cost with pLVADs highlight the importance of careful patient selection for its use. The decision regarding the need for mechanical support should be based on the patient's cardiac status, including functional class and systolic function, the cycle length of clinical and inducible VTs, hemodynamic status during VT, baseline renal and liver function,

myocardial substrate for VT, prior catheter ablations and reasons for prior ablation failure (such as inadequate activation/entrainment mapping caused by hemodynamic intolerance), and the depth of anesthesia. Although hemodynamic support may be beneficial in both ischemic and nonischemic cardiomyopathy, the benefit may be even greater in patients with nonischemic cardiomyopathy in whom substrate-based ablation is less effective. Patients with nondilated LV or significant LV hypertrophy are less likely to benefit from pLVAD. Furthermore, pLVADs should be avoided in patients with disproportionately severe right ventricular dysfunction or advanced pulmonary hypertension, as they may have worsening of their hemodynamic profile with pLVADs.[18]

SUMMARY

The use of percutaneous hemodynamic support devices during ablation of unstable VT in patients with structural heart disease seems safe and feasible. The pLVADs have shown efficacy in maintaining adequate end-organ perfusion during prolonged episodes of VT, thereby offering longer time for detailed activation and entrainment mapping. They may additionally improve the safety of the procedure by unloading the left ventricle during periods of sinus rhythm. Cerebral oximetry monitoring during pLVAD-supported VT ablation seems to have incremental benefit over other hemodynamic monitoring strategies in safely increasing the duration of VT tolerated during ablation. The combined strategy of pLVAD support and monitoring with cerebral oximetry has permitted a high rate of successful VT termination during ablation. The greatest hemodynamic benefit of pLVAD support may be in the setting of the fast unstable VTs. The potential benefits need to be weighed against the risk of complications, longer procedural time, and incremental cost associated with the pLVAD placement. Despite their ability to safely maintain VT for longer periods to assist detailed mapping of VT, most observational studies have not shown improvement long-term procedural success (compared with substrate-based ablation alone or with repetitive inductions and brief VT circuit mapping). The question of whether hemodynamic support during VT ablation translates to improved clinical outcomes needs to be evaluated by appropriately powered randomized trials.

REFERENCES

1. Palaniswamy C, Kolte D, Harikrishnan P, et al. Catheter ablation of postinfarction ventricular

tachycardia: ten-year trends in utilization, in-hospital complications, and in-hospital mortality in the United States. Heart Rhythm 2014;11(11):2056–63.

2. Stevenson WG, Khan H, Sager P, et al. Identification of reentry circuit sites during catheter mapping and radiofrequency ablation of ventricular tachycardia late after myocardial infarction. Circulation 1993;88: 1647–70.

3. Arenal A, Glez-Torrecilla E, Ortiz M, et al. Ablation of electrograms with an isolated, delayed component as treatment of unmappable monomorphic ventricular tachycardias in patients with structural heart disease. J Am Coll Cardiol 2003;41:81–92.

4. Marchlinski FE, Callans DJ, Gottlieb CD, et al. Linear ablation lesions for control of unmappable ventricular tachycardia in patients with ischemic and nonischemic cardiomyopathy. Circulation 2000;101: 1288–96.

5. Jaïs P, Maury P, Khairy P, et al. Elimination of local abnormal ventricular activities: a new end point for substrate modification in patients with scar-related ventricular tachycardia. Circulation 2012;125(18): 2184–96.

6. Di Biase L, Burkhardt JD, Lakkireddy D, et al. Ablation of stable VTs versus substrate ablation in ischemic cardiomyopathy: the VISTA randomized multicenter trial. J Am Coll Cardiol 2015;66(25): 2872–82.

7. Nakahara S, Tung R, Ramirez RJ, et al. Characterization of the arrhythmogenic substrate in ischemic and nonischemic cardiomyopathy implications for catheter ablation of hemodynamically unstable ventricular tachycardia. J Am Coll Cardiol 2010;55(21): 2355–65.

8. Sacher F, Tedrow UB, Field ME, et al. Ventricular tachycardia ablation: evolution of patients and procedures over 8 years. Circ Arrhythm Electrophysiol 2008;1(3):153–61.

9. Reynolds HR, Hochman JS. Cardiogenic shock: current concepts and improving outcomes. Circulation 2008;117:686–97.

10. Santangeli P, Muser D, Zado ES, et al. Acute hemodynamic decompensation during catheter ablation of scar-related ventricular tachycardia: incidence, predictors, and impact on mortality. Circ Arrhythm Electrophysiol 2015;8(1):68–75.

11. Miller MA, Dukkipati SR, Mittnacht AJ, et al. Activation and entrainment mapping of hemodynamically unstable ventricular tachycardia using a percutaneous left ventricular assist device. J Am Coll Cardiol 2011;58(13):1363–71.

12. De Backer D, Biston P, Devriendt J, et al. Comparison of dopamine and norepinephrine in the treatment of shock. N Engl J Med 2010;362(9): 779–89.

13. Ostadal P, Mlcek M, Holy F, et al. Direct comparison of percutaneous circulatory support systems in specific hemodynamic conditions in a porcine model. Circ Arrhythm Electrophysiol 2012;5(6): 1202–6.

14. Naidu SS. Novel percutaneous cardiac assist devices: the science of and indications for hemodynamic support. Circulation 2011;123(5): 533–43.

15. Mylonas I, Sakata Y, Salinger M, et al. The use of percutaneous suture-mediated closure for the management of 14 French femoral venous access. J Invasive Cardiol 2006;18(7):299–302.

16. Seyfarth M, Sibbing D, Bauer I, et al. A randomized clinical trial to evaluate the safety and efficacy of a percutaneous left ventricular assist device versus intra-aortic balloon pumping for treatment of cardiogenic shock caused by myocardial infarction. J Am Coll Cardiol 2008;52(19):1584–8.

17. Dixon SR, Henriques JP, Mauri L, et al. A prospective feasibility trial investigating the use of the Impella 2.5 system in patients undergoing high-risk percutaneous coronary intervention (The PROTECT I Trial): initial U.S. experience. JACC Cardiovasc Interv 2009;2(2):91–6.

18. Miller MA, Dukkipati SR, Koruth JS, et al. How to perform ventricular tachycardia ablation with a percutaneous left ventricular assist device. Heart Rhythm 2012;9(7):1168–76.

19. Carbucicchio C, Della Bella P, Fassini G, et al. Percutaneous cardiopulmonary support for catheter ablation of unstable ventricular arrhythmias in high-risk patients. Herz 2009;34(7):545–52.

20. Bunch TJ, Darby A, May HT, et al. Efficacy and safety of ventricular tachycardia ablation with mechanical circulatory support compared with substrate-based ablation techniques. Europace 2012;14(5):709–14.

21. Lu F, Eckman PM, Liao KK, et al. Catheter ablation of hemodynamically unstable ventricular tachycardia with mechanical circulatory support. Int J Cardiol 2013;168(4):3859–65.

22. Miller MA, Dukkipati SR, Chinitz JS, et al. Percutaneous hemodynamic support with Impella 2.5 during scar-related ventricular tachycardia ablation (PERMIT 1). Circ Arrhythm Electrophysiol 2013; 6(1):151–9.

23. Reddy YM, Chinitz L, Mansour M, et al. Percutaneous left ventricular assist devices in ventricular tachycardia ablation: multicenter experience. Circ Arrhythm Electrophysiol 2014;7(2):244–50.

24. Aryana A, Gearoid O'Neill P, Gregory D, et al. Procedural and clinical outcomes after catheter ablation of unstable ventricular tachycardia supported by a percutaneous left ventricular assist device. Heart Rhythm 2014;11(7):1122–30.

25. Novak V, Hajjar I. The relationship between blood pressure and cognitive function. Nat Rev Cardiol 2010;7(12):686–98.

26. Highton D, Elwell C, Smith M. Noninvasive cerebral oximetry: is there light at the end of the tunnel? Curr Opin Anaesthesiol 2010;23:576–81.

27. Tobias JD. Cerebral oximetry monitoring with near infrared spectroscopy detects alterations in oxygenation before pulse oximetry. J Intensive Care Med 2008;23(6):384–8.

28. Murkin JM, Arango M. Near-infrared spectroscopy as an index of brain and tissue oxygenation. Br J Anaesth 2009;103(Suppl 1):i3–13.

Ventricular Tachycardia Ablation Clinical Trials

 CrossMark

Jackson J. Liang, DO, Daniele Muser, MD, Pasquale Santangeli, MD, PhD*

KEYWORDS

- Ventricular tachycardia • Clinical trial • Catheter ablation • Outcome

KEY POINTS

- Catheter ablation is an effective treatment option to reduce ICD therapies in patients with ventricular tachycardia.
- To date, there have been limited data from prospective randomized clinical trials comparing efficacy of VT ablation versus antiarrhythmic drugs, and evaluating the effect of VT ablation on long-term mortality.
- There are several barriers to enrollment and completion of randomized clinical trials for ventricular tachycardia ablation.

INTRODUCTION

Ventricular tachycardia (VT) occurs most frequently in patients with structural heart disease, and implantable cardioverter defibrillators (ICDs) have been clearly shown to improve mortality in these patients by preventing death due to recurrent ventricular arrhythmias. However, ICDs do not prevent recurrent VT episodes, which may result in ICD shocks. Antiarrhythmic drugs (AADs) can be effective in preventing recurrent VT and reducing appropriate ICD shocks, but may be associated with significant long-term side effects and organ toxicities.

Radiofrequency (RF) catheter ablation of VT is an effective method to reduce VT recurrences and appropriate ICD therapies (both shocks and antitachycardia pacing [ATP]). Although the number of VT ablations performed on a yearly basis has gradually risen over the past decade,[1] patients with structural heart disease are still frequently referred fairly late in their disease course—particularly at institutions that do not routinely perform VT ablations. Data from a limited number of prospective randomized controlled trials (RCTs) have demonstrated the effectiveness of VT ablation in reducing recurrent VT, but these trials have not shown a clear improvement in patient-based hard clinical outcomes, including overall survival, health care utilization costs, and quality of life after ablation.[2] A recent meta-analysis examining the efficacy of catheter ablation versus AADs to prevent VT in patients with ICDs demonstrated that both treatment strategies are similarly effective in preventing recurrent VT, but neither strategy was associated with decreased mortality.[3] Interestingly, a reduction in recurrent VT with AADs was seen only among those treated with amiodarone, and amiodarone was also independently associated with increased mortality (odds ratio 3.36, 95% confidence interval [CI], 1.36–8.3; $P = .009$).

Standardization of Reporting Outcomes of Clinical Trials for Ventricular Tachycardia Ablation

There is a significant amount of diversity in the methodology and reporting of outcomes in studies

Electrophysiology Section, Division of Cardiology, Hospital of the University of Pennsylvania, 3400 Spruce Street, Philadelphia, PA 19104, USA
* Corresponding author. Hospital of the University of Pennsylvania, 9 Founders Pavilion – Cardiology, 3400 Spruce Street, Philadelphia, PA 19104.
E-mail address: Pasquale.santangeli@uphs.upenn.edu

Card Electrophysiol Clin 9 (2017) 153–165
http://dx.doi.org/10.1016/j.ccep.2016.10.012
1877-9182/17/© 2016 Elsevier Inc. All rights reserved.

for VT ablation, particularly among observational studies. Several variables may exist that can profoundly affect interpretability of results between studies, including heterogeneity of patient selection, arrhythmia severity (number of VT episodes, hemodynamic stability of VTs,), ablation strategies (ie, mapping strategies, extensive substrate vs limited ablation approaches, endocardial vs endocardial/epicardial approach, and so forth), and outcome reporting. In particular, there tends to be a wide variation in substrate-based ablation approaches between different operators and institutions. The 2009 VT ablation guidelines have proposed standards in an attempt to minimize heterogeneity of reporting results of clinical trials for VT ablation (**Box 1**).[4]

Systematic Review of Ventricular Tachycardia Ablation Clinical Trials

Using the search term "Ventricular tachycardia," the authors identified 270 clinical trials in the National Institutes of Health (NIH) database (clinicaltrials.gov) and 25 clinical trials in "circulatory domain" in the International Standard Randomised Controlled Trial Number (ISRCTN) registry. Upon review of these 295 studies, 18 of these were identified to be RCTs comparing ablation or catheter/surgical denervation procedure with placebo or medications (17 from NIH database, 1 from ISRCTN registry). Fifteen of the studies were for catheter ablation (an additional 4 were for catheter/surgical denervation procedures). Among the 15 catheter ablation trials, 4 have been completed, 3 are ongoing, 6 were prematurely terminated before completion, and 2 have unknown status. All 4 of the denervation trials are currently ongoing. **Table 1** lists the completed, ongoing, terminated clinical trials on catheter ablation or denervation for treatment of VT as well as those with unknown status.

Completed Randomized Control Trials

There have been 4 major prospective RCTs comparing catheter ablation with no ablation for VT in patients with ischemic cardiomyopathy (ICM), which are summarized in later discussion.

Substrate mapping and ablation in sinus rhythm to halt ventricular tachycardia

Published in 2007, the Substrate Mapping and Ablation in Sinus Rhythm to Halt Ventricular Tachycardia (SMASH-VT) study was the first large-scale RCT comparing catheter ablation with medical therapy.[5] It was a multicenter prospective RCT that initially enrolled patients with prior myocardial infarction (MI) who underwent

recent (within 6 months) ICD implantation for secondary prevention and later included those who received ICD for primary prevention but received an appropriate ICD therapy for a single episode of VT or ventricular fibrillation (VF). Importantly, patients who had been treated with class I or III AADs were excluded from this trial. Patients were randomized 1:1 to either ablation plus ICD or ICD plus standard medical therapy. Those in the ablation group were treated with primarily substrate-based endocardial ablation, although entrainment mapping was performed when VT was hemodynamically stable. The primary endpoint was survival from any appropriate ICD therapy (ATP or shock), and secondary endpoints were freedom from inappropriate ICD shock, death, and ICD storm ($\geq$3 shocks within a 24-hour period). A total of 128 patients were included (64 in the ablation group and 64 in the control group), and after 2 years of follow-up, patients randomized to VT ablation were significantly more likely than those in the control group to achieve freedom from any appropriate ICD therapy (shock or ATP) (88 vs 67%; hazard ratio [HR] 0.35, 95% CI, 0.15–0.78; P = .007). However, there was no significant difference in overall survival between groups (P = .29).

SMASH-VT enrolled relatively low-risk patients who had experienced a single episode of VT/VF and had not been previously treated with AADs and demonstrated that "prophylactic" substrate modification with catheter ablation in these patients can effectively decrease the likelihood of developing recurrent VT/VF requiring appropriate ICD therapy. Although the study was underpowered to show differences in mortality between groups, there did appear to be a trend toward mortality benefit in the ablation group (9 vs 17%; P = .29). One major limitation of the study was the omission of data on ICD programming, which could have influenced outcomes between groups. Importantly, the fact that the control group in SMASH-VT was not treated with AADs limits the relevance of the study results because no comparisons could be made on efficacy and safety between VT ablation versus AADs, including amiodarone.

Ventricular tachycardia ablation in coronary heart disease

The Ventricular Tachycardia Ablation in Coronary Heart Disease (VTACH) study was a prospective multicenter European RCT published in 2010 that compared ICD plus VT ablation with ICD alone.[6] Eligible patients were those with prior MI, with reduced left ventricular ejection fraction (<50%), and had stable VT, who qualified for

---

Box 1
Proposed standards for reporting results of catheter ablation for ventricular tachycardia

Baseline clinical characteristics
- Characteristics of spontaneous arrhythmias
  - Duration over which episodes of VT/VF have occurred
    - Number of episodes within preceding year, or other defined interval
    - Specify whether VT frequency is determined from an implanted device
  - Type of VT (monomorphic, polymorphic, sustained, stable, unstable), and method of termination
  - Indication of whether patients have previously failed AADs due to VT recurrences or inability to tolerate AADs
- Type and severity of underlying heart disease (including right and left ventricular function, presence of coronary artery disease)
- Significant comorbidities that may influence mortality
- Use of medications known to influence outcomes: AADs, beta-blockers, and other heart failure medications (ie, ACE inhibitors, aldosterone antagonists)

Mapping and ablation
- Protocol for VT initiation should be described in detail
- Mapping criteria for identification of ablation target
- Method of ablation (catheter used, energy source, power, duration of energy application)
- Endpoint of ablation and clear definition of acute procedural success
- Results of stimulation protocol repeated after ablation

Detection and reporting of VT recurrences
- Recurrences for patients with ICD
  - ICD interrogation should be obtained whenever symptoms suggest ICD therapy occurred, or at intervals sufficiently frequent to avoid ICD storage overload, and in the event of death
  - Because ICD storage data can be limited, recurrences should be categorized based on whether all diagnostic information for VT/VF episodes were available (including EGMs)
  - Data on specific ICD programming should be reported and, possibly, maintained uniform among patients enrolled in trials
- Recurrences for patients without ICDs
  - Assessment for symptomatic VT recurrences requires ECG documentation
  - Routine screening for asymptomatic slow VT at 6-month intervals

Follow-up and efficacy Endpoints
- VT recurrence: minimum follow-up duration of 6 to 12 months
- Mortality: minimum follow-up duration of 1 year
- VT recurrence defined as any VT episode lasting 30 seconds or more or requiring ICD intervention
- Reporting of the following efficacy measures is required:
  - Spontaneous recurrence of any sustained VT
  - Freedom from VT in absence of antiarrhythmic drug use (follow-up begins 5 half-lives after drug discontinuation, or 3 months after stopping amiodarone)
  - Death
- Other outcomes to be reported (if possible)
  - Number of VT recurrences during follow-up period
  - Recurrence of monomorphic VT (as opposed to VF or polymorphic VT)
  - Freedom from VT with previously ineffective antiarrhythmic therapy

- ○ Improvement in VT burden (ie, >75% decrease in VT frequency for 6-month monitoring period before and after ablation)
- ○ Quality of life
- ○ Cost-effectiveness

Complications

- All studies should include a complete reporting of major complications
- Major complications are defined as those resulting in permanent injury or death, or that require intervention for treatment, or that prolong or require hospitalization

Modified from Aliot EA, Stevenson WG, Almendral-Garrote JM, et al. EHRA/HRS expert consensus on catheter ablation of ventricular arrhythmias: developed in a partnership with the European Heart Rhythm Association (EHRA), a registered branch of the European Society of Cardiology (ESC), and the Heart Rhythm Society (HRS); in collaboration with the American College of Cardiology (ACC) and the American Heart Association (AHA). Heart Rhythm 2009;6:886–933; with permission.

secondary prevention ICD. Patients were randomized in a 1:1 fashion to VT ablation plus ICD versus ICD alone. Unlike SMASH-VT, the use of AADs was allowed in VTACH. Those in the ablation group underwent ablation guided by entrainment and activation mapping, as well as substrate modification, per operator discretion. ICD was then implanted in all patients (VF rate cutoff set at 200–220 beats per minute; VT zone with cutoff cycle length of 60 ms above the slowest documented VT, with ATP followed by shock). Primary endpoint in VTACH was time to first VT/VF recurrence. Enrollment began in August 2002, and follow-up was completed in January 2006. Overall, data for 107 patients were included for analysis (52 in ablation group, 55 in control group) with a mean follow-up duration of 22.5 ± 9 months. Median time to VT recurrence

Table 1
Clinical trials of interventional nonpharmacologic treatment of ventricular tachycardia

Clinical Trial	Clinical Trial Identifier	Current Status	Treatment
SMASH-VT[5]	ISRCTN62488166	Completed	Catheter ablation
VTACH[6]	NCT00919373	Completed	Catheter ablation
CALYPSO[7]	NCT01576042	Completed	Catheter ablation
VANISH[8]	NCT00905853	Completed	Catheter ablation
PARTITA[15]	NCT01547208	Ongoing	Catheter ablation
INTERVENE[16]	NCT02301390	Ongoing	Catheter ablation
BERLIN VT[17]	NCT02501005	Ongoing	Catheter ablation
VeTAMed[23]	NCT01798277	Terminated	Catheter ablation
ASPIRE[24]	NCT01557842	Terminated	Catheter ablation
STAR-VT[25]	NCT02130765	Terminated	Catheter ablation
CEASE-VT[26]	NCT01097330	Terminated	Catheter ablation
AVATAR[27]	NCT02114528	Terminated	Catheter ablation
ABLATION 4 ICD[28]	NCT00481377	Terminated	Catheter ablation
MANTRA-VT[29]	NCT02303639	Unknown	Catheter ablation
SMS[30]	NCT00170287	Unknown	Catheter ablation
PREVENT VT[31]	NCT01013714	Ongoing	Bilateral cardiac sympathectomy
RESCUE-VT[32]	NCT01747837	Ongoing	Renal denervation
RESET-VT[33]	NCT01858194	Ongoing	Renal denervation
Stellate Ganglion Resection[34]	NCT02646501	Ongoing	Stellate ganglion resection

was longer in the ablation group versus controls (18.6 vs 5.9 months), and long-term freedom from recurrent VT/VF was higher in the ablation group (47 vs 29%; HR 0.61, 95% CI, 0.37–0.99; P = .044). In addition, patients randomized to ablation were more likely to be free from cardiac rehospitalization (67 vs 45%; HR 0.55, 95% CI, 0.30–0.99), and had, on average, significantly lower burden of ICD shocks per patient-year (mean 0.6 ± 2.1 vs 3.4 ± 9.2 shocks; P = .018). There was no significant difference in overall mortality between groups (8.5 vs 8.6%; P = .68). The major take-away point of the VTACH study was that VT ablation reduces recurrent VT episodes and appropriate ICD therapies compared with no ablation. However, given the high (>50%) rates of VT recurrence in the ablation group during follow-up, VT ablation is inadequate as a stand-alone therapy (without ICD) in patients with VT after MI. The study results suggest that VT ablation, when performed, should be done so as an adjunctive treatment option to reduce ICD therapies in patients with VT.

Catheter ablation for ventricular tachycardia in patients with implantable cardioverter defibrillator trial

The Catheter Ablation for Ventricular Tachycardia in Patients with Implantable Cardioverter Defibrillator (CALYPSO) trial was a prospective RCT comparing early VT ablation with AADs in patients with ICM and ICDs who had received appropriate ICD therapies for VT.[7] Importantly, this multicenter pilot study excluded patients with any prior intolerance or contraindication to AADs. Patients were randomized in a 1:1 fashion to ablation versus AAD therapy. Patients randomized to ablation were treated with an ablation strategy targeting the clinical VT when able, and achievement of noninducibility of the clinical VT was used as the endpoint of the procedure. If the clinical VT could not be established, substrate-guided ablation was performed. The primary endpoint of the pilot study was feasibility to recruit, enroll, and complete follow-up in order to determine whether a larger clinical trial could be done. Secondary endpoints included death, time to first recurrent ICD therapy for VT, recurrent VT, treatment-related adverse events, and hospitalization for VT. Between May 2012 and February 2014 (when enrollment was terminated prematurely), the investigators screened 243 patients, only 27 of whom met enrollment criteria and agreed to participate (13 randomized to ablation, 14 to AADs). Of these, only 17 (71%) patients completed 6 months of follow-up. There were

no differences in the rate of VT recurrence at 6 months (62% vs 43%; P = NS) or overall mortality (15% vs 14%; P = NS) between those treated with ablation versus AADs.

Although enrollment for CALYPSO was terminated prematurely and the study was underpowered to detect differences between ablation and AAD therapy, the trial was valuable in that it revealed several obstacles to completing large RCTs comparing early ablation with AAD therapy. Difficulty with enrollment for CALYPSO was driven primarily by the fact that most patients with VT tended to be referred for ablation late in the disease process, after they have already failed 1 or more AAD. Surprisingly, only 8% of the patients in CALYPSO who failed screening were excluded due to refusal to participate in the trial. Thus, to maximize enrollment for large VT RCTs, the authors suggested that entry criteria for clinical trials should allow for prior use of AADs and that discussion with referring providers of patients with VT for potential VT ablation should be made early on in the disease process.

Ventricular tachycardia ablation versus escalated antiarrhythmic drug therapy in ischemic heart disease

Published in 2016, the Ventricular Tachycardia Ablation versus Escalated Antiarrhythmic Drug Therapy in Ischemic Heart Disease (VANISH) trial compared catheter ablation with escalation of AAD therapy in patients with ICM and an ICD with VT despite treatment with AAD therapy.[8] The trial was a multicenter RCT that enrolled patients at centers in Canada, Europe, the United States, and Australia. Inclusion criteria included prior MI with ICD placement and subsequent VT despite treatment with amiodarone or another class I or class III AAD within the past 6 months. Patients were randomized 1:1 to catheter ablation versus escalated AAD therapy. Patients randomized to the ablation group underwent catheter ablation within 14 days of randomization with targeting of mappable VTs using activation and entrainment mapping techniques, whereas unmappable VTs were targeted with pace-mapping and substrate ablation in sinus rhythm. Those randomized to the escalated AAD group were treated with either initiation of amiodarone (in those not on amiodarone) or amiodarone plus the addition of mexiletine (in those whose VT occurred while on amiodarone). The primary outcome measure in VANISH was a composite endpoint of all-cause mortality, VT storm, or appropriate ICD shock after 30-day treatment period. Overall, 259 patients were enrolled between July 2009 and November 2014 (132 randomized to ablation, 127 randomized to AAD escalation). After a mean follow-up duration of 28 months, the primary composite endpoint of death, VT storm, or appropriate ICD shock was less likely to occur in patients randomized to ablation versus AAD escalation (59.1% vs 68.5%; HR 0.72, 95% CI, 0.53–0.98; $P = .04$), and the difference was driven primarily by reduction in rates of appropriate ICD shocks and VT storm. There was no significant difference in mortalities between groups (27.3% vs 27.6%; HR 0.96, 95% CI, 0.60–1.53; $P = .86$). In regard to safety, those in the ablation group were more likely to have procedural complications (ie, major bleeding, vascular injury, cardiac perforation, and heart block), although treatment-related adverse events were actually more frequent in those randomized to escalated AAD therapy compared with ablation (51 vs 22; $P = .002$).

The major message of VANISH was that in relatively high-risk patients with ICM experiencing recurrent VT despite treatment with AADs, catheter ablation is superior to escalation of AADs in reducing the combined outcome of death, VT storm, or ICD shocks after 30 days. In addition, catheter ablation is less likely to cause treatment-attributed adverse events compared with escalation of AAD therapy.

Prospective Observational Trials

Cooled Radiofrequency Ablation System
The Cooled RF Ablation System clinical trial was a multicenter prospective nonrandomized observational study published in 2000.[9] The study included high-risk patients with VT and structural heart disease who underwent VT ablation across 18 institutions between September 1995 and December 1997. Patients were eligible for inclusion if they fulfilled all of the following criteria: (1) documented sustained monomorphic VT with 2 or more episodes within 2 months of enrollment; (2) spontaneous hemodynamically stable VT; (3) VT due to ICM; (4) previous ICD implantation; (5) failure of 2 or more AADs. Although the initial study design was as an RCT that randomized patients to catheter ablation versus medical therapy, it was eventually changed to a nonrandomized design due to poor enrollment. Patients were treated with an ablation strategy based primarily on entrainment mapping, activation mapping, and pace-mapping with a predetermined ablation endpoint of elimination of all mappable VTs. Acute study endpoint was elimination of all mappable VTs. The long-term efficacy outcome was defined as absence of any spontaneous sustained VT

during follow-up, whereas the safety outcome included in-hospital major or minor complications or procedural death. Overall, 146 patients were included (82% with ICM). Acute procedural success rate was 75%, and there was an 8% complication rate (2.7% procedural mortality). At 1 year, the VT recurrence rate was 56% and overall mortality was 25%.

Multicenter THERMOCOOL Ventricular Tachycardia Ablation Trial
The Multicenter THERMOCOOL VT Ablation Trial was a prospective observational trial that enrolled 231 patients with ICM and recurrent monomorphic VT.[10] This study preferentially enrolled high-risk patients with hemodynamically unstable and unmappable VTs and multiple VT morphologies. Patients were enrolled at 18 centers between February 1999 and December 2003 and underwent catheter ablation using an irrigated RF ablation catheter (NaviStar Thermocool; Biosense Webster, Diamond Bar, CA, USA) guided by entrainment, activation, and pace-mapping for mappable VTs and substrate-based ablation for unmappable VTs. The primary endpoint was freedom from any VT recurrence at 6 months. For those patients with incessant VT, success was defined as no recurrence of incessant VT. In this high-risk cohort, acute procedural success (noninducibility) was achieved in 49%, and the primary endpoint of freedom from recurrent VT (or recurrent incessant VT) was achieved in 53% of patients at 6 months. In those patients with recurrent VT, VT burden was significantly decreased, allowing for reduction or discontinuation of AADs in many patients. The 1-year mortality was 18%, and there was a 3% procedural mortality. Following the release of the study results, the US Food and Drug Administration approved the use of the open-irrigated catheter for VT ablation in patients with prior MI.

Postapproval THERMOCOOL ventricular tachycardia trial
After the approval of the Thermocool open-irrigated catheter, a prospective postapproval study was undertaken to monitor the long-term safety and effectiveness of ablation using the study catheter in patients with post-MI VT.[11] This prospective, nonrandomized, single-arm study enrolled patients between April 2007 and May 2009, continued patient follow-up through June 2012, and was published in 2015. Similar to the initial THERMOCOOL VT ablation trial, this study included high-risk patients with prior MI who had multiple episodes of sustained VT ($\geq$4 documented episodes in patients with ICD; $\geq$2

documented episodes within 2 months in patients without ICD; incessant VT; and/or spontaneous symptomatic VT despite AADs and ICD intervention). Mappable VTs were targeted with activation and entrainment mapping, whereas unmappable VT were treated with substrate-based ablation. A total of 249 patients were enrolled (29% of whom had undergone ≥1 previous VT ablation attempt). The safety analysis cohort comprised 233 patients, whereas the efficacy cohort comprised 224 patients. Acute procedural success (noninducibility) was achieved in 76% after index ablation. There was a 3.9% rate of acute procedural adverse events. Rates of all-cause mortality after 1-, 2-, and 3-years postablation were 13.4%, 18.8%, and 25.4%. At 6-months postablation, 62% of patients had no VT recurrences. Of those with recurrences, 64% had greater than 50% reduction of VT frequency. Importantly, there was a reduction of both amiodarone use and hospitalization out to 3 years (compared with preablation).

Euro–Ventricular Tachycardia

The Euro–Ventricular Tachycardia (Euro-VT) study was a multicenter, prospective, nonrandomized observational study published in 2010.[12] Similar to the Thermocool VT Ablation Trial, Euro-VT enrolled patients with ICM and multiple (≥4) episodes of symptomatic VT within 6 months of randomization or a history of VT storm and included patients with unmappable VT. A total of 63 consecutive patients were enrolled at 8 European institutions between November 1999 and January 2003 for ablation. Mappable VTs were targeted using an irrigated catheter, guided primarily by entrainment and activation mapping. Unmappable VTs were targeted with substrate-based ablation with one of the following ablation approaches: (1) linear ablation around infarct border zone including the target region; (2) series of lesions confined to the target region; and (3) multiple lines through a target region. Acute success in this high-risk population was achieved in 81%, and over a mean follow-up duration of 12 ± 3 months, 49% of patients had at least one VT recurrence. Importantly, among those with recurrent VT after ablation, there was a significant reduction of ICD therapies in 79%. There was a 1.5% major adverse event rate related to the ablation and a 5% rate of minor complications. Overall all-cause mortality at last follow-up was 8% after ablation.

Substrate versus clinical ventricular tachycardia ablation

In 2012, Di Biase and colleagues[13] compared the efficacy of an extensive combined endocardial/ epicardial "scar homogenization" substrate ablation approach with standard limited ablation for patients with ICM and electrical storm (≥3 ICD therapies within 24 hours). Ninety-two patients were included across 5 centers in a nonrandomized fashion (49 treated with limited ablation, 43 treated with scar homogenization) from March 2007 to August 2008. After mean follow-up of 25 ± 10 months, patients treated with scar homogenization were significantly less likely to have recurrent VT (19 vs 47%; $P = .006$).

Based on the promising results of their preliminary nonrandomized study, the authors performed the Ablation of Clinical Ventricular Tachycardia versus Addition of Substrate Ablation on the Long-Term Success Rate of VT Ablation (VISTA) trial.[14] Published in 2015, VISTA was a multicenter RCT comparing limited ablation targeting only clinical and mappable VTs versus extensive substrate-based ablation. Substrate-based ablation in the VISTA study involved empiric ablation to regions within the scar targeting any abnormal potentials in sinus rhythm. The procedural endpoint of this ablation strategy was abolishment of all abnormal potentials. If clinical VT remained inducible after endocardial ablation, epicardial mapping and ablation were considered as well. All AADs were discontinued after ablation in all patients and were reinitiated only for recurrent VT. Included patients had ICM and ICD with recurrent VT despite AADs. The primary efficacy endpoint of VISTA was any VT recurrence within 12 months. Secondary endpoints included periprocedural complications, 1-year mortality, and cardiac rehospitalization. A total of 118 patients were enrolled between April 2009 and July 2013 (58 randomized to substrate-based ablation; 60 to limited clinical ablation). Epicardial mapping and ablation were performed in 11.7% in the clinical ablation group and 10.3% in the substrate ablation group. All patients in both ablation groups were noninducible for the clinical VT at the end of the procedure. One year after ablation, patients treated with substrate-based ablation had a significantly lower rate of VT recurrence (15.5 vs 48.3%; HR for recurrence 0.26, 95% CI, 0.11–0.61; $P<.001$). Median time of recurrence was significantly lower in the substrate (vs clinical) ablation group (7.0 [interquartile range, IQR, 6.3–7.8] vs 2.5 [IQR, 1.2–8.6] months), and fewer patients in the substrate group remained on AADs after ablation (58 vs 12%; $P<.001$). Although there was no significant difference between groups with regards to mortality at 1 year (8.6 vs 15.0%; $P = .21$), those treated with substrate ablation were significantly less likely to require repeat hospitalization (12.1 vs 32%; $P = .014$).

ONGOING RANDOMIZED CONTROLLED TRIALS FOR CATHETER ABLATION OF VENTRICULAR TACHYCARDIA

PARTITA

The ongoing PARTITA trial is an RCT that aims to assess whether early ablation affects long-term prognosis in patients with ICD and VT.[15] The study began enrolling patients in September 2012 and is currently still recruiting patients. Patients with primary or secondary prevention ICD are eligible for inclusion, whereas patients who are already being treated with class I or III AADs are excluded. Patients are randomized to either immediate VT ablation after appropriate ICD shock or to wait until development of VT storm before ablation is performed. Goal enrollment is 590 patients, and the estimated study completion date is September 2018. The results of PARTITA should help to answer the question regarding whether early VT ablation results in superior outcomes.

Indian Trial of Endocardial Ventricular Substrate Ablation to Prevent Recurrent Ventricular Tachycardia Events

The Indian Trial of Endocardial Ventricular Substrate Ablation to Prevent Recurrent Ventricular Tachycardia Events (INTERVENE) is an ongoing RCT in India comparing amiodarone alone versus amiodarone plus catheter ablation for treatment of patients with VT in the setting of ICM.[16] Importantly, the trial will include only patients who qualify for secondary prevention ICD but are instead being treated with amiodarone because they cannot afford ICD. The study began in October 2009, and estimated study completion is December 2017 (estimated enrollment of 136 patients). Primary outcome is all-cause mortality after 24 months, and secondary outcome measures include death within 30 days, recurrent VT/VF, and change in left ventricular ejection fraction. It is hoped that this trial will serve as a representative model for the developing world.

Prevention of aBlation of vEntricular tachycaRdia in Patients with myocardiaL INfarction

The aBlation of vEntricular tachycaRdia in patients with myocardiaL INfarction (BERLIN VT) study is an RCT that aims to evaluate the impact of prophylactic VT ablation on all-cause mortality and hospital admissions for heart failure or VT/VF versus delayed VT ablation (after the third appropriate ICD shock).[17] The primary outcome measure is time to death or first cardiac hospitalization. Secondary outcomes include time to VT/VF,

appropriate and inappropriate ICD therapies, all-cause mortality, cardiac mortality, hospitalization, cardiac hospitalization, and quality of life. Enrollment began June 2015, and estimated study completion date is December 2018, with a goal enrollment of 208 patients.

Ventricular Tachycardia Ablation for Patients with Nonischemic Cardiomyopathy

Data examining efficacy and safety of VT ablation in patients with nonischemic cardiomyopathy come primarily from single- and multicenter retrospective studies, and to date, there have been no prospective RCTs in this population. Although patients with ICM tend to have predictable substrate at regions of scar from prior MI, the substrate in patients with NICM is quite heterogenous, depending on the underlying cause (ie, idiopathic dilated cardiomyopathy, arrhythmogenic right ventricular cardiomyopathy, hypertrophic cardiomyopathy, cardiac sarcoidosis, congenital heart disease, myocarditis, noncompaction cardiomyopathy). The distribution of abnormal substrate in nonischemic cardiomyopathy (NICM) tends to involve the basal "perivalvular" regions of the ventricles, and there is a higher likelihood of epicardial and intramural involvement. Long-term outcomes after ablation are quite variable, depending on the underlying cause of NICM. **Table 2** summarizes long-term outcomes in the major studies for VT ablation in patients with NICM.

Difficulty of Completing Ventricular Tachycardia Clinical Trials

There are several obstacles that complicate enrollment of patients and completion of VT ablation RCTs. First, primary care providers and general cardiologists may be unaware of available RCT opportunities for their patients with VT, or providers may be hesitant to enroll their patients due to fear of complications. Although certain patient risk factors may in fact predispose to worse outcomes, the authors' group and others have shown that VT ablation in the elderly (as an example) can be performed just as safely and effectively as in younger patients.[18–20] Although the number of VT ablations performed each year continues to increase, and despite the evidence that early VT ablation may result in improved outcomes,[21,22] contemporary studies such as CALYPSO suggest that most patients with VT continue to be referred for VT ablation late in their disease course as a "last resort" treatment option. Furthermore, electrophysiologists who work at institutions where ICDs are implanted but VT ablation is not routinely

Table 2
Clinical studies examining outcomes after VT ablation in patients with nonischemic cardiomyopathy

Author, Year	NICM Type	N	Follow-up (mo)	VT Recurrence (%)
Marchlinski et al,[35] 2000	DCM	7	8	43
Hsia et al,[36] 2003	DCM	19	22	74
Soejima et al,[37] 2004	DCM	28	9	36
Cesario et al,[38] 2006	DCM	8	12	25
Cano et al,[39] 2009	DCM	22	18	29
Schmidt et al,[40] 2010	DCM	16	12	47
Nakahara et al,[41] 2010	DCM	16	14	50
Kuhne et al,[42] 2010	DCM	24	18	57
Haqqani et al,[43] 2011	DCM	31	20	32
Vergara et al,[44] 2012	DCM	14	13	14
Muser et al,[45] 2016	DCM	282	60	31
Marchlinski et al,[46] 2004	ARVC	19	27	11
Verma et al,[47] 2005	ARVC	22	36	47
Yao et al,[48] 2007	ARVC	32	29	19
Dalal et al,[49] 2007	ARVC	24	32	91
Garcia et al,[50] 2009	ARVC	13	18	23
Bai et al,[51] 2011	ARVC	49	40	31
Philips et al,[52] 2012	ARVC	87	88	85
Müssigbrodt et al,[53] 2015	ARVC	28	19	47
Santangeli et al,[54] 2015	ARVC	62	56	29
Koplan et al,[55] 2006	CS	8	6	75
Jefic et al,[56] 2009	CS	9	10	44
Naruse et al,[57] 2014	CS	14	33	43
Kumar et al,[58] 2015	CS	21	58	86
Muser et al,[59] 2016	CS	31	30	60
Santangeli et al,[60] 2010	HCM	22	20	27
Dukkipati et al,[61] 2011	HCM	10	38	30
Gonska et al,[62] 1996	CHD	16	16	0
Furushima et al,[63] 2006	CHD	7	61	0
Zeppenfeld et al,[64] 2007	CHD	11	30	9
Kriebel et al,[65] 2007	CHD	8	35	25
Kapel et al,[66] 2015	CHD	34	46	12
van Zyl et al,[67] 2016	CHD	21	33	14
Kapel et al,[68] 2016	CHD	74	50	7
Dello Russo et al,[69] 2012	Myocarditis	20	28	10
Maccabelli et al,[70] 2014	Myocarditis	26	23	23

Abbreviations: ARVC, arrhythmogenic right ventricular cardiomyopathy; CS, cardiac sarcoidosis; DCM, dilated cardiomyopathy; HCM, hypertrophic cardiomyopathy.

Adapted from Liang JJ, Santangeli P, Callans DJ. Long-term outcomes of ventricular tachycardia ablation in different types of structural heart disease. Arrhythm Electrophysiol Rev 2015;4:177–83; with permission.

performed may be less likely to refer patients elsewhere to be treated with VT ablation. These patients may be more likely to be managed with AADs and adjustment of ICD programming. After patients are referred, there comes the issue of randomization. The "unknown factor" of being randomized to 2 very different treatment methods may deter patients from choosing to participate in RCTs. Similarly, patients who enroll and are randomized to the control arm may cross over and undergo VT ablation (or vice versa), affecting the study results—particularly in intention-to-treat analyses. Funding is a major limiting factor for VT ablation RCTs, which tend to be funded primarily by industry, although other organizations (ie, NIH, Canadian Institutes of Health Research) may provide assistance as well. Industry-supported RCTs generally require that procedures be performed using devices from a certain company for the clinical trial (ie, ICDs, catheters, mapping systems), introducing bias.

SUMMARY

Data examining the efficacy and safety of VT ablation from RCTs are lacking, in large part due to the difficulty with patient enrollment and completion of long-term studies. Published RCTs have demonstrated that catheter ablation is effective in reducing VT recurrences and ICD therapies in patients with ICM, although studies have been underpowered to detect mortality benefit. There has been no VT ablation RCTs in patients with NICM, an area in which there is a strong need for data. Future studies should aim to compare the efficacy and safety of VT ablation in all sorts of structural heart disease compared with AADs and to examine the optimal timing for VT ablation to optimize procedural success.

REFERENCES

1. Palaniswamy C, Kolte D, Harikrishnan P, et al. Catheter ablation of postinfarction ventricular tachycardia: ten-year trends in utilization, in-hospital complications, and in-hospital mortality in the United States. Heart Rhythm 2014;11:2056–63.
2. Liang JJ, Santangeli P, Callans DJ. Long-term outcomes of ventricular tachycardia ablation in different types of structural heart disease. Arrhythm Electrophysiol Rev 2015;4:177–83.
3. Santangeli P, Muser D, Maeda S, et al. Comparative effectiveness of antiarrhythmic drugs and catheter ablation for the prevention of recurrent ventricular tachycardia in patients with implantable cardioverter-defibrillators: a systematic review and meta-analysis of randomized controlled trials. Heart Rhythm 2016;13(7):1552–9.
4. Aliot EM, Stevenson WG, Almendral-Garrote JM, et al. EHRA/HRS Expert Consensus on catheter ablation of ventricular arrhythmias: developed in a partnership with the European Heart Rhythm Association (EHRA), a registered Branch of the European Society of Cardiology (ESC), and the Heart Rhythm Society (HRS); in collaboration with the American College of Cardiology (ACC) and the American Heart Association (AHA). Heart Rhythm 2009;6:886–933.
5. Reddy VY, Reynolds MR, Neuzil P, et al. Prophylactic catheter ablation for the prevention of defibrillator therapy. N Engl J Med 2007;357:2657–65.
6. Kuck KH, Schaumann A, Eckardt L, et al. Catheter ablation of stable ventricular tachycardia before defibrillator implantation in patients with coronary heart disease (VTACH): a multicentre randomised controlled trial. Lancet 2010;375:31–40.
7. Al-Khatib SM, Daubert JP, Anstrom KJ, et al. Catheter ablation for ventricular tachycardia in patients with an implantable cardioverter defibrillator (CALYPSO) pilot trial. J Cardiovasc Electrophysiol 2015;26:151–7.
8. Sapp JL, Wells GA, Parkash R, et al. Ventricular tachycardia ablation versus escalation of antiarrhythmic drugs. N Engl J Med 2016;375(2):111–21.
9. Calkins H, Epstein A, Packer D, et al. Catheter ablation of ventricular tachycardia in patients with structural heart disease using cooled radiofrequency energy: results of a prospective multicenter study. Cooled RF Multi Center Investigators Group. J Am Coll Cardiol 2000;35:1905–14.
10. Stevenson WG, Wilber DJ, Natale A, et al. Irrigated radiofrequency catheter ablation guided by electroanatomic mapping for recurrent ventricular tachycardia after myocardial infarction: the multicenter thermocool ventricular tachycardia ablation trial. Circulation 2008;118:2773–82.
11. Marchlinski FE, Haffajee CI, Beshai JF, et al. Long-term success of irrigated radiofrequency catheter ablation of sustained ventricular tachycardia: post-approval THERMOCOOL VT trial. J Am Coll Cardiol 2016;67:674–83.
12. Tanner H, Hindricks G, Volkmer M, et al. Catheter ablation of recurrent scar-related ventricular tachycardia using electroanatomical mapping and irrigated ablation technology: results of the prospective multicenter Euro-VT-study. J Cardiovasc Electrophysiol 2010;21:47–53.
13. Di Biase L, Santangeli P, Burkhardt DJ, et al. Endoepicardial homogenization of the scar versus limited substrate ablation for the treatment of electrical storms in patients with ischemic cardiomyopathy. J Am Coll Cardiol 2012;60:132–41.
14. Di Biase L, Burkhardt JD, Lakkireddy D, et al. Ablation of stable VTs versus substrate ablation in ischemic cardiomyopathy: the VISTA randomized multicenter trial. J Am Coll Cardiol 2015;66:2872–82.
15. Does timing of VT Ablation affect prognosis in patients with an implantable cardioverter-defibrillator? (PARTITA). Available at: https://clinicaltrialsgov/ct2/show/NCT01547208. Accessed June 11, 2016.
16. Indian trial of endocardial ventricular substrate ablation to prevent recurrent VT Events (INTERVENE). Available at: https://clinicaltrialsgov/ct2/show/NCT02301390. Accessed June 11, 2016.
17. Preventive aBlation of vEntricular tachycaRdia in patients with myocardiaL INfarction (BERLIN VT).

Available at: https://clinicaltrialsgov/ct2/show/NCT02501005. Accessed June 11, 2016.

18. Liang JJ, Khurshid S, Schaller RD, et al. Safety and efficacy of catheter ablation for ventricular tachycardia in elderly patients with structural heart disease. JACC Clin Electrophysiol 2015;1:52–8.

19. Inada K, Roberts-Thomson KC, Seiler J, et al. Mortality and safety of catheter ablation for antiarrhythmic drug-refractory ventricular tachycardia in elderly patients with coronary artery disease. Heart Rhythm 2010;7:740–4.

20. Barra S, Begley D, Heck P, et al. Ablation of ventricular tachycardia in the very elderly patient with cardiomyopathy: how old is too old? Can J Cardiol 2015;31:717–22.

21. Frankel DS, Mountantonakis SE, Robinson MR, et al. Ventricular tachycardia ablation remains treatment of last resort in structural heart disease: argument for earlier intervention. J Cardiovasc Electrophysiol 2011;22:1123–8.

22. Dinov B, Arya A, Bertagnolli L, et al. Early referral for ablation of scar-related ventricular tachycardia is associated with improved acute and long-term outcomes: results from the heart center of Leipzig ventricular tachycardia registry. Circ Arrhythm Electrophysiol 2014;7:1144–51.

23. Trial comparing ablation with medical therapy in patients with ventricular tachycardia (VeTAMed). Available at: https://clinicaltrialsgov/ct2/show/NCT01798277. Accessed June 11, 2016.

24. Early ablation therapy for the treatment of ischemic ventricular tachycardia in patients with implantable cardioverter defibrillators (ASPIRE). Available at: https://clinicaltrialsgov/ct2/show/NCT01557842. Accessed June 11, 2016.

25. Substrate targeted ablation using the flexability™ ablation catheter system for the reduction of ventricular tachycardia (STAR-VT). Available at: https://clinicaltrialsgov/ct2/show/NCT02130765. Accessed June 11, 2016.

26. Catheter ablation versus amiodarone for shock prophylaxis in defibrillator patients with ventricular tachycardia (CEASE-VT). Available at: https://clinicaltrialsgov/ct2/show/NCT01097330. Accessed June 11, 2016.

27. Anti-arrhythmic therapy vs catheter ablation as first line treatment for AICD shock prevention (AVATAR). Available at: https://clinicaltrialsgov/ct2/show/NCT02114528. Accessed June 11, 2016.

28. Ablation for ICD intervention reduction in patients with CAD (ABLATION 4 ICD). Available at: https://clinicaltrialsgov/ct2/show/NCT00481377. Accessed June 11, 2016.

29. Medical ANtiarrhythmic treatment or radiofrequency ablation in ischemic ventricular tachyarrhythmias (MANTRA-VT). Available at: https://clinicaltrialsgov/ct2/show/NCT02303639. Accessed June 11, 2016.

30. Substrate modification study in patients getting an implantable cardioverter defibrillator (ICD) (SMS). Available at: https://clinicaltrialsgov/ct2/show/NCT00170287. Accessed June 11, 2016.

31. Cardiac denervation surgery for prevention of ventricular tacharrhythmias (PREVENT VT). Available at: https://clinicaltrialsgov/ct2/show/NCT01013714. Accessed June 11, 2016.

32. REnal sympathetic denervation to sUpprEss ventricular tachyarrhythmias (RESCUE-VT). Available at: https://clinicaltrialsgov/ct2/show/NCT01747837. Accessed June 11, 2016.

33. REnal sympathetic dEnervaTion as an a adjunct to catheter-based VT ablation (RESET-VT). Available at: https://clinicaltrialsgov/ct2/show/NCT01858194. Accessed June 11, 2016.

34. Prospective randomized clinical trial for effect of stellate ganglion block in medically refractory ventricular tachycardia. Available at: https://clinicaltrialsgov/ct2/show/NCT02646501. Accessed June 11, 2016.

35. Marchlinski FE, Callans DJ, Gottlieb CD, et al. Linear ablation lesions for control of unmappable ventricular tachycardia in patients with ischemic and nonischemic cardiomyopathy. Circulation 2000;101:1288–96.

36. Hsia HH, Callans DJ, Marchlinski FE. Characterization of endocardial electrophysiological substrate in patients with nonischemic cardiomyopathy and monomorphic ventricular tachycardia. Circulation 2003;108:704–10.

37. Soejima K, Stevenson WG, Sapp JL, et al. Endocardial and epicardial radiofrequency ablation of ventricular tachycardia associated with dilated cardiomyopathy: the importance of low-voltage scars. J Am Coll Cardiol 2004;43:1834–42.

38. Cesario DA, Vaseghi M, Boyle NG, et al. Value of high-density endocardial and epicardial mapping for catheter ablation of hemodynamically unstable ventricular tachycardia. Heart Rhythm 2006;3:1–10.

39. Cano O, Hutchinson M, Lin D, et al. Electroanatomic substrate and ablation outcome for suspected epicardial ventricular tachycardia in left ventricular nonischemic cardiomyopathy. J Am Coll Cardiol 2009;54:799–808.

40. Schmidt B, Chun KR, Baensch D, et al. Catheter ablation for ventricular tachycardia after failed endocardial ablation: epicardial substrate or inappropriate endocardial ablation? Heart Rhythm 2010;7:1746–52.

41. Nakahara S, Tung R, Ramirez RJ, et al. Characterization of the arrhythmogenic substrate in ischemic and nonischemic cardiomyopathy implications for catheter ablation of hemodynamically unstable ventricular tachycardia. J Am Coll Cardiol 2010;55:2355–65.

42. Kuhne M, Abrams G, Sarrazin JF, et al. Isolated potentials and pace-mapping as guides for ablation of

ventricular tachycardia in various types of nonischemic cardiomyopathy. J Cardiovasc Electrophysiol 2010;21:1017–23.

43. Haqqani HM, Tschabrunn CM, Tzou WS, et al. Isolated septal substrate for ventricular tachycardia in nonischemic dilated cardiomyopathy: incidence, characterization, and implications. Heart Rhythm 2011;8:1169–76.

44. Vergara P, Trevisi N, Ricco A, et al. Late potentials abolition as an additional technique for reduction of arrhythmia recurrence in scar related ventricular tachycardia ablation. J Cardiovasc Electrophysiol 2012;23:621–7.

45. Muser D, Santangeli P, Castro S, et al. Long-term outcome after catheter ablation of ventricular tachycardia in patients with nonischemic dilated cardiomyopathy. Circ Arrhythm Electrophysiol 2016;9(10).

46. Marchlinski FE, Zado E, Dixit S, et al. Electroanatomic substrate and outcome of catheter ablative therapy for ventricular tachycardia in setting of right ventricular cardiomyopathy. Circulation 2004;110:2293–8.

47. Verma A, Kilicaslan F, Schweikert RA, et al. Short- and long-term success of substrate-based mapping and ablation of ventricular tachycardia in arrhythmogenic right ventricular dysplasia. Circulation 2005; 111:3209–16.

48. Yao YAN, Zhang SHU, He DS, et al. Radiofrequency ablation of the ventricular tachycardia with arrhythmogenic right ventricular cardiomyopathy using non-contact mapping. Pacing Clin Electrophysiol 2007;30:526–33.

49. Dalal D, Jain R, Tandri H, et al. Long-term efficacy of catheter ablation of ventricular tachycardia in patients with arrhythmogenic right ventricular dysplasia/cardiomyopathy. J Am Coll Cardiol 2007; 50:432–40.

50. Garcia FC, Bazan V, Zado ES, et al. Epicardial substrate and outcome with epicardial ablation of ventricular tachycardia in arrhythmogenic right ventricular cardiomyopathy/dysplasia. Circulation 2009;120:366–75.

51. Bai R, Di Biase L, Shivkumar K, et al. Ablation of ventricular arrhythmias in arrhythmogenic right ventricular dysplasia/cardiomyopathy: arrhythmia-free survival after endo-epicardial substrate based mapping and ablation. Circ Arrhythm Electrophysiol 2011;4:478–85.

52. Philips B, Madhavan S, James C, et al. Outcomes of catheter ablation of ventricular tachycardia in arrhythmogenic right ventricular dysplasia/cardiomyopathy. Circ Arrhythm Electrophysiol 2012;5:499–505.

53. Müssigbrodt A, Dinov B, Bertagnoli L, et al. Precordial QRS amplitude ratio predicts long-term outcome after catheter ablation of electrical storm due to ventricular tachycardias in patients with arrhythmogenic right ventricular cardiomyopathy. J Electrocardiol 2015;48:86–92.

54. Santangeli P, Zado ES, Supple GE, et al. Long-term outcome with catheter ablation of ventricular tachycardia in patients with arrhythmogenic right ventricular cardiomyopathy. Circ Arrhythm Electrophysiol 2015;8:1413–21.

55. Koplan BA, Soejima K, Baughman K, et al. Refractory ventricular tachycardia secondary to cardiac sarcoid: electrophysiologic characteristics, mapping, and ablation. Heart Rhythm 2006;3:924–9.

56. Jefic D, Joel B, Good E, et al. Role of radiofrequency catheter ablation of ventricular tachycardia in cardiac sarcoidosis: report from a multicenter registry. Heart Rhythm 2009;6:189–95.

57. Naruse Y, Sekiguchi Y, Nogami A, et al. Systematic treatment approach to ventricular tachycardia in cardiac sarcoidosis. Circ Arrhythm Electrophysiol 2014; 7:407–13.

58. Kumar S, Barbhaiya C, Nagashima K, et al. Ventricular tachycardia in cardiac sarcoidosis: characterization of ventricular substrate and outcomes of catheter ablation. Circ Arrhythm Electrophysiol 2015;8:87–93.

59. Muser D, Santangeli P, Pathak R, et al. Long-term outcomes of catheter ablation of ventricular tachycardia in patients with cardiac sarcoidosis. Circ Arrhythm Electrophysiol 2016;9(8).

60. Santangeli P, Di Biase L, Lakkireddy D, et al. Radiofrequency catheter ablation of ventricular arrhythmias in patients with hypertrophic cardiomyopathy: safety and feasibility. Heart Rhythm 2010;7:1036–42.

61. Dukkipati SR, d'Avila A, Soejima K, et al. Long-term outcomes of combined epicardial and endocardial ablation of monomorphic ventricular tachycardia related to hypertrophic cardiomyopathy. Circ Arrhythm Electrophysiol 2011;4:185–94.

62. Gonska BD, Cao K, Raab J, et al. Radiofrequency catheter ablation of right ventricular tachycardia late after repair of congenital heart defects. Circulation 1996;94:1902–8.

63. Furushima H, Chinushi M, Sugiura H, et al. Ventricular tachycardia late after repair of congenital heart disease: efficacy of combination therapy with radiofrequency catheter ablation and class III antiarrhythmic agents and long-term outcome. J Electrocardiol 2006;39:219–24.

64. Zeppenfeld K, Schalij MJ, Bartelings MM, et al. Catheter ablation of ventricular tachycardia after repair of congenital heart disease: electroanatomic identification of the critical right ventricular isthmus. Circulation 2007;116:2241–52.

65. Kriebel T, Saul JP, Schneider H, et al. Noncontact mapping and radiofrequency catheter ablation of fast and hemodynamically unstable ventricular tachycardia after surgical repair of tetralogy of Fallot. J Am Coll Cardiol 2007;50:2162–8.

66. Kapel GFL, Reichlin T, Wijnmaalen AP, et al. Re-entry using anatomically determined isthmuses: a curable

ventricular tachycardia in repaired congenital heart disease. Circ Arrhythm Electrophysiol 2015;8:102–9.

67. van Zyl M, Kapa S, Padmanabhan D, et al. Mechanism and outcomes of catheter ablation for ventricular tachycardia in adults with repaired congenital heart disease. Heart Rhythm 2016;13(7):1449–54.

68. Kapel GF, Sacher F, Dekkers OM, et al. Arrhythmogenic anatomical isthmuses identified by electroanatomical mapping are the substrate for ventricular tachycardia in repaired tetralogy of Fallot. Eur Heart J 2016. [Epub ahead of print].

69. Dello Russo A, Casella M, Pieroni M, et al. Drug-refractory ventricular tachycardias after myocarditis: endocardial and epicardial radiofrequency catheter ablation. Circ Arrhythm Electrophysiol 2012;5:492–8.

70. Maccabelli G, Tsiachris D, Silberbauer J, et al. Imaging and epicardial substrate ablation of ventricular tachycardia in patients late after myocarditis. Europace 2014;16:1363–72.

Moving?

Make sure your subscription moves with you!

To notify us of your new address, find your **Clinics Account Number** (located on your mailing label above your name), and contact customer service at:

Email: journalscustomerservice-usa@elsevier.com

800-654-2452 (subscribers in the U.S. & Canada)
314-447-8871 (subscribers outside of the U.S. & Canada)

Fax number: 314-447-8029

Elsevier Health Sciences Division
Subscription Customer Service
3251 Riverport Lane
Maryland Heights, MO 63043

ELSEVIER

Moving?

Make sure your subscription moves with you!

To notify us of your new address, find your Clinics Account Number (located on your mailing label above your name), and contact customer service at:

Email: journalscustomerservice-usa@elsevier.com

800-654-2452 (subscribers in the U.S. & Canada)
314-447-8871 (subscribers outside of the U.S. & Canada)

Fax number: 314-447-8029

Elsevier Health Sciences Division
Subscription Customer Service
3251 Riverport Lane
Maryland Heights, MO 63043

To ensure uninterrupted delivery of your subscription, please notify us at least 4 weeks in advance of move.

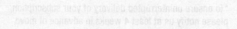

Printed and bound by CPI Group (UK) Ltd, Croydon, CR0 4YY

03/10/2024

01040302-0017